Clinical Medicine and the Nervous System
Series Consulting Editor: Michael Swash

Syndromes that have an underlying neurological basis are common problems in many different specialties. Clinical Medicine and the Nervous System is a series of monographs concerned with the diagnosis and management of clinical problems due primarily to neurological disease, or to a neurological complication of another disorder. Thus the series is particularly concerned with those neurological syndromes that may present in different contexts, often to specialists without special expertise in neurology. Since the range of clinical practice embraced by neurologists is wide, the books in this series will appeal to many different specialists in addition to neurologists and neurosurgeons. It is the aim of the series to produce individual volumes that are succinct, informative and complete in themselves, and that provide sufficient practical discussion of the issues to prove useful in the diagnosis, investigation and management of patients. Important advances in basic mechanisms of disease are emphasized as they are relevant to clinical practice. In particular, individual volumes in the series will be useful especially to neurologists, neurosurgeons, physicians in internal medicine, oncologists, paediatricians, neuro-radiologists, rehabilitationists, otorhinolaryngologists and ophthalmologists, and to those in training in these specialties.

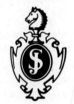

Diseases of the Spinal Cord

Edmund Critchley and Andrew Eisen (Eds.)

With 88 Figures

Springer-Verlag
London Berlin Heidelberg New York
Paris Tokyo Hong Kong
Barcelona Budapest

Edmund Critchley, DM, FRCP
Consultant Neurologist, Department of Neurology, Royal
Preston Hospital, Sharoe Green Lane, Preston, Lancashire
PR2 4HT, UK

Andrew Eisen, MD, FRCP(C)
Professor of Medicine (Neurology), University of British
Columbia, and Head of the Neuromuscular Disease Unit,
Vancouver General Hospital, Vancouver, British Columbia, V5Z
4E3, Canada

Consulting Editor

Michael Swash, MD, FRCP, MRCPath
Consultant Neurologist, Neurology Department, The London
Hospital, Whitechapel, London E1 1BB

Cover illustration: Ch. 23, Fig. 5. Intradural tumour:
neurofibroma with cord and root compression – conus medullaris

ISBN 3-540-19684-6 Springer-Verlag Berlin Heidelberg New York
ISBN 0-387-19684-6 Springer-Verlag New York Berlin Heidelberg

British Library Cataloguing in Publication Data
Disease of the spinal cord. – (Clinical medicine and the nervous system)
  I. Critchley, Edmund II. Eisen, Andrew III. Series 616.73
ISBN 3-540-19684-6

Library of Congress Cataloging-in-Publication Data
Diseases of the spinal cord/edited by Edmund Critchley and Andrew
  Eisen.
    p.   cm.—(Clinical medicine and the nervous system)
  Includes index.
  ISBN 3-540-19684-6 (alk. paper).—ISBN 0-387-19684-6 (alk. paper)
    1. Spinal cord – Diseases. I. Critchley, E.M.R. (Edmund Michael R.)
II. Eisen, Andrew, 1936–   . III. Series.
  [DNLM: 1. Spinal Cord Diseases. WL 400 D611]
RC400.D52   1992
616.8'3—dc20
DNLM/DLC   91-5079
for Library of Congress   CIP

Typeset by Best-set Typesetter Ltd., Hong Kong
2128/3830-543210 Printed on acid-free paper

Consulting Editor's Foreword

The spinal cord is a long structure, consisting of white and grey matter, that not only serves to provide a neural connection between the brain and the body, but also contains neural circuits that are organized segmentally and that are responsive to central and peripheral sensory input. Thus the spinal cord is capable of some behavioural activity that is of clinical significance, and that is more evident when higher modulation is disturbed. The released activity of spasticity, and the disturbances of bladder and bowel control that occur in patients with spinal cord lesions are examples. The spinal cord is well protected within its bony canal but is, nonetheless, susceptible to compression by degenerative joint or bone disease, or by neoplasm. Spinal cord compression is a common clinical problem that is not always easy to recognize. However, it is particularly important because of the good results of appropriate treatment and the unfortunate consequences should the diagnosis be missed. Many other medical and surgical disorders affect the spinal cord, including vascular disease, decompression sickness, degenerative disorders and multiple sclerosis.

In this book Dr. Critchley and Dr. Eisen, and their collaborators, chosen for their expertise and experience in spinal cord disorders, have gathered together descriptions of the symptoms and signs of spinal cord disease. They have planned the book in relation to the underlying causes of spinal cord syndromes, and have carefully considered the methods of clinical assessment and diagnosis in current use, including the well-established and newer clinical neurophysiological and imaging techniques. Accurate diagnosis is an essential prerequisite to adequate clinical management. Diseases of the spinal cord and their clinical manifestations deserve to be better understood and better managed in clinical practice. This book will serve to address this aim.

The Royal London Hospital   Michael Swash
May 1991

Preface

Publication of a textbook of diseases of the spinal cord is born of necessity: to correct the low standards of diagnosis and management of spinal cord problems in the past and the neglect of the subject in the teaching of neurology and neurosurgery. In fact, many of the older neurologists felt it beneath their dignity to teach on such a mundane subject as the spinal cord.

The purpose of the present volume is to provide a clinical guide appealing to all those involved in spinal cord problems whatever their experience or designation. Exciting advances, especially in the application of neuroradiological and neurophysiological techniques, justify a fresh enthusiasm for this aspect of neurological endeavour. With the support of these new diagnostic facilities many neurologists and neurosurgeons have developed a research interest in disorders of the spinal cord and nerve roots and this is reflected in the chapters in which contributors elaborate on features they feel important for the optimum management of patients. Controversies are not ignored and among the special topics discussed are diving injuries, disorders of the conus, paraplegia and rehabilitation.

Nonetheless, the primary aim is to provide a sound and comprehensive manual for the clinician, valuable for learning, review and reference. Early chapters include the application of basic sciences, knowledge of neuropathology and diagnostic techniques at the bedside, but where necessary more specific details of the underlying anatomy and physiology are re-emphasized in the clinical chapters, as for example in that concerned with spinal and neural compression, in order to give a holistic view of the clinician's approach to the problem posed.

Preston, Lancashire   Edmund Critchley
Vancouver, British Columbia   Andrew Eisen

Contents

Contributors

M.J. Aminoff, MD, FRCP
Professor of Neurology, School of Medicine, University of
California, San Francisco, California 94143-0114, USA

E.M.R. Critchley, DM, FRCP
Consultant Neurologist, Royal Preston Hospital, Sharoe Green
Lane, Preston, Lancashire PR2 4HT, UK

C.H.G. Davis, FRCS
Consultant Neurosurgeon, Royal Preston Hospital, Sharoe
Green Lane, Preston, Lancashire PR2 4HT, UK

J.P.R. Dick, PhD, MRCP
Consultant Neurologist, The Royal London Hospital,
Whitechapel, London E1 1BB, UK

A.A. Eisen, MD, FRCP(C)
Professor of Medicine (Neurology), University of British
Columbia, and Head of the Neuromuscular Disease Unit,
Vancouver General Hospital, Vancouver, British
Columbia, V5Z 4E3, Canada

F.J. Eismont, MD
Professor of Orthopedics and Rehabilitation, Neurological
Surgery and Co-Director of the Acute Spinal Cord Injury
Service, University of Miami School of Medicine/Jackson
Memorial Hospital, 8004 Rosenstiel Medical Science Building,
Miami, Florida 33136, USA

D.I. Graham, FRCPath, FRCP
Professor of Neuropathology, Southern General Hospital, 1345
Govan Road, Glasgow G51 4TF, UK

B.A. Green, MD
Professor of Neurological Surgery, Orthopedics and
Rehabilitation, and Co-Director of the Acute Spinal Cord Injury
Service, University of Miami School of Medicine/Jackson
Memorial Hospital, Attending Physician at the Veterans
Administration Hospital, President and Director of Clinical
Research at the Miami Project to Cure Paralysis, 1501 NW 9th
Avenue, Miami, Florida 33136, USA

N.T. Gurusinghe, FRCSE
Consultant Neurosurgeon, Royal Preston Hospital, Sharoe
Green Lane, Preston, Lancashire PR2 4HT, UK

M.T. Isaac, MRCPath, MRCPsych
Senior Registrar in Psychiatry, The Bethlem Royal Hospital and
The Maudsley Hospital, Denmark Hill, London SE5 8AZ, UK

H.J. Landy, MD
Assistant Professor of Neurological Surgery, University of Miami
School of Medicine/Jackson Memorial Hospital, 1501 NW 9th
Avenue, Miami, Florida 33136, USA

J.S. Lapointe, MD, FRCP(C)
Associate Professor of Radiology, University of British
Columbia, Neuroradiologist, Vancouver General Hospital,
Vancouver, British Columbia, V5Z 4E3, Canada

R.A. Metcalfe, MD, MRCP
Consultant Neurologist, Southern General Hospital, 1345 Govan
Road, Glasgow G51 4TF, UK

J.D. Mitchell, MD, FRCPG
Consultant Neurologist, Royal Preston Hospital, Sharoe Green
Lane, Preston, Lancashire PR2 4HT, UK

M.J. Noronha, FRCP, FRCPE
Consultant Paediatric Neurologist, Royal Manchester Children's
Hospital, Pendlebury, Manchester M27 1HA, UK

R.R. Pearson, MD, MFOM, RN
Surgeon Captain, HMS Saker, BFPO 2. (Home address: 1509
Allview Drive, Potomac, Maryland 20854, USA)

B. Pentland, BSc, MB, FRCPE
Consultant Neurologist, Astley Ainslie Hospital, Grange Loan,
Edinburgh EH9 2HL, UK

M.S. Schwartz, MD
Consultant Neurophysiologist, Atkinson Morley's Hospital,
Copse Hill, Wimbledon, London SW20 0NE, UK

M. Swash, MD, FRCP, FRCPath
Consultant Neurologist, Department of Neurology, Section of
Neurological Sciences, The Royal London Hospital,
Whitechapel, London E1 1BB, UK

K.A. Tucci, MD
Chief Resident, Department of Neurological Surgery, University
of Miami School of Medicine/Jackson Memorial Hospital, 1501
NW 9th Avenue, Miami, Florida 33136, USA

C.U. Velmurugendran, MD, DM, FIMSA
Professor of Neurology, Institute of Neurology, Madras Medical
College and Government General Hospital, Madras, 600 003
India

R.J. Weber, MD
Professor and Chairman, Department of Physical Medicine and
Rehabilitation, SUNY Health Science Center, 750 East Adams
Street, Syracuse, NY 13210, USA

Chapter 1

Introduction

E.M.R. Critchley and A.A. Eisen

The first separate treatise on the spinal cord, *Anatome Medullae Spinalis et Nervorum* (Gerard Blasius, Amsterdam, C. Commelinum), was published in 1666. The separate origin of the anterior and posterior roots, dorsal root ganglia and the differentiation between the grey and white matter of the spinal cord were illustrated. Despite this early description, the spinal cord has remained, until recently, the Cinderella of the nervous system, receiving relatively scanty attention.

In adults, the spinal cord is approximately 40 cm long and extends from the foramen magnum to the lower margin of the body of the first lumbar vertebra. For a long time the ability to localize lesions longitudinally within the spinal cord has been very limited. Sir David Ferrier's "golden guinea test" (now all but forgotten) used a guinea coin to demonstrate the upper limit of spinal compression. If a coin is run down the back of the spine, a wheal is produced in the skin above the level of the lesion, but at most a white mark occurs below the lesion when sweating and vital reactions are in abeyance (Critchley 1957).

It required the Second World War and the pioneering efforts of Sir Ludwig Guttmann (Guttmann 1946) to change the traditionally nihilistic view of spinal cord trauma and other lesions. The following four decades have witnessed the feasibility of inducing functional spinal cord regeneration (Aguayo 1987) and innovative biomedical engineering has made it possible for the paraplegic to "walk" (Marsolais and Kobetic 1983; Petrofsky and Phillips 1983; Weber 1987).

The basic anatomical unit at each spinal level, the simple reflex arc, belies the complex circuitry and operation of the spinal cord which is constantly being extended and refined (Ashby 1987). A great deal of signal processing takes place within the cord; the substrate for many motor programmes ranging from simple reflexes to the complex patterns required, for example, in walking.

Spinal protection by its membranes, the skin, the musculature of the back and the bony vertebral column is exceptional. They form important defences against trauma, infection, neoplasia, autoimmune disease and iatrogenic insult but are also factors rendering the spinal cord so inaccessible to direct clinical examination.

Investigative approaches to spinal cord disease have also been limited. For years one could do little more than interpret the results of CSF analysis via a lumbar puncture needle. Myelography permitted limited visualization of the outline of the cord, which has been marginally enhanced by CT scanning and selective angiography. MRI was a quantum leap in cord imaging (see Lapointe, this volume) but still leaves us largely in ignorance of the physiological, pathological and biochemical behaviour of the cord in response to disease.

Many cord lesions are not radiologically visible. In this respect motor and somatosensory evoked potentials can be helpful (Eisen and Aminoff 1986; Eisen and Shtybel 1990). However, these neurophysiological tests do not have the localizing ability of imaging techniques. Furthermore they are unable to discriminate between different types of pathology or disease.

Symptomatology

The essence of history taking in suspected spinal cord disease does not differ from that for other conditions affecting the nervous system. A full description of the circumstances of the onset of symptoms can help enormously in diagnosis particularly when the onset is abrupt. Even though clinicians pride themselves that, faced with a neurological problem, they can correctly make the diagnosis based upon history alone in approximately 80% of patients, such diagnostic prowess falls far below the norm when considering disorders affecting the spinal cord. A few examples will suffice.

1. Regardless whether trauma has been sustained at work, in road traffic accidents or during sport, bony and/or neural damage involving the cervical or dorsolumbar spine is frequently overlooked. Failure to recognize the extent of such injury – or even its presence – all too often precipitates avoidable neurological deficit or death at initial handling of the patient (Rubin and Fielding 1983; Ravichandran and Silver 1984).

In sports injuries a head-on tackle, as with "spearing" in American football, may result in a fracture of the lower cervical spine. Flexion or hyperextension injuries occur in rucks (collapsed scrums) or mauls. Whiplash injury is a result of the head jolted forwards and backwards in a road traffic accident. A twisting injury during lifting may suggest acute disc prolapse with consequent radicular pain and inability to straighten up immediately. It is useful to discover exactly how the patient was able to move from the scene of an accident or abrupt injury. What help was required? Conversely, with certain injuries such as whiplash, symptoms may be minimal at first but develop after a few hours.

2. The history of a "crick in the neck" with burning pain across the shoulders following minor trauma is easily misinterpreted as due to a root lesion despite unrestricted neck movement. Such patients, who are more likely to have neuralgic amyotrophy (paralytic brachial neuritis) or syringomyelia, not infrequently undergo inappropriate and unsuccessful neck traction.

3. Any number of explanations of spastic weakness of the legs may be offered before the possibility of cord compression is finally recognized. The gradual, subacute onset of spasticity in the lower limbs should always raise the possibility of spinal cord compression.

Early symptoms include a feeling of heaviness in the legs and the complaint that walking, an automatic event, now requires conscious effort. After a set distance the feet may begin to drag, the toes may catch with a tendency to trip.

The inner aspects of the toe caps of shoes may wear excessively. Investigation to exclude spinal compression should be considered before a definite sensory level is established or sphincter problems ensue.

The sudden onset of a paraparesis recognized for the first time when attempting to get out of bed can occur with spinal compression but is more usually an indication of a thrombotic lesion. Spinal multiple sclerosis may be suggested if, in addition to evidence of spasticity, the feet tend to kick out involuntarily, or unilateral symptoms are accompanied by bilateral signs.

4. Vascular accidents involving the cord often create diagnostic confusion. The symptoms of a spinal subarachnoid haemorrhage are not as readily manifest as those of an intracranial bleed. Thrombotic lesions of the cord, especially occurring in the elderly or as a consequence of blood loss, may be overlooked; as may the protean symptoms ascribable to the presence of ar-teriovenous malformations. In fact, arteriovenous malformations of the spinal cord and dura are as often discovered by accident as by anticipation.

It may be hard to differentiate cord compression from transverse myelitis and recurrent episodes at the same site may indicate the possibility of an arteriovenous malformation. A spinal subarachnoid haemorrhage may occur with symptoms developing acutely at one level, with other symptoms such as headache and lower back pain coursing into the legs, encountered several hours later.

5. Not every dorsal or girdle pain is the result of a prolapsed intervertebral disc or due to shingles.

6. Spinal meningitis at the extremes of life may escape detection unless specifically considered and sought for. Typical events heralding the acute phase of poliomyelitis and other enteroviruses – vomiting, diarrhoea or con-stipation followed by a mild temperature and a meningitic reaction – are easily overlooked.

Physical Signs

The examination provides the framework required to formulate a diagnosis, establish the level of the lesion and provide confirmatory evidence of the nature of the insult and the pathological changes found. Non-neurological physical signs provide information about the state of the overlying tissues and the likelihood of spinal cord pathology. Minor degrees of dysraphism include the presence of bifid vertebral spines, dermoids, dimpling and portwine stains. Deformities of the neck and the region of the foramen magnum such as platybasia, a short or webbed neck, torticollis, or Sprengel's deformity of the scapula, may be associated with abnormal or fused vertebrae and Arnold-Chiari malformation. If spastic paraparesis or ataxia is accompanied by the presence of kyphoscoliosis and sometimes clubbed feet, the patient is more likely to have a hereditary rather than an acquired neurological disorder. About 60%–90% of congenital and between 35%–90% of acquired spinal cord disorders have associated scoliosis (Dickson 1986). A wedged vertebra may occur with a variety of inherited conditions and with Paget's disease of the spine, but acute wedging of vertebrae more commonly suggests vertebral collapse. This may cause spinal cord compression, for example in the presence of carcinomatous deposits, tuberculosis, or an epidural abscess.

Two signs, in particular, indicate acute embarrassment of the cervical spinal cord following trauma. The adoption of a cock robin tilt or posture due to post-traumatic torticollis is indicative of a Jefferson fracture and fragmentation of the ring of the atlas caused by axial compression. The actual fracture may be fairly stable but in 50% of cases it is accompanied by fractures of the odontoid or the so-called hangman's fracture separating the body of the axis from the C2–3 facet joints.

Paradoxical neurogenic ventilation is an ominous sign of a high spinal cord lesion with paralysis of the phrenic nerve (C3,4,5) and diaphragm. Respiratory support becomes the immediate priority. There is paradoxical distension of the abdomen during inspiration with indrawing of damaged segments of the chest wall. In this situation stimulation of the phrenic nerve and assessment of phrenic nerve conduction, as well as needle EMG of the diaphragm, is useful for documenting the presence or otherwise of nerve–muscle continuity. Lesser cervical injuries may be recognized at times by careful palpation before attempting to move the patient. Lesions affecting the anterior quadrants of the spinal cord at C2–4 may impair the autonomic control of respiration whilst leaving intact voluntary control, thus giving rise to the situation wherein respiration is unimpaired in the alert state but fails when the patient becomes drowsy (Ondine's curse). Ventilatory problems also arise with lower cervical and high dorsal lesions as these are associated with small ventilatory capacity and inability to cough with a risk of atelectasis and decreased arterial P_{O_2} even if the CO_2 tension is maintained.

Anatomical localization within the spinal cord may be determined by piecing together, as it were on a grid, signs of vertical and horizontal dysfunction. The vertical manifestations are the less complex. Upper motor neurone signs indicate involvement of the pyramidal, or corticospinal, tracts at any level between cortex and anterior horn cells. Extrapyramidal features negate spinal disease, indicating a lesion rostral to the medulla.

Truncal ataxia and minor cerebellar signs may be mimicked by the presence of lower motor neurone weakness, loss of proprioceptive function, or damage to Clarke's column (the nucleus dorsalis) located at the base of the posterior horns and extending from T1 to L4. Sensory signs can involve end-organ dysfunction, the peripheral nerve, or spinal tracts. Whereas peripheral nerve disease is usually associated with a graded glove and stocking distribution, a distinct upper limit is usual with spinal dysfunction. This is often accompanied, if the lesion is intrinsic, by sacral sparing or suspended sensory loss. Dissociated sensory loss may occur with predominantly spinothalamic (pain and temperature) or dorsal column (proprioception, light touch and vibration) impairment; or, as is typical in Hansen's disease, with selective involvement of the larger fibres of the posterior root ganglia.

An intriguing sign worthy of careful analysis is the presence of pseudo-athetosis. Slow wandering movements of the outstretched fingers occur when the arms are extended and the eyes closed. Unlike true athetotic movements, these movements are readily suppressed when the patient is able to watch his hands. Unilateral involvement can occur with a lesion of the parietal lobe but usually pseudoathetosis is seen bilaterally with tabetic softening of the dorsal columns, or with compression of the dorsal columns as by cerebellar ectopia at the foramen magnum, carcinomatous meningitis or cervical spondylosis. It can occur, but is rare, as a result of interruption of the dorsal columns in multiple sclerosis and here it may remit spontaneously (Bickerstaff 1980).

Another cause of pseudoathetosis is sensory neuronopathy (Asbury 1987). The lesion is of the primary afferent neurone having its cell body in the dorsal root ganglia lying within the intervertebral foramina. Sensory neuronopathies can be difficult to interpret. Degeneration of the central process occurs with lesions that are proximal to the dorsal root. In this situation electrophysiological studies are helpful. Peripheral compound sensory nerve action potentials (SNAPs) are normal, but spinal or cortical evoked potentials (SEPs) are prolonged, small or absent. Several toxic and metabolic abnormalities affecting the primary sensory neurone induce a distal axonopathy with dying-back of both the peripheral and central arms of the neurone. When this happens both the peripheral SNAP and SEP are abnormal (Thomas 1982).

Sensory neuronopathies (acute or chronic) are, as a group, less common than other conditions affecting the peripheral or central components of the sensory axon. They affect the cell body directly with subsequent dying-forward of both its central and peripheral arms. Sensory neuronopathies are distinguishable from sensory neuropathies by the global, rather than distal, distribution of sensory loss, total areflexia and absence of recordable SNAPs in the face of normal compound muscle action potentials (Asbury 1987). The chronic variety is most usually associated with an underlying cancer. The much rarer acute forms originally occurred in association with antibiotic therapy but more recently cases without apparent cause have been described.

Among the classical tests of sensory loss is the Romberg test which is a test of postural instability, only apparent following closure of the eyes. Although it is used as a supportive test confirming the presence of vertigo, it is essentially a test of the integrity of the proprioceptive pathways transmitted via the dorsal columns. Romberg's test is of little value in the assessment of ataxia as an ataxic lesion due to cerebellar dysfunction is invariably present when the eyes are open, though worsened by eye closure.

Upward extension of the spinal lesion into the medulla oblongata is usually confirmed by cranial nerve involvement. The presence of wasting and fasciculation of the tongue, an increased jaw jerk, or a spastic bulbar palsy, may obviate the need to perform a myelogram, as for example in the differential diagnosis of motor neurone disease. Abnormal visual evoked potentials may differentiate spinal multiple sclerosis from familial spastic paraparesis. Nystagmus is the only cranial nerve sign about which there is some anatomical dispute. The vestibulospinal tract, involved in the righting reflexes, descends as low as C5 where synapses are found with anterior horn cells. The tract also contains some ascending fibres and it is theoretically possible that nystagmus can arise due to a defect of afferent impulses from the cervical spine (Biemond and De Jong 1969). In clinical practice, when nystagmus is seen in conjunction with cervical cord disease, as with syringomyelia, craniovertebral anomalies or a tumour, the disorder has invariably involved structures rostral to the foramen magnum (Spillane 1968). Down beating nystagmus more prominent on lateral gaze (Ross Russell and Wiles 1985) is characteristic of lesions in the neighbourhood of the foramen magnum, especially in cases of Chiari malformation (Barnett et al. 1973). Foramen magnum lesions may also be accompanied by tingling and sensory loss confined to the finger ends. With larger lesions, such as a high cervical cyst, pin-prick and vibration sensation may be altered over the nape of the neck. Priapism may sometimes occur with high cervical lesions, e.g. following an atlanto-axial dislocation or hangman's fracture. It can occasionally prove a useful diagnostic pointer in the event of sudden, unexplained collapse.

Patchy demyelination affecting the dorsal columns may result in Lhermitte's phenomenon whereby flexion or hyperextension of the neck is accompanied by a shower of electric sensations with a definite radiation: down the back, into the legs, into the arms or occasionally down the sternum or upwards to the head. These symptoms may be mentioned spontaneously or can be elicited by direct questioning. Occasionally they may present for the first time as a sign – the Barber's chair sign – with apparent discomfort when the patient is asked to flex the neck in the course of a neurological examination. The commonest cause in young people is multiple sclerosis, and in the elderly cervical spondylosis. But it may be an early sign of subacute combined degeneration of the cord, occur with pyridoxine excess, after intrathecal administration of vincristine, with cervical cord tumours or as a feature of radiation myelopathy. When Lhermitte's phenomenon follows neck trauma such as whiplash injury, there is often a latent period of about three months and the symptoms may remit spontaneously after a further three to six months.

Cervical spondylosis may present with neck stiffness, as a radiculopathy, as a myelopathy or as a combination of these. Neck movements should be examined as part of the routine neurological examination: at first as actively performed movements of flexion, extension, rotation and lateral flexion (bending the neck towards the shoulder), and then passively, gently repeating the same movement but holding the head for a moment at the extreme of each movement to check whether this elicits any particular complaint from the patient.

Myelopathy usually takes the form of spasticity and long tract signs in the lower limbs. Compressive lesions of the cervical spinal cord usually produce proximal leg weakness and impaired vibration in the feet. However, cases with predominant hand involvement also occur. Usually sensory loss dominates. It is often global (glove distribution) and may extend proximally as far as the elbow (Voskuhl and Hinton 1990). The most likely mechanism is ischaemia of the intrinsic border areas of collateralization between the superficial pial network and the central arterial supply to the cervical cord. Venous stagnation may also play a role.

The presence of radiculopathy, representing the horizontal parameter of spinal cord involvement, can be recognized by means of: (a) lower motor neurone signs, (b) segmental sensory loss and (c) altered reflex activity over the C5,6,7 segments. Wasting and even fasciculation may be observed proximally in the arms. Unilateral neurogenic wasting of the small muscles of the hands, if not due to a combined median/ulnar palsy usually indicates a lesion of the C8 or T1 myotome, either a radiculopathy or anterior horn cell disease. Occasionally, lesions rostral to C8 such as anterior spinal artery thrombosis or insufficiency can cause wasting of the muscles of the hands. Rarely, mid and high cervical cord compression from cervical spondylosis may also result in hand wasting (Goodridge et al. 1987).

The power of each group of muscles is checked noting their segmental references. Likewise, segmental sensory loss to light touch, pin-prick and temperature may be examined. Loss or diminution of reflex activity accompanied by weakness or wasting suggests a lower motor neurone lesion at that segmental level. However, the reflex may also be diminished if there is sensory impairment involving afferent nerve fibres. Compression of the afferent fibres as from osteophyte formation may result in the reflex being lost.

With the arm reflexes, there is some overlap of segments between muscle groups. Thus percussion of the biceps tendon excites C5,6 (chiefly 5) and at the same time evokes a slight response from the triceps muscle C6,7 (chiefly 7), but the resulting contraction produces predominant flexion of the elbow. The spread of a reflex vibratory wave after percussion is enhanced in the presence of spasticity so that there is reflex excitation of other segments and muscle groups due to alpha motor neurone hyperexcitability affecting other muscle spindles. Thus activating the supinator jerk C5,6 (chiefly 6) may also elicit finger flexion C8 and contractions of the brachioradialis, biceps and triceps. In the presence of an efferent radiculopathy, where a disc or osteophyte obstructs the emergent roots at the exit foramen, spread of the reflex to unblocked segments causes other muscles to contract thus producing an inverted response.

The finding of segmental sensory loss provides an indication of root involvement but not of the site of interference. However, once the afferent sensory fibres enter the spinal cord, they become dissociated: those subserving light touch and proprioception pass upwards in the ipsilateral dorsal columns, whereas those subserving pain and temperature enter the posterolateral aspect of the cord, travel upwards for two or three segments, and then cross the midline to the opposite anterolateral spinothalamic tract. An intrinsic lesion such as a cyst or solid tumour in the ventral part of the cord may have no pressure effect upon the dorsal columns or upon the afferent ipsilateral spinothalamic tract; it will almost certainly damage the crossing spinothalamic fibres to right and left (but not necessarily in a symmetrical fashion), and will encroach upon the more deeply situated contralateral spinothalamic fibres in the ascending anterolateral spinothalamic tract. Within this tract there will be relative sparing of the more superficial anterolateral fibres which entered the spinal cord at the lowest level. If the intrinsic lesion is a central syrinx in the neighbourhood of the central canal the result will be bilateral impairment of spinothalamic sensation with a sharp, distinct upper level and a less distinct lower level, producing dissociated and suspended sensory loss. A suspended sensory loss is a sign of an intrinsic lesion: sacral sparing is a less definite sign of an intrinsic lesion and can occur with extrinsic lesions also.

A traumatic, infiltrative or compressive lesion affecting one side of the spinal cord will produce a Brown-Séquard syndrome. A pure hemisection is rarely seen but the concept is useful in diagnosis. Disruption of the anterolateral spinothalamic tract will produce loss of temperature and pain sensation over the opposite side of the body nearly up to the level of the lesion. Disruption of the dorsal columns will result in an ipsilateral sensory loss to light touch and joint position sensation as high as the upper level of the lesion, with an ipsilateral band of total sensory loss over a few segments just below the upper level of the lesion. The plantar reflex on the ipsilateral side will be briskly extensor due to corticospinal tract involvement: that on the contralateral side will be silent because of loss of nociceptive sensation. More commonly an incomplete lesion is seen in clinical practice, usually with bilateral spasticity.

When this is so, the ipsilateral plantar reflex will be briskly extensor and the contralateral reflex less certain with a sluggish extensor response.

References

Aguayo AJ (1987) Peripheral nerve transplants used to test the regenerative capacities of central nervous system neurons. Twelfth Annual Edward H. Lambert Lecture; AAEM 34th Annual Meeting, Oct 15–17, Custom Printing Inc, Rochester, Minnesota, pp 7–25

Asbury AK (1987) Sensory neuropathy. Semin Neurol 7:58–66

Ashby P (1987) Clinical neurophysiology of the spinal cord. In: Brown WF, Bolton CF (eds) Clinical electromyography. Butterworths, Boston, Toronto, pp 453–482

Barnett HJM, Foster JB, Hudgson P (1973) Syringomyelia. Saunders, London

Bickerstaff ER (1980) Neurological examination in clinical practice, 4th edn. Blackwell, Oxford

Biemond A, De Jong JMBV (1969) On cervical nystagmus and related disorders. Brain 92: 437–452

Critchley EMR (1957) Sir David Ferrier. King's College Hospital Gazette 36:243–250

Dickson JH (1986) Pathogenesis and treatment of scoliosis in neuromuscular diseases. In: Dimitrrijevic MR, Kakulas BA, Vrbova G (eds) Recent advances in restorative neurology, vol 2. progressive neuromuscular disorders. Karger, Basel, pp 11–14

Eisen A, Aminoff MJ (1986) Somatosensory evoked potentials. In: Aminoff MJ (ed) Electrodiagnosis in clinical neurology. Churchill Livingstone, Edinburgh, pp 535–573

Eisen A, Shtybel W (1990) Clinical experience with transcranial magnetic stimulation. AAEM Minimonograph. Muscle Nerve 13:1330–1343

Goodridge AE, Feasby TE, Ebers GC, Brown WF, Rice GPA (1987) Hand wasting due to mid-cervical spinal cord compression. Can J Neurol Sci 14:309–311

Guttmann L (1946) Rehabilitation after injuries to the spinal cord and cauda equina. Br J Phys Med 9:162–180

Marsolais EB, Kobetic R (1983) Functional walking in paralysed patients. Clin Orthop Operations 175:30–36

Petrofsky JS, Phillips CA (1983) Computer controlled walking in the paralysed individual. J Neurol Orthop Surg 4:153–164

Ravichandran G, Silver JR (1984) Recognition of spinal cord injury. Hospital Update 10:77–86

Ross Russell RW, Wiles CM (1985) Neurology: integrated clinical science. Heinemann, London

Rubin BD, Fielding JW (1983) Neurological sequelae of cervical cord trauma. Bull Los Angeles Neurol Soc 45:36–40

Spillane JD (1968) An atlas of clinical neurology. Oxford University Press, Oxford, p 16

Thomas PK (1982) Selective vulnerability of the centrifugal and centripetal axons of primary sensory neurons. Muscle Nerve 5(9S):S117–121

Voskuhl RR, Hinton RC (1990) Sensory impairment in the hands secondary to spondylotic compression of the cervical spinal cord. Arch Neurol 47:309–311

Weber RJ (1987) Functional electric stimulation. AAEM, Didactic Program, 34th Annual Meeting. Custom Printing Inc, pp 29–32

Chapter 2

Anatomy as a Key to Function of the Spinal Cord

M.T. Isaac

Various aspects of the topographical anatomy of the spinal cord are discussed in their appropriate chapters in relation to disc disease, tumours, meningitis and vascular pathology. The purpose of the present chapter is to outline the tracts of the human spinal cord with respect to their plasticity and probable function, and to describe something of the function of the grey matter of the cord as understood from anatomical, microelectrode and biochemical studies.

In cross-section the cord can be divided into eight sectors; or two halves composed of quadrants. In Fig. 2.1, the white matter on the right is divided into quadrants, while the left half of the diagram is intended to illustrate the

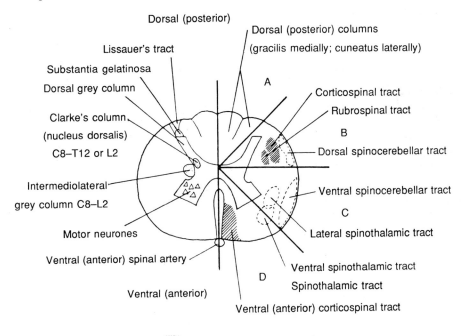

Descending tracts hatched

Fig. 2.1. Spinal cord: diagrammatic cross-section of representative section. (Reproduced with permission from J.H. Adams and D.I. Graham, *An introduction to neuropathology*, Churchill Livingstone, Edinburgh, 1988.)

main features within the grey matter. The transverse section shown is taken at a "representative" level. There is, however, much longitudinal variation in sectional appearance. Thus the proportion of grey to white matter is greater in the more caudal regions and less as one proceeds rostrally due to the addition of motor tracts terminating in the region of the anterior horn cells and the sequential increase in the number of sensory tracts entering the cord. The cord tapers as it descends caudally but bulges in the cervicothoracic and thoracolumbar areas, becoming more oval in cross-section, to encompass intraneurally the extensions of the limbs. A less apparent widening between the C8 to L2 segments is due to the prominence of the intermediolateral column of grey matter which contains the thoracolumbar sympathetic outflow.

The *ascending dorsal* columns of white matter contain fibres principally concerned with pressure discrimination, joint sensation, touch and vibration. Somatotopic representation is fairly precise, with axons from more caudal areas arranged towards the midline. Axons in the ascending columns synapse in the sensory nuclei of the medulla oblongata and, as medial lemnisci, provide considerable input to the contralateral cerebral cortex.

The *anterolateral* white matter systems are known also as "spinothalamic"; though in fact only about one-third of the fibres form terminal arborizations in the thalamus. These columns are concerned predominantly with the sensory modalities of temperature, pain, touch and deep pressure. Localization is less exact with a serial arrangement of modalities laterally to medially. Substantial variation is found in somatotopic alignment within the anterolateral white matter systems; thus the boundaries of the dermatomes associated with dorsal column sensation do not correspond with those for the "spinothalamic" sensations of temperature, pain, etc.

The spinothalamic tract is segmentally laminated. Fibres joining the spinal cord synapse within the grey matter of the dorsal horns. The ascending fibres, arising within the region of the substantia gelatinosa, decussate within 1–2 segments after entry and are added on to the contralateral spinothalamic tract in an orderly way, caudorostrally. Therefore the longest fibres will be sacral, superficial and somewhat dorsal to the more rostrally derived fibres. A central lesion, such as a syrinx, is likely to affect particularly the decussating fibres and the innermost ascending fibres with a resulting bilateral, segmental, and suspended loss of pain and temperature sensation. *Cordotomy* for intractable pain involves the operative sectioning of the anterolateral columns. Unless the cordotomy is made sufficiently deep, fibres from the upper segments may escape and analgesia will be achieved at a lower segment level than intended.

An interesting refinement of this description is offered by Merrill (1974) who showed that expiratory axons (largely derived from the ventral respiratory group in the brainstem) form a discrete and constant bundle within the ventrolateral white matter. Inspiratory axons are more lateral and do not form a discrete bundle (Nakayama and Baumgarten 1964), at least in the cat. Interruption of expiratory tracts may be of significance in *"Ondine's curse"* (Severinghaus and Mitchell 1962) where long periods of apnoea occur when awake unless the patient makes a purposeful voluntary effort to override the apnoea.

The *spinocerebellar* tracts convey proprioceptive information. Approximately 50% of fibres in the ventral tract cross the midline within 1–2 segments of entry and recross at the level of the superior cerebellar peduncle. The remaining ventral tract fibres and virtually all fibres of the dorsal spinocerebellar tracts retain their ipsilateral array and ultimately reach the anterior lobe of the cerebellum, via the inferior cerebellar peduncle. The main sensory input to the spinocerebellar tracts is derived from sensory fibres which synapse in Clarke's column (the nucleus dorsalis) between C8–L2 and in the cuneate nucleus of the medulla oblongata.

The *descending corticospinal* tracts arise from the somatomotor cortex in Broadman's area 4 in the frontal lobes and probably derive from the large pyramidal (Betz) cells in that area. Many constituent fibres are received from other parts of the premotor area and the parietal lobe (especially the somatosensory cortex). The precise origin of all the fibres is not entirely clear. The tracts proceed without interruption to synapse in the ventral (anterior) horns of the grey matter. About 85%–90% of fibres forming the so-called pyramidal tracts decussate in the lower medulla and form the lateral corticospinal tracts, whilst the ipsilateral fibres form the anterior corticospinal tracts. Approximately three-quarters of the fibres are myelinated, and a proportion of these carry antidromic (caudorostral) impulses. Thus, although most axons in the corticospinal tract convey motor impulses from their cortical origin, some intraspinal modulation undoubtedly occurs. The lateral corticospinal tract diminishes in size as it descends and vanishes at the level of S3–4. The developed corticospinal system is not a feature of non-primates, and its phylogenetic youth is thought to be reflected in the tract's presumed function in the facilitation of fine movements of the hands and feet. This assumed role fails to explain the number of clinical reports of preserved fine movements in subjects in whom the corticospinal tract has been interrupted.

Conventionally, the corticospinal tracts are described as *pyramidal* and the remaining descending tracts as *extrapyramidal*. Such a separation is not justified either structurally (the pyramids of the medulla also contain corticobulbar fibres to the cranial nerve nuclei), or functionally. Although it is true that the other descending tracts – vestibulospinal, rubrospinal, reticulospinal – form intermediate synapses outside the spinal grey matter, they can not be shown to have a unique function. They are dependent on afferent modulation, both intra- and supraspinal and probably form an indissoluble functional unity with other tracts. The role of intermediate synapses and the demonstration and analysis of the fact that descending tracts contain ascending fibres and vice versa have been subjects of considerable attention.

The *rubrospinal* tract, which derives from both large and small cells in the red nucleus of the midbrain, runs the whole length of the cord in cats and monkeys but is often regarded as negligible in man, petering out around the level of the lower cervical or upper thoracic spinal segments. Whether this dismissive view is entirely justified or not remains to be established. The rubrospinal tract and the red nucleus both display a crude somatotopic representation, with hindlimb territories represented in the ventrolateral region and forelimb territories in the dorsomedial region. In broad functional terms, both corticospinal and rubrospinal tracts (together with the medullary reticulospinal tract) facilitate flexor movements and inhibit extensor movements. The *olivospinal* tract present in the upper cervical region appears to be part of a circuit of descending and ascending fibres associated with the inferior olivary nucleus of the medulla. A diffuse sytem of descending autonomic fibres does not form a clearly defined tract.

Almost by way of introduction to the *grey matter* organization of the spinal cord, mention should be made of the *tract of Lissauer* (1886), often described as the dorsolateral tract. It is formed by bifurcating ascending and descending small myelinated and unmyelinated fibres of the dorsal root region. The tract appears to contain fibres from small neurones of the substantia gelatinosa and conveys impulses from proprioceptive fibres for a few segments. The term "tract" is perhaps an exaggeration, since the fibres form a few, not always easily discernible, strands. Nevertheless, their intimacy with the substantia gelatinosa merits their mention in any discussion of the structure and function of this region.

The major impetus for the study of the grey matter of the spinal cord came from the work of Rexed (1952, 1954) on the architectonics of the spinal cord in the cat. Rexed analysed the size, packing density and cellular morphology, assorting the spinal grey matter into nine laminae (a tenth is added by some authorities). These are conventionally numbered I–IX (X) and run more or less parallel with the dorsal and ventral boundaries of the grey matter. Since Rexed's initial observations, the laminae have been minutely examined, and innovative techniques of studying individual neurones using iontophoretically applied vital dyes, such as Procion Orange, Red and Yellow, have allowed deeper analysis of the fine details of grey matter architectonics.

Rexed's laminae I–V (or VI) comprise the *dorsal horn* of grey matter, and laminae (VI) VII–IX the *ventral horn*. Lamina I is thin, fibrous and poorly defined; laminae II and III comprise the *substantia gelatinosa*, whilst lamina IV (probably III as well) roughly comprises the *nucleus proprius* of the cord. Laminae V and VI contain a mixed population of cells which are most obvious at the levels of the *limbs' extensions*. Lamina VII contains the *intermediolateral* and *Clarke's columns*; lamina VIII forms a heterogenous anatomical transition zone containing *proprioceptive* fibres, and lamina IX has a complex arrangement of cell columns, the most prominant of which are the large cell bodies of *alpha motor neurones*, together with the smaller perikarya of *gamma efferents* (to muscle spindles) and numerous interneurones. Some of the latter are probably inhibitory in function (cf. Renshaw cells). Such identification is to some extent tentative since, with relatively few exceptions, they do not have the typical (Golgi type II) morphology held to be characteristic of inhibitory cells elsewhere in the central nervous system.

Detailed attention has been paid to the *substantia gelatinosa* in relation to the reception and modulation of painful stimuli. Melzack and Wall (1965) identified the substantia gelatinosa of laminae II and III of the dorsal horn as occupying a pivotal position in the processing of nociceptive information. Their model has been critically reviewed by Nathan (1976) but, nonetheless, has proved of considerable and continuing heuristic value in the discussion of pain mechanisms. They postulated that neurones in the substantia gelatinosa receive stimulatory and inhibitory impulses from small and large diameter afferent fibres, respectively. This information is then used to inhibit, probably presynaptically, the "pain-exciting" afferent impulses to grey matter laminae projecting thence to the spinothalamic/anterolateral ascending tracts. The whole system is subject to higher level (supraspinal) modification. The substantia gelatinosa is thus conceived as a gate governing to some extent the intensity of nociceptive stimuli.

The presence of ascending and descending exchanges of information is of critical conceptual importance. The substantia gelatinosa is regarded by Melzack

(1989) as part of a *"neuromatrix"* which he envisages as a plastic supraspinal calculus into which is fed proprioceptive and other sensorimotor patterns derived from spinally mediated neural inputs. Melzack (1990) conjectures that this "neuromatrix" ultimately provides an "anatomical substratum of the physical self" at cortical level; is partly genetically determined; functions as a form of epigenetic functional algorithm and provides, among other things, a conceptual framework for thinking about the phenomenon of phantom limb pain. (A more general discussion of phantom limb pain and Melzack's hypothesis is presented in the next chapter.)

The cytoarchitectonics of the substantia gelatinosa are well described. Widely arborizing dendritic networks from lamina I and deep fibres from Lissauer's tract intermesh in lamina II with some of the dorsal root afferents and axonal terminations. From the radial array of interneurones in lamina II, axonal connections deliver terminal collaterals to the subjacent laminae III, IV and V, forming synaptic contacts. However, most neuronal connections of the substantia gelatinosa remain intralaminar. Axodendritic interaction also occurs with cells in the deeper laminae. These cells participate in the formation of complex glomerular synapses, sending recurrent axons to the substantia gelatinosa.

A further biochemical dimension to this arrangement has been indicated by recent immunohistochemical studies of neuropeptides. Prominent among these is *substance P*, which contributes to the humoral microenvironment in the substantia gelatinosa in its resting state; but the release of substance P is increased by noxious, rather than by non-noxious stimuli (Duggan et al. 1988). Even so, the presence of substance P alongside endogenous opioids, such as met-enkephalin (Senba et al. 1988), lends support to the view that substance P has a crucial role in modifying nociceptive stimuli in the "gate control" of pain.

There are other questions concerning the role of substance P. In addition to its abundant presence in the substantia gelatinosa, substance P is also found in considerable quantities within other grey matter laminae. Dietl et al. (1989) found that it was present in both the preganglionic (autonomic) neurones of the intermediolateral columns and in lamina X in association with motor neurones. Furthermore the immunoreactivity of substance P is decreased in motor neurone disease (amyotrophic lateral sclerosis) (Dietl et al. 1989). A whole range of neuroactive substances such as 5-hydroxytryptamine, bradykinin, cholecystokinin, neuropeptide Y, somatostatin and thyrotropin releasing factor have been localized within the substantia gelatinosa and, at some time or other, all these have been implicated in pain control. It is presumed that many of these chemicals act over short diffusion distances as neuromodulators, released from excitable cells in response to low (microvolt) voltage dendritic changes, rather than action potentials (millivolt) (Guillemin 1977).

References

Adams JH, Graham DI (1988) An introduction to neuropathology. Churchill Livingstone, Edinburgh, p 14

Dietl MM, Sanchez M, Probst A, Palacios JM (1989) Substance P receptors in the human spinal cord: decrease in amyotrophic lateral sclerosis. Brain Res 483:39–49

Duggan AW, Hendry IA, Morton CR, Zhao ZQ (1988) Cutaneous stimuli releasing immunoreactive substance P in the dorsal horn of the cat. Brain Res 451:261–273

Guillemin R (1977) The significance of hypothalamic peptides: IV. Looking to the future. Recent Prog Horm Res 33:9–18

Melzack R (1989) Phantom limbs, the self and the brain (DO Hebb Memorial Lecture). Can J Psychol 30:1–16

Melzack R (1990) Phantom limbs and the concept of a neuromatrix. Trends Neurosci 13:88–92

Melzack R, Wall PD (1965) Pain mechanisms: a new theory. Science 150:971–979

Merrill EG (1974) Finding a respiratory function for the medullar respiratory neurons. In: Bellairs R, Gray EG (eds) Essays on the nervous system. Clarendon Press, Oxford, pp 451–486

Nakayama S, von Baumgarten R (1964) Lokaliserung absteigender Atmungsbahnenim Rukenmark der Katze mittels antidromer Reizung. Pflugers Archiv 281:231–244

Nathan PW (1976) The gate control theory of pain: a critical review. Brain 99:123–158

Rexed B (1952) The cytoarchitectonic organisation of the spinal cord in the cat. J Comp Neurol 96:415–495

Rexed B (1954) A cytoarchitectonic atlas of the spinal cord in the cat. J Comp Neurol 100: 297–379

Senba E, Yanaihara C, Yanaihara N, Tohyama M (1988) Co-localisation of substance P and met-enkephalin-Arg 6-Gly 7-Leu 8 in the intraspinal neurons of the rat, with special reference to the neurons of the substantia gelatinosa. Brain Res 453:110–116

Severinghaus JW, Mitchell RA (1962) Ondine's curse – failure of respiratory centre automaticity while awake. Clin Res 10:122

Chapter 3

Spinal Modulation of Noxious Stimuli

E.M.R. Critchley and M.T. Isaac

Pain is an imprecise symptom that achieves recognition as a percept within the mind. The central appreciation of pain involves the cerebral cortex, and probably also the lower end of the thalamus and upper end of the midbrain. There are both an organic component – an unpleasant experience primarily associated with physical damage and often described in terms relating to injury (Merskey and Spear 1967) – and a psychological component as interpretation takes place only in the mind, and the information recorded there is entirely personal, a private matter that cannot be shared by anyone else or described in terms that mean the same thing to another person (Mehta 1973). It is learnt from childhood onwards and the expression of that symptom is often governed by memory of previous occasions when it occurred.

At the spinal level we can refer to pain mechanisms, i.e., the processing of information whereby noxious stimuli and tissue injury at the periphery are translated centrally into awareness of pain (Fig. 3.1).

Somatic Sensibility

Normal sensibility depends on temporal and spatial summation and this fact is particularly important for the appreciation of pain (Nathan 1976). Sherrington (quoted by Denny-Brown et al. 1973) showed that any single spot on the trunk is innervated by nerve fibres running into many neighbouring posterior roots. Thus, as part of the process of full, normal sensibility, the stimulus–response is enhanced by an overlap of fibres from neighbouring dorsal roots providing, at spinal level, a background of polysynaptic facilitation.

Historically, the many hypotheses used to explain the transmission of the various modalities of sensation from the periphery to the spinal cord can be grouped into two major theories. The stimulus-specificity theory originally depended on the finding of specific nerve endings in hairy skin. The neurones from which they arise, selectively transmit touch, cold or warmth, but if excessively stimulated give rise to nociceptive sensations. However, non-hairy skin such as that covering the human back is devoid of distinctive end-organs and the human cornea contains only one kind of nerve ending (Lele and Weddell 1956). Even so both these areas are capable of transmitting the full

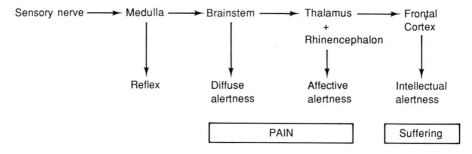

Fig. 3.1.   Central regulation and integration. (From Charpentier 1968.)

range of sensory modalities. The alternative, and not mutually incompatible, pattern theory is that the pattern of discharge from any given fibre could at one time contribute towards the sensation of touch, and at another towards the experience of pain, cold or warmth (Sinclair 1981). Both theories – stimulus-specificity and pattern – have had to be modified in the light of recent research. The hypothesis that all primary afferents respond to pain is questionable. Individual primary afferents are sharply tuned so that they respond well to a certain kind of stimulus and poorly to others, irrespective of the size of their fibres (Hoffert 1989).

Although the types of fibres stimulated are important, the division of afferent nerves into two groups, fast conducting medullated A fibres usually associated with specific nerve endings, and slower conducting unmyelinated C fibres, is too simplistic. C fibres also constitute a major pathway for impulses generated by various innocuous stimuli (Douglas and Ritchie 1957). Individual C fibres are sensitive to only certain stimuli; and these fibres have most amazingly different thresholds (Iggo 1965). It is now accepted that large numbers of nociceptive A delta and C fibres are present in peripheral nerves and many of these specialized fibres respond only to intense stimulation (Wall 1978).

Discrete stimulation at a single site, as for example on the skin of the trunk, will trigger impulses which are transmitted both by fast medullated fibres and by slower conducting unmyelinated fibres. If a noxious stimulus is used, additional bursts of impulses will be triggered by tissue damage with release of nociceptive chemical substances. Injury will be followed by local tenderness, primary hyperaesthesia, which is to be explained by the sensitization of previously high threshold endings to the products of tissue breakdown (Wall 1978). The kind of pain experienced depends not only on groups and sizes of afferent fibres but also on the arrangement of fibres in the tissues, on the layer that is stimulated and on the actual structure stimulated (Keele and Armstrong 1964).

It is also accepted, as was first shown by Rivers and Head (1908), that a reduction in the number of peripheral nerve fibres could cause a change in the character of a sensation, apart from a diminution in its intensity. Noordenbos (1959) found that post-herpetic neuralgia was associated with a selective loss of large fibres. This finding, since modified even for post-herpetic neuralgia, was originally incorporated into the gate control theory of Melzack and Wall (1965) (Fig. 3.2). It was assumed that the input of small fibres was inhibitory on the

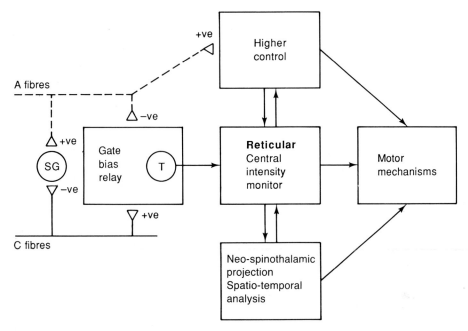

Fig. 3.2. The gate control theory. (From Melzack and Wall 1965.)

substantia gelatinosa and that of large fibres excitatory. Wall (1978) is more circumspect: merely stating that cells in the spinal cord, which are excited by injury signals, are also facilitated or inhibited by other peripheral nerve fibres which carry information about innocuous events. Most neuropathies manifest themselves as an irritative process followed by a destructive one, or else are destructive from the start (Sinclair 1981). Despite the fact that some neuropathies selectively affect large fibres and others small fibres, there is no consistent relationship between the size of fibres which are lost and the painfulness or otherwise of the condition. In Friedreich's ataxia and the polyneuropathy of renal failure, there is large fibre loss without pain. Thallium neuropathy and Fabry's disease are painful conditions associated with loss of small fibres.

The Dorsal Root Entry Zone

The spinal cord has a dual role with respect to noxious stimuli: an immediate reflex avoidance response, i.e., of the trunk away from the stimulus, and the modulation and transmission of impulses to alert the sensorium (Fig. 3.3). Withdrawal of a limb probably involves more complex reflexes without requiring prior awareness of the act. The dorsal root terminals are areas of convergence of sensory information of somatic, visceral and sympathetic origin. This fact has clinical importance in the understanding of referred pain and of the role of the autonomic nervous system in pain relief.

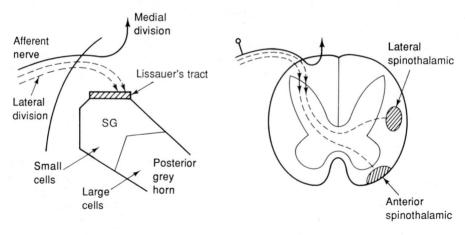

Spinothalamic tracts

Fig. 3.3.   Spinal nociceptive pathways. SG, substantia gelatinosa.

Uncertainty exists about the exact location of modulating mechanisms within the spinal cord, the identity of the cord cells which respond to injury and transmit the impulses onward (T or transmission cells), the relative importance of presynaptic and postsynaptic inhibition in determining the input of the T cells from the periphery, and the presumed role of the substantia gelatinosa (British Medical Journal Leading Article 1978). However, certain facts are known concerning the dorsal root entry zone, the most important being that the number of impulses received from the periphery far exceeds those transmitted rostrally. It is apparent that some selection and modulation of impulses occur in this area. Such modulation would appear to be in part electrical and in part chemical.

Matthews (1934) and Barron and Matthews (1935, 1938) studied the electrical activity originating in the neurones of the posterior horns. The initial finding of a discharge conducted antidromically beyond the ganglia to the periphery in muscular and cutaneous nerves has received little subsequent attention (Nathan 1976). Of greater significance was the finding of slow potential changes spreading along the dorsal roots by a mechanism apparently identical with electrotonic spread and involving depolarization of afferent fibres near their terminals in the grey matter. The degree of depolarization had the effect of partially or intermittently blocking afferent impulses. Hongo et al. (1968) also found evidence of postsynaptic inhibition, but their work has not been widely substantiated whereas presynaptic inhibition has been extensively examined.

The dorsal root potential appears to be subject to various influences:

1. The on-going activity which precedes any new stimulus
2. Descending fibres with both facilitatory and inhibitory effects from the brain and segmental interneurones. Descending fibres from the periaqueductal grey matter have been shown to inhibit the response of lamina V cells of the substantia gelatinosa to noxious stimuli (Oliveras et al. 1974)
3. Spread of activity within the substantia gelatinosa and Lissauer's tract operative over several segments (Wall 1959, 1962)

4. The stimulus evoked activity and the relative balance of activity between different fibre systems

Although everything points to the role of the substantia gelatinosa in the modulation of nociceptive impulses the function of the various laminae is far from clear. There are two areas of particular interest.

A large number of cells in lamina V respond to both myelinated and un-myelinated nociceptive afferents, and are affected by the presence of narcotic and anaesthetic agents. Their receptive fields are complex with some cells responding to high threshold visceral afferents and also to low threshold afferents from skin (Wall 1978). Some cells project to the opposite ventral white matter and some to the thalamus.

The surface of the substantia gelatinosa contains a few cells which only respond to nociceptive afferents. Denny-Brown et al. (1973) regard these marginal cells as a region of equilibrium of neural activity in which the arrival of an impulse from any one point greatly lowers the threshold for the synapse of the axon involved and of topographically related afferents. "The mechanism provides for a combination of temporal and spatial summation."

The modulation of noxious and innocuous sensory stimuli within the sub-stantia gelatinosa is helped by the presence of opiate receptors, including both morphine and met-enkephalin receptors. These receptors have several roles: inhibiting the release of putative nociceptive transmitters such as substance P from the primary afferent terminals, decreasing the excitability of postsynaptic cells, interfering with the activity of the excitatory nociceptive neurotransmitters, or hyperpolarizing cells and neighbouring dendrites (Haigler 1987).

Within the laminae of the substantia efferent axons run up and down the neuraxis in small closed loops or chains in contact with other gelatinosa cells. However, most of those relating to pain sensation travel for three segments or so in Lissauer's tract before crossing over and ascending in the anterolateral tract to the thalamus. It is not known how impulses that converge on cells in the substantia gelatinosa eventually reach the spinothalamic tracts which are situated deeper within the cord.

Pain transmission is best considered within the general framework of dis-criminative and non-discriminative sensations (Fig. 3.4). Several ascending tracts are involved. The limbic system has a role in gating or modulating the impulses. Short spinospinal interneurones may eventually reach the reticular formation. And the more rapidly ascending pain pathways are not rigidly confined within the spinothalamic tract.

Clinical Aspects of Pain Sensibility at Spinal Level

Congenital Analgesia

1. *Complete insensitivity to pain* may be a feature of congenital neuropathies, usually with a virtual absence of small primary afferent fibres in the sensory pathways. Many of these are associated with autonomic nervous system in-volvement which may manifest itself by disturbances in sweating and tempera-ture control (Swanson et al. 1965).

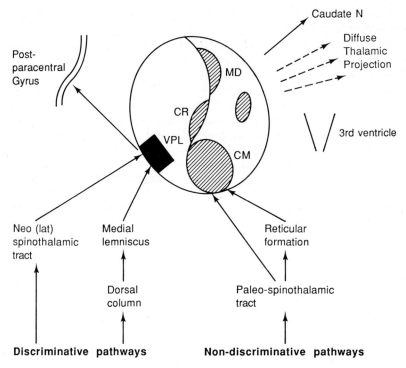

Fig. 3.4. Thalamic pain projection system. ■ ventroposterior lateral nucleus; ▨ intralaminar and parafascicular nuclei.

2. *Pain asymbolia or agnosia* is a condition in which noxious stimuli are felt but the psychiatric reaction to the sensation is absent. This impairment is usually the result of an acquired lesion involving the dominant parietal lobe, but Osuntokua et al. (1968) have described two half-siblings with congenital pain asymbolia and auditory imperception.

3. *Congenital universal indifference to pain* may occur as an inherited disorder. At about the third year of life the child appears not to guard against injury. Even though deep pain is also affected, there is no demonstrable structural damage to the nervous system. Many patients show evidence of repeated self-mutilation, and about 28% are mentally retarded (Thrush 1973; McMurray 1975). Dehen et al. (1979) suggest that the condition may be a manifestation of an overactive endogenous opioid system.

Referred Pain

Disordered localization of pain occurs in three circumstances:

1. Pain derived from a hollow viscus may be experienced in a comparatively remote cutaneous area. The classical example is pain in the shoulder due to lesion under the diaphragm.

2. Pain from non-visceral structures such as muscle, bone or bood vessels is usually misinterpreted as coming from other deep tissues, but never from the skin. This is true of anginal pain which may be transmitted to the jaw and down the left arm.

3. In association with peripheral nerve or spinal injury with areas of dysaesthesia, cutaneous stimulation may be associated with an unusual area of cutaneous "reference". A good example of this phenomenon is afforded by the paraesthesiae of Tinel's sign. The word synaesthesia has a special and distinctive meaning with respect to spinal injury or amputation of limbs. Abnormal spread of sensation can occur and the term, synchiria, is applied when a stimulus such as a pin-prick applied to the unaffected side produces an unpleasant sensation bilaterally. When this occurs unilaterally affecting the "mirror point" on the opposite side of the body it is known as "allochiria" (Obersteiner, 1882). Stimulation of an anaesthetic zone of a succesful cordotomy may produce a sensation of pain either on the same side just above the "level" or else on the opposite side. Other terms used include allaesthesia and synaesthesialgia. A somewhat similar phenomenon was described by Bender (1945) and Henson (1949) whereby simultaneous stimulation of the "mirror point" may either enhance or extinguish the sensory response to a stimulus applied within an area of altered sensibility.

The explanation of referred pain lies in the convergence of somatic and sympathetic impulses into the same sensory pool. The localization of visceral pain is diffuse and reference is often made to a presumed body-schema based on the dermatomal site of embryonic development. Cutaneous hyperalgesia may be present at the side of the referred pain. Infiltration of this trigger area with local anaesthetic agents can bring partial relief of symptoms. Alternatively, counter-irritants may crowd out the impulses from visceral afferents.

Persistent Pathological Pain States

Spontaneous pain may arise as a result of disordered function at spinal level. Several explanations have been proposed for these central pain syndromes. Livingston (1943) postulated a multisynaptic afferent system of short spinospinal fibres capable of setting up reverberating circuits if interfered with pathologically (Fig. 3.5). Gerard (1951) proposed that a peripheral nerve lesion could bring about a temporary loss of sensory control of firing in spinal cord

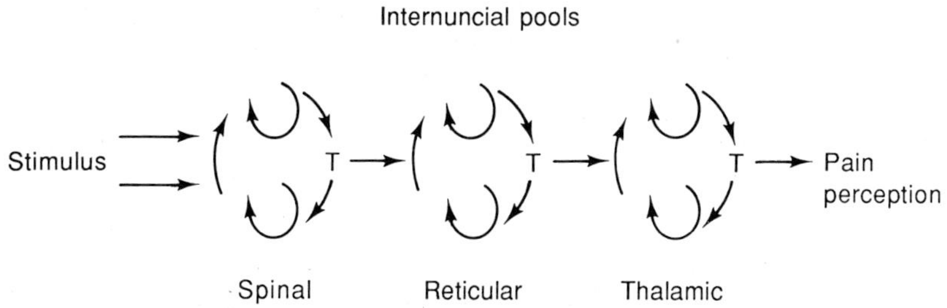

Internuncial pools

Fig. 3.5. Reverberating circuits. (From Livingston 1943.)

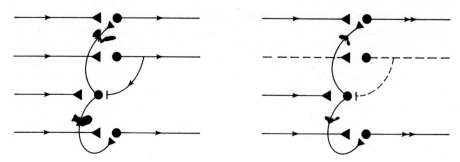

Fig. 3.6. Disruption of firing sequences. (From Gerard 1951.)

internuncial neurones (Fig. 3.6). These may then begin to fire in synchrony; and such synchronous firing could recruit additional units, could move along in the grey matter, and could be maintained by impulses different from and feebler than those needed to initiate it. Melzack (1972) suggested that excessive or otherwise abnormal stimulation can bring about a prolonged bias in the activity of the gate mechanism. Other properties of the "gate" – that it may be influenced by activity in spatially distant areas of the nervous system, and affected by brain mechanisms underlying psychological processes such as memory and emotion – may also serve to prolong this bias.

Causalgia

Causalgia originally denoted a burning quality in pain (Mitchell et al. 1864) and came to be used to describe a painful syndrome commonly found in wartime traumatic casualties. It may also arise in conjunction with fractures, sprains, crush injuries and relatively minor trauma (British Medical Journal Leading Article 1971), occurring in 2%–5% of people who sustain peripheral nerve injury. The severe and persistent unpleasant burning sensations are notoriously resistant to most forms of surgical and medical treatment.

Intense pain begins almost immediately after the accident, but occasionally is delayed for weeks or months. The pain may be spontaneous but may be aggravated or precipitated by touch, movement or psychological factors. New pains and trigger zones may spread unpredictably to other parts of the body where no pathology exists. Autonomic manifestations inevitably coexist with the peripheral injury. The limb may show typical skin changes with tightness, redness and sweating. Involuntary jerky movements may occur. If the pain is severe enough to prevent the full use of the limb, trophic changes appear in the skin and nails, and the bones become osteoporotic. Patients become demoralized by the persistence and severity of symptoms and the failure of treatment to control them (Mehta 1973).

Neuralgic Pains

Unpleasant explosive pains can occur in relation to many clinical conditions such as lesions of the thalamus, tabes dorsalis, mesencephalic tractotomy, lesions of the lemniscal system and post-herpetic neuralgia (Sinclair 1981). Some pains may be continuous but others spontaneous and paroxysmal. There may be a raised threshold for all forms of cutaneous sensibility with a painful over-reaction to such stimuli as are able to cross the threshold. The lesions are often infective or degenerative and judging from clinical observation the essential condition for the production of this syndrome at whatever level is a certain degree of incompleteness of the lesion (Symonds 1931).

Phantom Limbs

Phantom limb sensations occur in practically every patient following traumatic amputation of a limb, can occur following brachial plexus avulsion without loss of a limb, and are experienced in paraplegics following spinal injury. Phantoms are rare in those with mutilating diseases such as leprosy or gangrene (Frederiks 1980) or in children under the age of four years, but are almost invariable in adults following trauma (Simmel 1956, 1962). A phantom may last for years, and even when lost may be recovered under stress (Weddell and Sinclair 1947).

The most comprehensive studies of phantom limbs have tended to follow wartime experiences, as with the excellent study of 73 Israeli male soldiers injured in the Yom Kippur War of October 1973 (Carlen et al. 1978). All experienced an illusory awareness of the missing part. With time the phantom tended to weaken in intensity and the limb to telescope in towards the stump until the digits of the phantom merged into its substance. A painful phantom is less likely to shrink in size with the passage of time and may remain, continuing to cripple and oppress. Thus 5%–10% of patients suffered disagreeable sensations, variously described as cramp, shooting, burning and crushing. Phantom pains tend to develop in those who suffered pain in the limb for some time prior to amputation and may closely resemble in quality and localization the pain that was present before amputation. Thus burning pains generally follow irritant wounds and emergency amputation, sometimes freezing the phantom in distorted attitudes such as that occupied at the time of the accident. Pain emanates from pressure on specially sensitive areas, trigger zones which are situated initially in the injured part but gradually spread to other areas of the body which are healthy and unrelated to the injury; so much so that urination, defaecation and ejaculation may be accompanied by a burning sensation in both the phantom and the stump end.

Stump pain occurs in about 43% of amputees and is an ill-defined and painful muscle cramp occurring in the whole stump which will sometimes twitch or jerk spasmodically entirely beyond the control of the unfortunate patient. Drug-induced dyskinesias may even affect a phantom limb (Jankovic and Glass 1985). Painful neuromas may be present at the nerve ends. The overlying skin can become exquisitely tender to touch and undergo vasomotor changes of causalgic type. These symptoms occur independently or in addition to phantom limb pain.

In normal subjects, local anaesthesia of peripheral nerves, loss of sensation in a limb as in the Guillain-Barre syndrome, or avulsion of the brachial plexus may all generate phantom limb sensations, which would appear to indicate that the phantom can be generated centrally in the absence of neural impulses from affected dermatomes. This does not mean that the periphery is irrelevant to all phantoms, as electrical stimulation of the stump invariably exaggerates the phantom.

The phantom phenomena of paraplegics differ from those of amputees. Whereas the vividness of the phantom is obvious from discussion with any amputee, a similar complaint may be hard to elicit from a paraplegic. Boss (1951) cites two patients with arm and mid-thoracic amputations in whom the arm phantom was obvious while the lower body phantom required considerable concentration to describe. Paraplegics with complete cord section may feel as though their bodies caudal to the transection are missing entirely. Some paraplegics experience phantom feelings within a few days, but others note such feelings after several months have elapsed. In contrast to the detail with which a phantom limb is described, paraplegics cannot truly sense details but talk of a bizarre continuity or a vague awareness. Telescoping does not occur and painful phenomena are absent.

Phantom phenomena affecting other organs have also been described, e.g. following enucleation, tooth extraction, facial mutilation, castration or mastectomy (Frederiks 1980). In contrast to the 100% occurrence of phantom phenomena following limb amputation such phenomena – phantom pain and non-painful phantom sensations – rarely affect more than 20%–30% of those who undergo mutilation or amputation at other sites (Kroner et al. 1989).

The Origin of Phantom Phenomena

Controversy exists between those who hold Melzack's hypothesis of a central neuromatrix (1989) or a central generating mechanism for pain (Melzack and Loeser 1978) and others who suggest that phantom phenomena arise peripherally or at spinal level. Dimond (1980) sees the spinal cord (1) as a part of the brain extended longitudinally, (2) as having a localizing function at its different levels, (3) as relating to many psychological processes not usually thought to be associated with it and (4) as having an effect upon higher mental functions, including sexual libido, dreaming and emotional expressiveness. "It is clear that the cord speaks to the rest of the brain in ways we barely understand at present."

Centrally, phantom phenomena can be associated with schizophrenia (Ames 1984), parietal lesions, thalamic stimulation or epilepsy (Hecaen and de Ajurriaguerra 1952); and altered or abolished by ECT, vascular accidents, intoxication or vestibular stimulation (Frederiks 1980). Phantom limbs can arise from spinal cord lesions (Riddoch 1941; Berger and Gerstenbrand 1981), or be modified or abolished by cordotomy or section of posterior roots. That an interaction occurs between brain and spinal cord has been admirably summarized by Russell (1970): "Almost all amputees experience phantom limb sensations but these vary so widely as to indicate that the relationship between periphery and brain is variable according perhaps to personality, natural interest in giving attention to bodily sensations, previous occupation and the general threshold of the individual to pain, injury and other menacing situations. In other words, the individual's reaction to the effects of amputation partly depends on how the CNS has been trained during that person's life".

Treatment of Pain Syndromes

Two lines of treatment are of primary importance: recognition and treatment of the psychological effects of the trauma, and removal, as far as is possible, of any focus of irritation. Psychological aspects include adequate relief of pain in the acute stages, counselling, antidepressants, analgesics and thymoleptic drugs which alter the threshold of awareness of pain. Neuralgic pains, in particular, may not respond to conventional analgesics except in doses causing drowsiness, which may be unacceptable to the patient or to a normal life-style.

Cleansing the site of trauma is best illustrated by phantom limb and stump pain. Surgical debridement of the area, removing foci of infection, removing jagged structures, ensuring that all viable tissues have an adequate blood supply, and sectioning neuromas can bring much relief. Physiotherapy is vital for the relief of symptoms in a traumatized limb. Active treatment encouraging relaxation, reducing spasticity, putting the limb through passive movements and later encouraging the full range of motion exercises can prevent joints becoming fixed and contractures developing. Traditionally, pain in the stump can be alleviated by hitting trigger areas with a blunt hammer. Ultrasound, transcutaneous electrical stimulation and vibrators can all achieve the same effect. Only rarely do phantom limbs fail to respond to apparently complete peripheral anaesthesia (Carlen et al. 1978).

With referred pain, infiltration of hyperalgesic areas is also effective. Causalgias may be helped by sympathetic nerve blockade (Loh and Nathan 1978), so much so that they have been called sympathetic-maintained pains (Portenoy 1989). Surgical sympathectomies, however, are unsatisfactory as failure to bring relief may be accompanied by further spread of the pain to previously unaffected areas. Nerve blockade is probably more useful diag-nostically and prognostically than therapeutically. Peripheral nerve section is rarely of lasting help and where pain is relieved, memory of pain soon passes and the patient may find any dysaesthesia of the overlying skin equally unacceptable.

Counter-irritation is a household remedy for deep pain, but nobody knows how it works (Sinclair 1981). The modern pundits have given it a new acronym, DNIC (diffuse noxious inhibitory control) for the phenomenon in which the application of a focal noxious stimulus yields analgesia in a unrelated region of the body (Portenoy 1989). Topical capsaicin is advocated for the relief of post-herpetic neuralgia but the results are variable and some neurosurgeons believe that the patient should be heavily sedated before the drug is applied. Equally helpful but equally unexplained are the neuroaugmentative techniques of acupuncture, percutaneous stimulation and dorsal column stimulation (Sweet and Wepsic 1974). The assumption is that they all modify the bias of the "gate" (Melzack and Wall 1965). There is additional evidence that acupuncture and low frequency transcutaneous electrical stimulation (TENS) also stimulate the activity of endorphin systems within the substantia gelatinosa (Mayer et al. 1977). In contrast, an endorphinergic mechanism does not appear to be essential in the analgesia produced by high-frequency peripheral stimulation (Chapman and Benedetti 1977).

Rhizotomies, or section of dorsal root entry zones, have been used to bring 50% relief following spinal cord injury, but are of little value in the control of

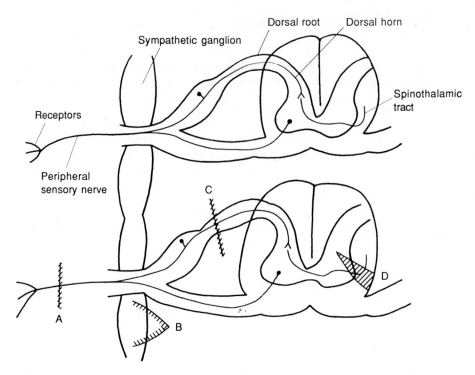

Fig. 3.7. Neurosurgical procedures for pain relief. A, neurectomy; B, sympathectomy; C, rhizotomy; D, cordotomy.

diffuse pain or predominantly sacral pain. Friedman and Nashold (1986) suggest that the best results are obtained when several roots are sectioned above a unilateral lesion. However an alternative explanation of the fact that section of the dorsal roots may not relieve pain (Coggeshall et al. 1975) may lie in the recognition that the spinal roots – and particularly the ventral root in man – contain a mixture of sensory and motor fibres. Sykes and Coggeshall (1973) found that one-third of the fibres of the ventral root are unmyelinated and presumably of sensory origin. This finding directly contradicts the early 19th century concept formulated by Bell (1811) and Magendie (1822) whereby the sensory and motor functions are discrete and localized to the dorsal and ventral roots respectively.

Chemical rhizotomy using intrathecal phenol, chlorocresol or silver nitrate is an exacting technique which can bring relief of severe pain or spasticity and can be repeated as necessary (Maher 1955). Relief of pain is unaccompanied by substantial alterations in other sensory modalities, but sphincter disturbances can arise if the patient is not skilfully positioned.

Section of the anterolateral tracts – cordotomy – can be performed percutaneously under X-ray control but should be reserved for patients with malignant disease or a limited life expectancy (Fig. 3.7). A unilateral cordotomy performed at C2–3 will relieve pain in 70%–75% of patients, raising the threshold to pain by 40%–50%. Complications include numbness below the lesion, muscle weakness in the legs, loss of bladder and rectal control, impotence and an unstable blood pressure. If a bilateral cordotomy is required the second operation should be performed at C5–6 in order to avoid respiratory distress. The fact that pain perception returns despite the irreversible nature of the neurosurgical operation is of great theoretical importance, and would indicate that the relationship of pain perception to its preferred spinal cord projection system is plastic (Hoffert 1989).

References

Ames D (1984) Self-shooting of a phantom head. Br J Psychiatry 145:193–194

Barron DH, Matthews BHC (1935) Intermittent conduction in the spinal cord. J Physiol (Lond) 85:73–103

Barron DH, Matthews BHC (1938) The interpretation of potential changes in the spinal cord. J Physiol (Lond) 92:272–321

Bell C (1811) Idea of a new anatomy of the brain. Strahan and Preston, London

Bender MB (1945) Extinction and precipitation of cutaneous sensation. Arch Neurol Psychiatry 54:1–9

Berger M, Gerstenbrand R (1981) Phantom illusions with spinal cord lesions. In: Siegfried I, Zimmerman M (eds) Phantom and stump pain. Springer-Verlag, Berlin, pp 66–73

Boss E (1951) Phantom limbs of patients after spinal cord injury. Arch Neurol Psychiatry 66: 610–631

British Medical Journal (1971) Causalgia. Br Med J i:64 (leading article)

British Medical Journal (1978) The gate control theory of pain. Br Med J ii:586–587 (leading article)

Carlen PL, Wall PD, Nadvoma H, Steinbeck T (1978) Phantom limbs and related phenomena in recent traumatic amputations. Neurology 28:211–217

Chapman RN, Benedetti I (1977) Analgesia following transcutaneous electrical stimulation and its partial reversal by a narcotic antagonist. Life Sci 21:1645–1648

Charpentier J (1968) Analysis and measurement of pain in animals: a new conception of pain. In: Soulairac A, Cahn J, Charpentier J (eds) Pain. Proc Int Symposium on Pain, Paris, 1967. Academic Press, London and New York, pp 171–200

Coggeshall RE, Applebaum ML, Fazen M, Stubbs TB, Sykes MT (1975) A review of the Bell-Magendie hypothesis. Brain 98:157–166

Dehen H, Willer JC, Cambier J (1979) Congenital indifference to pain and endogenous morphine-like system. In: Bonica JJ, Liebeskind JC, Albe-Fessard DG (eds) Advances in pain research and therapy, vol 3. Raven Press, New York, pp 553–557

Denny-Brown D, Kirk EJ, Yanagisawa N (1973) The tract of Lissauer in relation to sensory transmission in the dorsal horn of spinal cord in the macaque monkey. J Comp Neurol 151: 175–200

Dimond SJ (1980) Neuropsychology. Butterworths, London, pp 520–521

Douglas WW, Ritchie JM (1957) Non-medullated fibres in the saphenous nerve which signal touch. J Physiol (Lond) 139:385–399

Frederiks JAM (1980) Phantom limb and phantom limb pain. In: Vinken PJ, Bruyn GW, Klawans HL (eds) Handbook of clinical neurology 45. Elsevier, Amsterdam, pp 395–404

Friedman AH, Nashold BS (1986) DREZ lesions for relief of pain related to spinal cord injury. J Neurosurg 65:465–469

Gerard RW (1951) A new theory of causalgic pain. Anesthesiology 12:1–10

Haigler HJ (1987) Neurophysiological effects of opiates in the CNS. Monogr Neurolog Soc 13:132–160

Hecaen H, de Ajurriaguerra J (1952) Méconnaissance et hallucinations corporelles. Masson et Cie, Paris

Henson RA (1949) On thalamic dysaesthesiae and their suppression by bilateral stimulation. Brain 72:576–598

Hoffert MJ (1989) The neurophysiology of pain. Neurolog Clin 7:183–204

Hongo T, Jankowska E, Lundberg A (1968) Postsynaptic excitation and inhibition for primary afferents in neurons of the spinocervical tract. J Physiol (Lond) 199:569–592

Iggo A (1965) The peripheral mechanisms of cutaneous sensation. In: Curtis DR, McIntyre AK (eds) Studies in physiology. Springer, Berlin, pp 92–100

Jankovic J, Glass JP (1985) Metoclopramide-induced phantom dyskinesia. Neurology 35:432–435

Keele CA, Armstrong D (1964) Substances producing pain and itch. Arnold, London

Kroner K, Krebs B, Skov J, Jorgensen HS (1989) Immediate and long-term phantom breast syndrome after mastectomy: incidence, clinical characteristics and relationship to pre-mastectomy breast pain. Pain 36:327–334

Lele PP, Weddell G (1956) The relationship between neurohistology and corneal sensibility. Brain 79:119–154

Livingston WK (1943) Pain mechanisms. Macmillan, New York

Loh L, Nathan PW (1978) Painful peripheral states and sympathetic blocks. J Neurol Neurosurg Psychiatry 41:664–671

Magendie F (1822) Experiences sur les fonctions des racines des nerfs rachidiens. J Physiol Exp 2:276–279

Maher RM (1955) Relief of pain in incurable cancer. Lancet 1:18–20

Matthews BHC (1934) Impulses leaving the spinal cord by dorsal roots. J Physiol (Lond) 81:29–31P

Mayer DJ, Price DD, Rafii A (1977) Antagonism of acupuncture analgesia in man by the narcotic antagonist naloxone. Brain Res 121:368–372

McMurray GA (1975) Theories of pain and congenital universal insensitivity to pain. Can J Psychol 29:302–315

Mehta M (1973) Intractable pain. Saunders, London

Melzack R (1972) Mechanisms of pathological pain. In: Critchley M, O'Leary JL, Jennett B (eds) Scientific foundations of neurology. Heinemann, London, pp 153–165

Melzack R (1989) Phantom limbs, the self and the brain. DO Hebb Memorial Lecture. Can Psychol 30:1–16

Melzack R, Loeser JD (1978) Phantom body pain in paraplegics: evidence for a central "pattern generating mechanism" for pain. Pain 4:195–210

Melzack R, Wall PD (1965) Pain mechanisms: a new theory. Science 150:971–979

Merskey H, Spear FG (1967) Pain: psychological and psychiatric aspects. Ballière Tindall, Cassell, London

Mitchell SW, Morehouse GR, Keen WW (1864) Gunshot wounds and other injuries of nerves. Lippincott, Philadelphia

Nathan PW (1976) The gate-control theory of pain: a critical review. Brain 99:123–158

Noordenbos W (1959) Pain. Elsevier, Amsterdam

Obersteiner H (1882) On allochiria, a peculiar sensory disorder. Brain 4:153–163

Oliveras JL, Redjemi JM, Guilbaud G, Liebeskind JC (1974) Behavioural and electrophysiological evidence of pain inhibition from midbrain stimulation in the cat. Exper Brain Res 20:32–44

Osuntokua BO, Odeku EL, Luzzato L (1968) Congenital pain asymbolia and auditory imperception. J Neurol Neurosurg Psychiatry 31:291–296

Portenoy RK (1989) Mechanisms of clinical pain: observations and speculations. Neurolog Clin 7:205–230

Riddoch G (1941) Phantom limbs and body schema. Brain 64:197–222

Rivers WHR, Head H (1908) A human experiment in nerve division. Brain 31:323–450

Russell WR (1970) Neurological sequelae of amputation. Br J Hosp Med 4:607–609

Simmel ML (1956) On phantom limbs. Arch Neurol Psychiatry 75:637–647

Simmel ML (1962) Phantom experiences following amputation in childhood. J Neurol Neurosurg Psychiatry 25:69–78

Sinclair D (1981) Mechanisms of cutaneous sensation. Oxford University Press, Oxford

Swanson AG, Buchan GC, Alvord EC (1965) Anatomic changes in congenital insensitivity to pain. Am Med Assoc Arch Neurol 12:12–18

Sweet WH, Wepsic JG (1974) Stimulation of the posterior columns of the spinal cord for pain control: indications, technique and results. Clin Neurosurg 21:278–320

Sykes MT, Coggeshall RE (1973) Unmyelinated fibres in the human L4 and L5 ventral roots. Brain Res 63:490–495

Symonds CP (1931) The physiology of painful sensation. Lancet 2:723–726

Thrush DC (1973) Congenital insensitivity to pain – a clinical, genetic and neurophysiological study of four children from the same family. Brain 96:369–386

Wall PD (1959) Repetitive discharge of neurones. J Neurophysiol 22:305–320

Wall PD (1962) The origin of a spinal cord slow potential. J Physiol (Lond) 164:508–526

Wall PD (1978) The gate control theory of pain mechanisms – a re-examination and a re-statement. Brain 101:1–18

Weddell G, Sinclair D (1947) Pins and needles, observations on some of the sensations aroused in a limb by the application of pressure. J Neurol Neurosurg Psychiatry 10:26–46

Chapter 4

Spasticity

M.T. Isaac

The segmental structure of the spinal cord provides the framework for reflex equilibration of the state of tension within muscle groups at rest and during purposeful, voluntary and involuntary movement. Muscle stretch reflexes control the state of contraction not only of each particular muscle but are additionally responsible for coordinating the tonicity of agonists and antagonists over several adjacent segments. Each muscle receives a dual innervation.

Large, myelinated alpha motor neurones tonically activate the muscle bulk, controlling its length and degree of contraction at rest and producing active contraction or relaxation during initiation and performance of movement. A separate system of gamma efferent fibres, also arising from the grey matter of the anterior horns, controls flow of movement and finer adjustment of the state of muscle tension by modifying the length and contraction of muscle spindles situated within the muscle bellies. For practical purposes the effect of a third system of beta motor neurones which impinge on both extrafusal muscle fibres and intrafusal fibres of the muscle spindles can be ignored.

The afferent half of the reflex arc is provided by: (a) type Ib fibres arising from Golgi stretch receptors in the tendons, (b) medium-sized, myelinated Ia afferent fibres activated by "dynamic" gamma efferents and projecting directly on to homonymous alpha motor neurones, and (c) thinner, myelinated group II fibres activated by "static" gamma efferents, projecting via interneurones on to the flexor motor neurones of the same segment. Thus the balance of alpha and gamma motor neurone activity is sustained by an elaborate segmental meshwork of facilitatory and inhibitory synapses and interneurones coordinated from above by the tonic influence of extrapyramidal pathways with the cerebellar influence directed for the most part on to dynamic gamma efferents acting upon muscle spindles.

At rest, tonic activity of lower motor neurones is maintained at a relatively slow rate of firing in comparison to the assorted hyperactive afferent inflow. Only when impulses relayed by corticospinal pathways call forth a flurry of activity in the initiation of movement do activated lower motor neurones respond with a dramatic alteration in firing rate. Anterior horn cells must be repetitively stimulated in order to sustain a high firing rate; otherwise the pattern of discharge is dampened by the inhibitory synapse activity of Renshaw cells which arise from branches of the main axon of the lower motor neurone. In the rare syndrome of the isolated lower motor neurone, continuous autonomous firing of the anterior horn cell can result in wasting and fasciculating, spastic muscles.

Spinal cord dysfunction, except in the acute stage of spinal shock, results in muscle hypertonicity; whereas damage to the integrity of the lower motor neurone produces flaccidity. The various forms of hypertonia are important clinically and need to be assessed quantitatively as well as qualitatively so that response to treatment can be graded accurately.

Tone is assessed at rest with the patient as fully relaxed as possible by observing the response to muscle stretch when the limb is passively manipulated, preferably across two different joints in order to minimize the effect of any voluntary or involuntary participation by the patient. It has also been found useful to measure the excitability curve of tendon jerks or H reflexes (Delwaide et al. 1980), the interaction between tendon jerks, H reflexes and vibratory reflexes (Ashby et al. 1980), and the interaction between stretch reflexes and volitional control (Neilsen 1972).

With voluntary or hysterical hypertonia the degree of rigidity is proportional to the observer's efforts to move the limb and both flexors and extensors are equally involved.

The plastic rigidity of an extrapyramidal lesion results in a relatively constant quantum of resistance to passive stretching which always yields to a slightly greater force. If the limb is totally supported and relaxed, the rigidity can disappear allowing unimpeded passive movement within a small range of 5–10°. Over a larger range motor units are recruited into contraction by stretching but drop out again one by one as other units are recruited.

With dystonia, posture is maintained by exaggerated muscle tone, not in an intermediate state between flexion and extension but at an extreme degree of one or the other.

By contrast, when a spastic muscle is stretched more and more motor units are recruited until a peak of resistance is reached. Thereafter, the exhausted motor units suddenly cease to function with an immediate loss of further resistance – the clasp knife response. In many respects this is an inelegant and sometimes painful test but there are other pathognomonic properties of spastic muscles:

1. The resistance to stretch seen in spasticity is velocity dependent, i.e. resistance is increased with faster stretching movements and will be variable through a range of velocities.
2. Resistance is greatest when muscle stretch is first attempted and fades with further stretching.
3. Tone and resistance vary between flexor and extensor muscle groups being greatest in the lower limb extensors and upper limb flexors.
4. Spasticity is accompanied by upper motor neurone signs including exaggerated deep tendon reflexes and clonus.

The pattern of spasticity is dependent upon the level of upper motor neurone impairment (Dimitrijevic 1985). The mildest form with spinal cord injury results in muscle hypertonia predominantly affecting the flexor muscle groups with a selective increase in phasic stretch reflexes. With more severe and diffuse spinal lesions, tonic stretch reflexes, synkinetic reflexes, marked clonus, and paraplegia in extension may occur. Decerebrate rigidity is the hallmark of extensive brainstem lesions with enhancement of tonic stretch reflexes and extensor hypertonicity.

A hemispheric lesion, whether cortical or capsular, produces a spastic hemiparesis with hypertonia of the flexor muscles of the arm and extensor muscles of the legs and a corresponding weakness of the antagonistic extensors and flexor muscle groups respectively.

In all forms of spasticity tonic activity of the anterior horn cells is accompanied by an increased sensitivity to peripheral afferent input. There is a lowered threshold for the activation of withdrawal reflexes. Proprioceptive afferents from the tension receptors and muscle spindles enhance the degree of spasticity. Furthermore, exteroceptive afferents from other tissues will also influence the state of muscle tension.

In clinical practice this means that the degree of spasticity in a particular patient can be markedly increased by distension of a viscus, infection or irritation. Examples include: a full bladder due to urinary retention, a loaded colon, burns and scalds, pressure sores and decubitus ulcers, irritation from ingrowing toe-nails, the presence of fractures, pockets of infection, interdigital tinea, and cystitis.

The treatment of spasticity must begin by asking the question why it has occurred. Otherwise there is a tendency to overlook the possibility of an expanding lesion or spinal cord compression. Next, one should eliminate all treatable causes of exteroceptive stimulation of the reflex arc and, thirdly, every attempt should be made to keep the patient or the limb mobile.

The profusion of available drugs is a reminder that the results of medication are rarely totally successful and may be limited by tolerance, loss of effectiveness, concomitant weakness or unwanted side-actions. Selective tenotomies and peripheral neurectomies may be performed to prevent the development of contractures and abnormal postures. However, the mainstay of interventional treatment is the reduction of the influx of afferent stimulation to the spinal cord by nerve blockade, posterior rhizotomies, or through the use of intrathecal drugs such as phenol or chlorocresol.

References

Ashby P, Verrier M, Carleton S, Somerville J (1980). Vibratory inhibition of the monosynaptic reflex and presynaptic inhibition in man. In: Feldman RG, Young RR, Koella WP (eds) Spasticity: disordered motor control. Chicago Year Book Medical Publications, pp 335–344

Delwaide PJ, Martinelli P, Crenna P (1980) Clinical neurophysiological measurement of spinal reflex activity. In: Feldman RG, Young RR, Koella WP (eds) Spasticity: disordered motor control. Chicago Year Book Medical Publications, pp 345–371

Dimitrijevic MR (1985) Spasticity. In: Swash M, Kennard C (eds) Scientific basis of clinical neurology. Churchill Livingstone, Edinburgh, pp 108–115

Neilsen PD (1972) Interaction between voluntary contraction and tonic stretch reflex transmission in normal and spastic patients. J Neurol Neurosurg Psychiatry 35:853–860

Chapter 5

Hazards of Lumbar Puncture

J.P.R. Dick

With the wider availability of computed brain tomography (CT) not only is it possible to predict which patients are likely to suffer adverse effects from lumbar puncture (LP) (Gower et al. 1987) but it has also become unnecessary to puncture several categories of patient who required this investigation in the pre-CT era. Thus LP is unnecessary both in patients with an intracranial mass lesion and in the majority of patients with aneurysmal subarachnoid haemorrhage (SAH, Macdonald and Mendelow 1988). Indeed, it is probably unwise to LP some patients with SAH as there is evidence that prolonged CSF drainage leads to an increased risk of aneurysmal rupture (Hasan et al. 1989). However, LP is essential in the management of CNS infection and valuable in excluding SAH, so long as it is done within 21 days of the ictus (Walton 1956; Vermeulen et al. 1983); in addition, it is useful in the investigation of certain vascular, toxic, inflammatory, degenerative and immunological disorders of the CNS.

Two urgent indications for LP remain: suspected purulent or carcinomatous meningitis and suspected spinal cord compression due to epidural disease (malignant or infective), which requires myelography. At tertiary referral centres the latter indication will become less pressing with the wider use of MR imaging (Berns et al. 1989).

However, even in these circumstances care needs to be taken as certain categories of patient may fare poorly with LP. For instance, it is recognized that cardiac arrest may occur during LP in infants with cardiopulmonary disease (Margolis and Cook 1973) and in infants with severe meningitis, death from LP is still reported (Harper et al. 1985). It may be better to treat first and base a bacteriological diagnosis on clinical grounds and blood culture (Harper et al. 1985; Shapiro et al. 1986).

Complications of the Technique

Spinal anaesthesia has provided useful data on the incidence of traumatic complications from LP in experienced hands. Dripps and Vandam (1951) reported that complications were rare and were usually related to the dural puncture rather than the anaesthetic agent. They attributed complications to three processes: trauma, changes in CSF pressure and infection. They sent questionnaires to 6147 patients who had had spinal anaesthesia over the period 1948–1951. Of the 90% who replied, 13% had had electric shock sensations radiating down one leg at the time of puncture (root trauma) and 1% had experienced subsequent tinnitus which resolved spontaneously. This concurs with data from a neurological centre (Brem et al. 1981) where 11 of 175 patients developed traumatic complications of LP. Of 637 patients who had had 16 G needles (Dripps and Vandam 1951), 22% had post-LP headache and 5 of these had had horizontal diplopia which recovered spontaneously over 3 weeks to 9 months. None of their cases suffered infective complications.

Trauma

Weber and Weingarden (1979) have shown that EMG abnormalities occur in 40% of cases following myelography. They were not associated with significant symptomatology and disappeared by the fourth post-myelogram day. Although the incidence of even minor traumatic complications is low in experienced hands – 10% according to Dripps and Vandam (1951) – rarely a nerve root may be transected (Young and Burney 1971) and this has been associated with Sudeck's atrophy (Morettin and Wilson 1970). On withdrawal of the spinal needle, the stylet should be replaced as it is possible to aspirate a nerve root and draw it through the dura (Trupp 1977). It is important to have a stylet that fits flush with its casing as there are reports of intradural epidermoid tumours, resulting from the proliferation of epithelial cells originally introduced at LP (Tabaddor and Lamorgese 1975).

Trauma and Associated Bleeding

Traumatic haemorrhage occurs not infrequently with LP. This is usually minimal, occurs because sharp needles transgress the subarachnoid space and traumatize the rich collection of veins in the ventral epidural space and will complicate cellular analysis of the CSF (Petito and Plum 1974). Excessive bleeding may occur in patients with angiomatous malformations, with hae-matological disorders, particularly thrombocytopenia (Edelson et al. 1974) and in patients receiving anticoagulants (Harik et al. 1971). In contrast to intra-cranial haemorrhage, traumatic haemorrhage into the spinal canal occurs in the extradural space more commonly than the subdural space. This is because the dura is attached to the inner table of the calvarium in the skull but is separated from the vertebrae by a venous plexus and loosely arranged fatty tissue. It is this venous plexus which is most often traumatized by the LP needle.

Haemorrhage into Extradural Space

This may occur after minor trauma, such as straining or turning over in bed (Dawson 1963) or may follow LP, particularly in patients on anticoagulant therapy (Harik et al. 1971). It is associated with severe local pain, may cause acute cord compression and is slightly commoner in the thoracic region (Harik et al. 1971). No structural lesion is found in many cases (angiomatous malformation ablated) while angiomatous lesions are found in others. Extradural angiomatous malformations may be associated with vertebral angiomata and are less common than intradural ones. Odom (1960) analysed 32 cases of extradural haemorrhage some of whom were associated with polycythaemia rubra vera (PRV), haemophilia and anticoagulant therapy. He noted that the onset of pain occurred after stooping in a considerable number. The clinical urgency is similar to that of spinal epidural abscess. Decompressive laminectomy, with adequate supplies of blood for transfusion, is urgent (Findlay 1987). Preoperative plain films should be inspected for a vertebral angiomatous malformation, and dura, spinal cord and evacuated clot for evidence of angiomata.

Haemorrhage into Subdural Space

This is extremely rare (Edelson et al. 1974) and in those cases in which subdural blood but no subarachnoid or extradural blood has been demonstrated post mortem, it has been suggested that the haematoma resulted from blood tracking out from the subarachnoid space (Masdeu et al. 1979). These authors have provided anatomical evidence that the initial haemorrhage was of a radicular artery and argue that any subarachnoid blood would have been cleared by CSF hydrodynamics.

Haemorrhage into Subarachnoid Space

This arises as a result of trauma to radicular arteries (Masdeu et al. 1979) and may cause an acute spinal cord or cauda equina syndrome, particularly in those on anticoagulants. Brem et al. (1981) reviewed their experience of LP in patients who were put immediately onto heparin: 3 of 175 patients developed paraparesis, of whom 2 had a subarachnoid haematoma, in 1 the LP had been acellular.

It is important, therefore, to consider carefully the indications for spinal puncture in patients with a coagulopathy (leukaemia, thrombocytopenia, liver disease, anticoagulation) and, if appropriate, to cover the procedure with haemostatic agents.

Pressure Changes

Removal of CSF from the lumbar theca will cause a pressure gradient between intracranial and spinal compartments; this may simply cause a low pressure intracranial headache or can have more significant consequences. These occur in patients with raised intracranial pressure (ICP) when LP may cause herniation of the hindbrain through the foramen magnum. It is essential therefore to judge in which patients ICP is raised. Before CT this was judged to be present if there was papilloedema or a depressed level of consciousness; now CT criteria also can be used (Gower et al. 1987).

Duffy (1969) reported a 40% mortality in 30 patients who underwent LP during the investigation of intracranial mass lesions. In half the deterioration occurred immediately after the procedure and in the rest it occurred within 12 hours. Those with brain abscess did particularly badly. This high mortality from LP in patients with intracranial mass lesions has been confirmed by other reports (Connolly 1982). For intraspinal mass lesions Hollis et al. (1986) reported a 14% risk of "spinal" coning if LP was performed below a spinal block; as a result when myelography is performed for a suspected spinal tumour a lateral cervical puncture should be performed.

Post-LP Headache

Post-LP headache occurs in 13%–32% of cases (Hilton-Jones 1984). Tourtelotte et al. (1964) reported a 32% incidence in unselected cases of LP performed for diagnostic purposes but lower figures were quoted for spinal anaesthesia (18% obstetric, 13% non-obstetric). The headache, probably due to venous dilatation consequent on CSF hypotension, is exacerbated by jugular compression and is abolished by re-injecting fluid. An identical headache occurs if sufficient CSF (25 ml) is removed initially and it is thought that a continuing leak of CSF through the dural tear causes significant CSF loss to cause headache. As a result most studies have suggested that to minimize dural trauma a small diameter spinal needle should be used (22 G) and the bevel of the needle should be inserted in the vertical plane as the dural fibres run rostrocaudal (Hilton-Jones 1984).

Infection

Rarely, infection may follow LP in an intervertebral disc (Feinbloom and Halaby 1966), the epidural space (Rangell and Glassman 1945), the spinal cord (Rifaat et al. 1973), the vertebral body (Bergman et al. 1983) or the meninges (Eng and Seligman 1981; Teele et al. 1981; Harper et al. 1985; Shapiro et al. 1986). All are uncommon (Dripps and VanDam 1951) though there is doubt as to the frequency of post-LP meningitis.

Dickson (1944) pointed out that in a centrifugalized specimen of CSF it was not uncommon to see a cylindrical fragment of skin, punched out by the exploring needle, incidental squamous cells from the skin and associated commensal staphylococci, and cartilage or bone marrow cells. Infection may be introduced directly, as above, or by causing a small haematoma which may act as a "locus minoris residentiae". Teele et al. (1981) analysed the course of 277 episodes of bacteraemia in infants seen at one institution from 1971–1980. They were usually sent home with or without antibiotic therapy. An LP (having less than 8 mononuclear cells, less than 1 polymorph and a normal sugar level) was performed in 46 patients at initial presentation, but not in 231. Seven of the 46 developed meningitis but this occurred in only 2 of the 231 patients. They argued that LP had been instrumental in the development of meningitis in the 7 children all of whom were under 18 months of age. This concurred with laboratory data from Petersdorf et al. (1962) who had demonstrated in the dog that dural puncture in the presence of a high grade bacteraemia might lead to meningitis. However, Eng and Seligman (1981) suggested it was rare to develop LP-induced meningitis in adults. They analysed 1089 cases of bacteraemia seen over one year at a single institution. Of these, 200 cases had an LP within 3 days of the blood culture, 30 having meningitis. Of the 170 cases with a normal LP, 3 subsequently developed infected CSF. They found a 14% incidence of meningitis amongst those with bacteraemia due to *Neisseria meningitidis*, *Haemophilus influenzae* and *Streptococcus pneumoniae* and argued that previous reports of LP-induced meningitis may have been an expression of the high "spontaneous" potential of these organisms to cause meningitis. This latter point was emphasized by Shapiro et al. (1986) who calculated an 85.6% chance of developing meningitis "spontaneously" in association with meningococcal septicaemia.

References

Bergman I, Wald ER, Meyer JD, Painter MJ (1983) Epidural abscess and vertebral osteomyelitis following serial lumbar punctures. Pediatrics 72:476–480

Berns DH, Blaser SJ, Modic MT (1989) Magnetic resonance imaging of the spine. Clin Orthop 244:78–100

Brem S, Hafler DA, Van Uitert RL, Ruff RL, Reichert WH (1981) A hazard of lumbar puncture resulting in reversible paraplegia. N Engl J Med 304:1020–1021

Connolly ES (1982) Spinal cord tumours in adults. In: Youmans JR (ed) Neurological surgery. Saunders, Philadelphia, p 3200

Dawson BH (1963) Paraplegia due to spinal epidural haematoma. J Neurol Neurosurg Psychiatry 26:171–173

Dickson WEC (1944) The cerebrospinal fluid in meningitis. Postgrad Med J 20:69–74

Dripps RD, VanDam LD (1951) Hazards of lumbar puncture. JAMA 147:1118–1121

Duffy GP (1969) Lumbar puncture in the presence of raised intracranial pressure. Br Med J i:407–409

Edelson RN, Chernik NL, Posner JB (1974) Spinal subdural hematoma complicating lumbar puncture: occurrence in thrombocytopenic patients. Arch Neurol 31:134–137

Eng RHK, Seligman SJ (1981) Lumbar puncture induced meningitis. JAMA 245:1456–1459

Feinbloom RI, Halaby FA (1966) Acute pyogenic spondylitis in infancy: a case report to emphasize the potential risk in lumbar puncture. Clin Pediatr 5:683–684

Findlay GFG (1987) Compression and vascular disorders of the spinal cord. In: Miller JD (ed) Northfields surgery of the central nervous system. Blackwell Scientific, Oxford, pp 707–759

Gower DJ, Baker AL, Bell WO, Ball MR (1987) Contraindications to lumbar puncture as defined by computed cranial tomography. J Neurol Neurosurg Psychiatry 50:1071–1074

Harik SI, Raichle ME, Reis DJ (1971) Spontaneously remitting spinal epidural hematoma in a patient on anticoagulants. N Engl J Med 284:1355–1357

Harper JR, Lorber J, Hillas Smith G (1985) Timing of lumbar puncture in severe childhood meningitis. Br Med J 291:651–652, 1123–1124

Hasan D, Vermeulen M, Wijdicks EFM, Hijdra A, Van Gijn J (1989) Management problems in acute hydrocephalus after subarachnoid haemorrhage. Stroke 20:747–753

Hilton-Jones D (1984) What is post lumbar puncture headache and is it avoidable? In: Warlow C, Garfield J (eds) Dilemmas in the management of the neurological patient. Churchill Livingstone, Edinburgh, pp 144–158

Hollis PH, Malis LI, Zappula RA (1986) Neurological deterioration after lumbar puncture block
    below complete spinal subarachnoid block. J Neurosurg 64:253–256
Macdonald A, Mendelow AD (1988) Xanthochromia revisited: a re-evaluation of lumbar puncture
    and CT scanning in the diagnosis of subarachnoid haemorrhage. J Neurol Neurosurg Psychiatry
    51:342–344
Margolis CZ, Cook CD (1973) The risk of lumbar puncture in pediatric patients with cardiac
    and/or pulmonary disease. Pediatrics 51:562–564
Masdeu JC, Breuer AC, Schoene WC (1979) Spinal subarachnoid hematoma: clue to source of
    bleeding in traumatic lumbar puncture. Neurology 29:872–876
Morettin LB, Wilson M (1970) Severe reflex algodystrophy (Sudeck's atrophy) as a complication
    of myelography: report of two cases. AJR 110:156–158
Odom GL (1960) Clin Neurosurg 8:197
Petersdorf RG, Swarner DR, Garcia M (1962) Studies on the pathogenesis of meningitis. II
    Development of meningitis during pneumococcal bacteremia J Clin Invest 41:320–327
Petito F, Plum F (1974) The lumbar puncture. N Engl J Med 290:224–226 (editorial)
Rangel L, Glassman F (1945) Acute spinal epidural abscess as a complication of lumbar puncture.
    J Nerv Ment Dis 102:8–18
Rifaat M, el Shafei I, Samra K (1973) Intramedullary spinal abscess following lumbar puncture:
    case report. J Neurosurg 38:366–367
Shapiro D, Aaron N, Wald E (1986) Risk factors for the development of bacterial meningitis
    among children with occult bacteremia J Pediatr 109:15–19
Tabaddor K, Lamorgese JR (1975) Lumbar epidermoid cyst following single lumbar puncture. J
    Bone Joint Surg 57A:1168–1169
Teele DW, Dashevsky B, Rakusan T, Klein JO (1981) Meningitis after lumbar puncture in
    children with bacteremia. N Engl J Med 305:1079–1081
Tourtelotte WW, Haerer AF, Heller GL, Sommers JE (1964) Post lumbar puncture headache.
    Thomas, Illinois
Trupp M (1977) Stylet injury syndrome. JAMA 237:2524
Vermeulen M, Van Gijn J, Blijenberg BG (1983) Spectrophotometric analysis of CSF after
    subarachnoid haemorrhage. Limitations in the diagnosis of rebleeding. Neurology 33:112–114
Walton JN (1956) Subarachnoid haemorrhage. Churchill Livingstone, Edinburgh
Weber RJ, Weingarden SI (1979) Electromyographic abnormalities following myelography. Arch
    Neurol 36, 588–589
Young DA, Burney RE (1971) Complications of myelography: transection and withdrawal of a
    nerve filament by the needle. N Engl J Med 285:156–157

Chapter 6

Neuropathology

D.I. Graham

Introduction

The tissue of the spinal cord is similar to that of the brain and is made up of two main types consisting of highly specialized nerve cells (neurones) with their processes and neuroglial cells (Lantos 1990a). Both of these are of neuro-ectodermal origin in contrast to the second main type of tissue which comprises the meninges, the blood vessels and their supporting connective tissue. These together with phagocytic cells are derived from mesoderm. Whereas some of the diseases affecting the spinal cord are similar to those seen in other organs, e.g. inflammation, vascular disease and tumours, others are primarily diseases of the neurone affecting its cell body, its axon or its myelin sheath, or the neuroglial cells or the blood vessels. It, therefore, follows that because the constituent cells of the spinal cord are similar to those found elsewhere in the nervous system, the disease processes and tissue reactions in response to them are similar to those found elsewhere in the brain (Hughes 1978; Duchen 1985; Esiri and Oppenheimer 1989; Lantos 1990b). However, the prevalence of the various disease processes in the spinal cord differs from that found elsewhere in the brain.

Applied Anatomy

The dura mater acts as the periosteum to the spinal canal, but it can be stripped from the vertebrae by haemorrhage or abscess formation into the potential extradural space. The dura and the outer surface of the arachnoid are normally in contact but the subdural space can more readily be distended by blood or pus than the extradural space. The arachnoid forms a continuous sheet in contact with the dura while the pia follows the contours of the spinal cord. Between the pia and arachnoid is the subarachnoid space traversed by delicate trabeculae of connective tissue that divide it up into a series of intercommunicating spaces filled with CSF. The major spinal arteries and veins run in the subarachnoid space, and from the artery small vessels pass into the spinal cord. As an artery penetrates the spinal cord, it carries with it a potential perivascular space (often known as the Virchow-Robin space) which is separated from the substance of the spinal cord by a cuff of astrocytic foot processes.

Micro-organisms and their toxins readily spread throughout the subarachnoid space which may become filled with inflammatory exudate. Examination of the CSF often provides valuable information about diseases of the nervous system. Specimens are ordinarily obtained by lumbar puncture during the course of which the pressure of the CSF should always be measured. Normal CSF is clear and colourless and does not coagulate and has a specific gravity of 1.006. It contains 0.15–0.45 g/l protein, 2.8–4.4 mmol/l glucose and approximately 128 mmol/l sodium and 128 mmol/l chloride. A few lymphocytes and monocytes may be seen in normal fluid but rarely more than 4 per millilitre.

Reactions of the Tissues of the Spinal Cord to Disease

Neurones

The neurone is one of the most complex and specialized cells in the body and since it is incapable of dividing after the first few weeks of extrauterine life any damage involving loss is structurally irreversible. A detailed understanding of the structure and function of neurones requires the application of multiple methods which show that they are made up of the perikaryon or cell body from which extend the dendrites and the axon. The perikarya are the main component of grey matter in which they tend to have characteristic arrangements. A conspicuous feature in the perikarya is the presence of Nissl granules rich in RNA, that are composed of stacks of rough endoplasmic reticulum and intervening groups of free ribosomes. Special staining techniques demonstrate the cytoskeleton in the cytoplasm comprising principally neurofilaments and microtubules. Mitochondria are numerous in dendrites and in the presynaptic region. Lysosomes are also found and a particularly characteristic feature in large neurones, such as those found in the ventral horns of the spinal cord, is their content of lipofuscin. Various substances (neurotransmitters, proteins and organelles) are relayed in fast and slow phases of axoplasmic flow from the cell body along the axons and dendrites to synapses. There is also a retrograde axoplasmic flow of material from the periphery towards the perikaryon.

The reactions of neurones take several forms. Central chromatolysis occurs in the perikaryon between 5 to 8 days after the axon has been cut. At first the cell body becomes swollen and spherical. The nucleus becomes eccentric and the Nissl granules break down into dustlike particles which may persist at the margin of the cell. Cytoplasm becomes pale and homogeneous. This response to injury has recently been shown to be accompanied by an increase in protein synthesis. It is, therefore, considered to be a regenerative phenomenon. When it is due to damage to a spinal nerve central chromatolysis is sometimes reversible. By contrast, effective regeneration does not occur in the CNS and retrograde degeneration of the axon results so that following axonal transection the proximal ends of the severed axon swell to form axonal bulbs: these may be found within 3 to 6 hours of injury, may persist for up to 60 days and are thought to be due to continuance of axoplasmic flow in both directions (Nauta and Gygax 1954; Fink and Heimer 1967; Vaughn et al. 1970; Vaughn and Pease 1970).

Neurones require a constant supply of oxygen and glucose and if this is inadequate they undergo a series of changes referred to as the ischaemic cell process. Mitochondria become swollen, the perikaryon shrinks and often becomes triangular in shape. Nissl granules disappear and cytoplasm becomes intensely eosinophilic and the nucleus pyknotic. A characteristic feature of recent neuronal necrosis is the presence of small dark granules known as encrustations on the surface of the perikaryon and its dendrites. Dead neurones are removed by phagocytes. Moderate neuronal loss is very difficult to recognize histologically unless there are also some reactive changes in the neuroglia. Not all neurones in the CNS are equally vulnerable to the effects of hypoxia, there being a pattern of selective vulnerability. Within the rank order of vulnerability some of the most resistant cells to the ischaemic cell process are those found in the dorsal and ventral horns of the spinal cord.

There are many other less common changes in neurones. For example, inclusion bodies may be found in certain virus infections and in many of the slowly progressive degenerative diseases such as motor neurone disease. In some of the inborn errors of metabolism the cytoplasm of neurones becomes distended with lipid-laden lysosomes.

When the cell body of a myelinated neurone is irreversibly damaged its axon and myelin sheath break down by the process of Wallerian degeneration (see below). Another form of degeneration is transynaptic atrophy which occurs in neurones whose principal afferent connections have been destroyed: an example is in the nucleus gracilis and nucleus cuneatus when the posterior columns of the spinal cord have undergone degeneration.

Neuroglia

These include astrocytes, oligodendrocytes and ependymal cells.

Damage to the spinal cord whatever its cause is invariably accompanied by hypertrophy and hyperplasia of astrocytic processes referred to as gliosis or astrocytosis. Within a day or so of tissue damage astrocytes begin to divide, this response being associated with the production of large amounts of glial fibrillary protein. Characteristically gliosed tissue is firmer than normal and tends to appear grey and translucent as in plaques of multiple sclerosis. Usually the glial fibres are laid down in an irregular manner and in areas of long-standing gliosis Rosenthal fibres and granular bodies may be seen. These are eosinophilic structures which may be round, oval or elongated ranging in size from 10 to 40 µm. Another type of astrocytic response is seen in oedematous white matter when the cell body enlarges, becomes rounded and acquires an eosinophilic homogeneous cytoplasm and the nucleus becomes eccentric. These cells are known as gemistocytic astrocytes and have been found in the white matter within as little as 6 hours after the onset of acute oedema: they are seen also in relation to tumours and infarcts. Even though gliosis is the principal response of the CNS to injury in certain circumstances when there has been tissue necrosis, there is often a mixed glial and fibroblastic response referred to as a glio-mesodermal reaction. This is most frequently seen in subacute and chronic abscesses. Basophilic circular bodies known as corpora amylaceae accumulate and the brain tissue is firmer than normal and may have a grey translucent appearance.

Oligodendrocytes are small cells with darkly staining nuclei resembling that of a lymphocyte. They are often numerous and are seen as perineuronal satellites in the grey matter and as rows of closely apposed nuclei between bundles of myelinated nerve fibres – the interfascicular oligodendroglia. Oligodendrocytes play an important role in both the formation and maintenance of myelin and loss of the interfascicular oligodendrocyte in some of the demyelinating diseases appears to precede obvious degeneration of myelin.

A single layer of ependymal cells lines the central canal of the spinal cord. They are columnar and have a ciliated free (luminal) surface immediately deep to which there is a line of small oval bodies known as blepharoplasts. Ependymal cells show few reactive changes. If the central canal becomes distended then the ependyma is stretched and then broken, but the cells do not proliferate to fill the defects.

Microglia

These respond rapidly to any noxious process, but it is not yet clear what proportion of reactive microglia are derived from microglia already present in the CNS and what proportion from circulating monocytes. In the process of neuronophagia, phagocytes engulf and eventually digest irreversibly damaged neurones. Initially microglia become elongated and their processes are more apparent: they are referred to as rod cells. When brain tissue is destroyed the microglia act as phagocytes: the cell becomes enlarged and rounded, the nucleus eccentric and the cytoplasm filled with ingested material, usually the breakdown products of myelin: these cells – lipid phagocytes – are sudanophilic and react strongly for acid phosphatase. They are most commonly seen in relation to vascular disease and in recent plaques of demyelination. Microglia also ingest the breakdown products of haemoglobin when they are referred to as siderophages and stain positively with Perls' Prussian blue reaction. Small clusters of reactive microglia are frequently seen throughout the CNS in patients with a bacteraemia.

Transverse Lesions of the Spinal Cord

Various specific disorders of the spine and spinal cord are described elsewhere, but it is appropriate at this stage to describe the events that take place when there is either partial or complete interruption of the cord. For example, acute transverse lesions may be due to trauma, usually a fracture dislocation of the vertebrae, infarction when the circulation of the anterior spinal artery is compromised, haemorrhage usually as a result of vascular malformation, or acute demyelination as in neuromyelitis optica. However, transverse lesions may also develop as a result of slowly progressive pathology, such as pressure on the cord by tumours. Although much less common than formerly, infections such as tuberculosis (Fig. 6.1), brucellosis and other bacterial infections that may cause cord compression include *E. coli* and staphylococcal infections. Compression may also occur as a result of metabolic bone disease.

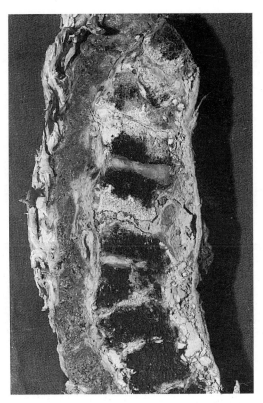

Fig. 6.1. Tuberculosis of spine. Sagittal section of the vertebral column that has led to angular curvature of the spine and cold abscess formation.

Following partial or total interruption of the cord in addition to local damage, an inevitable consequence is the development of ascending and descending Wallerian degeneration in the interrupted tracts of the spinal cord. The distribution of the degenerative processes and its time course in the long tracts can be studied by one of two main staining techniques that are used to demonstrate the loss of myelin. First, there is the Marchi technique to demonstrate recent breakdown of myelin within the preceding 2 to 3 months: the unsaturated fatty acids formed during this process are stained black, while normal myelin remains unstained (Smith 1951; Smith et al. 1956). Additional histological techniques that yield useful information about the state of myelin breakdown include Sudan IV, Sudan Black or Oil Red O in frozen sections. Myelin sheaths break up into ellipsoids and gradually the products of degeneration are taken up by phagocytes, a process that may be seen after 6 to 8 weeks. Gradually the amount of Marchi positive material diminishes, but it may remain in affected tracts for many months or even several years and it becomes resistant to prolonged fixation in formalin. The degenerative process is accompanied by an astrocytosis which gradually increases over several weeks and may still be evident some 6 to 12 months later. The second technique is one used for showing the long-term consequences of myelin degeneration by revealing the

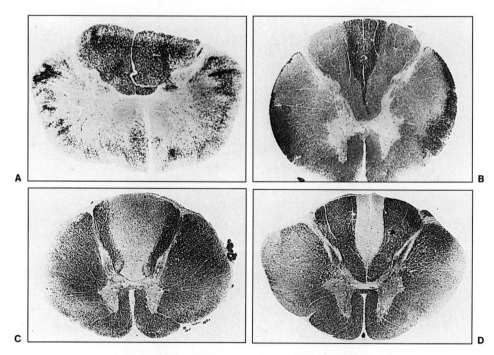

Fig. 6.2A–D. **A** Thoracic cord above lesion. The whole of the posterior columns and antero-lateral ascending tracts are degenerating. Marchi. **B** Cervical region. There are fewer degenerating fibres because of the inflow of fibres above the level of the lesion. Marchi. **C** Thoracic cord above the lesion. Weigert-Pal. **D** Cervical region. Degeneration appears to be confined to the gracile tracts. Weigert-Pal. (Figs. 6.2A–D reproduced with permission from *Muir's textbook of pathology*, 12th edn. J.R. Anderson (ed), Edward Arnold, London 1985.)

demyelinated areas by their failure to stain with conventional stains, e.g. Luxol fast blue and by the Weigert-Pal method and its modifications.

Ascending Degeneration

The pattern following a transverse lesion in the lower thoracic spine is shown in Figs. 6.2A–D. In the section taken a few segments above the lesion (Fig. 6.2A) degeneration is seen in the posterior columns (with the exception of the small area dorsal to the grey commissure where there are chiefly commissural fibres) and the spinothalamic and spinocerebellar tracts. In the cervical region the degeneration of the posterior columns is virtually confined to the gracile tracts (Fig. 6.2B). Because the cuneate tract is composed of ascending fibres that have joined the cord above the level of the lesion, anatomical studies have shown that the degenerative process in the posterior columns ascends up to the cuneate and gracile nuclei in the medulla. On the other hand, ascending degeneration in the spinocerebellar tracts extends up to the inferior cerebellar peduncle and into the cerebellum and in the anterior spinocerebellar tracts to the middle lobe of the cerebellum. The long-term consequences of this degeneration are well seen in Figs. 6.2C and 6.2D where there is a pallor of staining due to loss of myelin in the posterior columns.

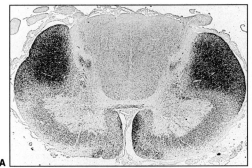
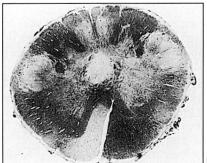
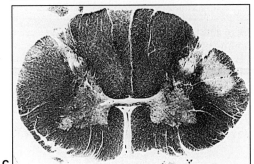

Fig. 6.3A–C. Wallerian degeneration. **A** Descending degeneration below level of lesion. There is degenerating myelin (dark area) in the lateral and anterior white columns. Marchi. (Reproduced with permission from J.H. Adams and D.I. Graham, *An introduction to neuropathology*, Churchill Livingstone, Edinburgh, 1988.) **B** Wallerian degeneration – medulla. The pyramid on one side is degenerated. Weigert-Pal. **C** Wallerian degeneration – thoracic region. The crossed pyramidal tract on one side is degenerated. Weigert-Pal. (Figs. 6.3B and 6.3C reproduced with permission from *Muir's textbook of pathology*, 12th edn. J.R. Anderson (ed), Edward Arnold, London, 1985.)

Descending Degeneration

In a section taken distal to a transverse lesion of the cord marked degeneration is seen in the crossed (lateral) and uncrossed (anterior pyramidal) tracts unless the lesion is low in the cord where the uncrossed tract is no longer present (Fig. 6.3A).

A different pattern of descending degeneration is seen following a lesion, either in the brain stem or in one internal capsule, which results in retrograde degeneration of the corticospinal tract. In these situations there is degeneration of the crossed pyramidal tract on the opposite side (Fig. 6.3B) and of the uncrossed pyramidal tract on the same side. As the uncrossed pyramidal tract does not usually extend below the upper thoracic segments, its degeneration will not be seen in sections of the lower thoracic cord (Fig. 6.3C).

Spinal Injury

It has been estimated that within the United Kingdom each year between 13 and 27 per million of population suffer from serious paralysis following injury of the spinal cord and that there is an even higher prevalence if cases of sudden death after accident are included (Hughes 1974, 1984). Injuries may be classified as either non-missile or missile. The former result from subluxations and fracture/dislocations of the vertebral column, and in civilian practice almost half of all new cases of spinal injury result from motor car or motor cycle accidents, with 30% being due to falls and the remainder being due to sporting injuries. The vertebrae may return to a normal position when the fracture/dislocation is said to be stable. If the damaged vertebrae are still capable of moving the fracture is unstable and any undue movement to the injured patient may intensify damage to the spinal cord. Missile injuries are caused by such objects as bullets or other missiles and may be caused by a stab wound. Some two-thirds of the patients are less than 40 years of age and some 90% are men.

The cervical spine at the level of C5–6 vertebrae and the thoracic spine are injured most commonly in road traffic accidents, whereas the lumbar spine is damaged most commonly in crush injuries of the type seen in mining accidents or after falls.

As with head injuries trauma to the spinal cord may be closed or open (penetrating). There are various mechanisms which include a combination of flexion, rotation, extension and compression. An extension injury is usually due to hyperextension of the mid-cervical vertebrae which causes a separation and dislocation of intervertebral discs, local haemorrhage and possible rupture of the longitudinal ligament. If there is excessive flexion of the cervical spine, there is compression of the vertebral bodies, parts of which may be displaced posteriorly causing damage to the spinal cord. The spinal canal may be narrowed by fracture/dislocation due to rotation and in patients with compressive fractures fragments of bone may be displaced backwards into the spinal canal or, if the spinal column is angulated acutely, stretching and compression of the theca and cord may result. Open injuries to the cord may result from missiles such as bullets and associated bony fragments which may lodge in the cord or in the case of high velocity missiles may cause severe damage to the cord by pressure changes resulting from shock waves. In civilian practice the cord may be injured by a stab wound especially if the knife enters the spinal canal antero-laterally.

Pathology of Spinal Cord Trauma

If possible, X-rays should be available to the pathologist at the time of the autopsy to allow an accurate assessment of bony lesions and location of any missile. It is essential during the post-mortem procedures to remove a block of the vertebral column extending for at least two or three vertebrae above and below the level of the injury. The specimen should then be fixed and, following laminectomy, the cord should be removed from the vertebral canal or the specimen can be cut with a band saw in the mid-sagittal plane to demonstrate the damaged vertebrae and spinal cord (Fig. 6.4A).

In cases of mild injury, where there is only temporary neurological dysfunction, the term concussion is used as it is presumed that structural abnormalities are minimal: indeed the external surface of the cord may be normal. In more severe injuries there is contusion of the cord, the extent and severity of which will vary from case to case, and in many there is extradural, subdural or subarachnoid haemorrhage. The lesion is characterized by haemorrhagic necrosis at the site of trauma, transverse sections revealing a centrally placed fusiform mass (traumatic haematomyelia) which tapers to the end of one or more

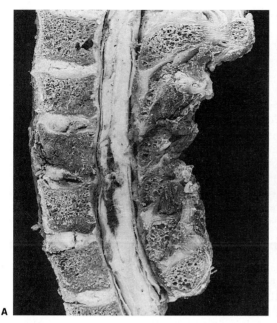

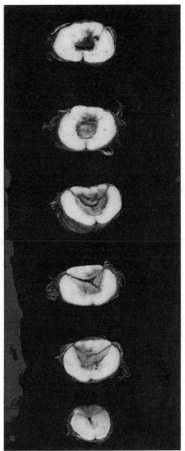

Fig. 6.4. A Spinal injury. There is a traumatic haematomyelia in relation to a fracture of the cervical
spine. (Reproduced with permission from J.H. Adams
and D.I. Graham, *An introduction to neuropathology*,
Churchill Livingstone, Edinburgh, 1988.) **B** Transverse
sections through traumatic haematomyelia in relation to
fracture of the cervical spine.

segments above and below the site of injury (Fig. 6.4B). Histologically there is
swelling, necrosis and petechial haemorrhage formation and silver impregnation
techniques reveal axonal swellings and bulb formation. Myelin sheaths become
swollen and disintegrate and within a few days of injury there is infiltration by
polymorphonuclear leucocytes. Gradually the swelling of the cord subsides and
small haemorrhages are absorbed and the necrotic tissue is gradually removed
by large numbers of macrophages. Eventually a cavity is formed, margins of
which are delineated by an astrocytosis in which iron pigment may be found.

In severe cases affected segments are replaced by what is predominantly an
astrocytic scar. If the injury involved root entry zones then regenerating axons
in Schwann cells may invade the cord and although effective axonal regeneration
does not occur, the appearances in some cases are similar to those of an
amputation neuroma. A late consequence of injury is the development of
Wallerian degeneration in both ascending and descending fibre tracts (see
above). Sometimes a longitudinally disposed cavity (post-traumatic syringomyelia) may track upwards to the medulla or downwards from the damaged
segment (Rossier et al. 1985).

Injury to the Spinal Cord and Roots Caused by Diseases of the Spine

Disease or malformation of the spine may cause local or widespread pressure either on the blood supply to the cord or the cord itself. The presentation may be acute or chronic and the histological changes in the cord depend upon the duration of the compression. The clinical effects depend to a considerable extent on the rate of development of the compressive lesion which may extend over many months or can produce paraplegia within a few days with more rapidly expanding lesions. If the lesion becomes large enough it will interfere with the blood supply to the cord at the level of the compression and if surgery is delayed there is frequently irreparable structural damage.

Many of the causes of cord compression are dealt with in more detail in the appropriate chapters. In brief, however, tumours are a common cause of compression of both the spinal cord and its nerve roots. Most commonly these are metastatic carcinoma, lymphoma and myeloma. Primary bone tumours, meningioma, schwannomas and neurofibromas may also present in this way. Compression may also develop as a result of various inflammatory diseases. *Staphylococcus aureus* is one of the more common organisms which may cause either a localized abscess or suppuration which may track through the epidural or subdural space. Tuberculosis of the spine (Pott's disease) presents most frequently in the cervical and thoracic vertebrae. The disease invariably starts as tuberculous osteitis of the vertebral bodies before spreading into the para-vertebral tissues then to the adjacent epidural or subdural spaces to form a cold abscess. If kyphosis develops the cord is likely to be damaged due to compression by granulation tissue, through angulation of the spine or by interference with the vascular supply. Other inflammatory causes of cord pressure include abscess due to *Brucella abortus* and metastatic abscess due to *Escherichia coli* in association with chronic urinary tract infection.

Prolapsed Intervertebral Disc

This condition is due to herniation of the central part of the disc which consists of soft cellular fibrocartilage forming the nucleus pulposus through part of the annulus fibrosus which is a ring of much firmer fibrocartilage attached directly to the margin of the vertebral bodies. The nucleus pulposus develops from the notochord and forms the central portion of the disc: it often lies eccentrically because the ring of the annulus fibrosus is thicker anteriorly than posteriorly, whereas in childhood the nucleus pulposus constitutes by far the greater part of the disc. With advancing years its bulk is reduced by an encroaching enlarge-ment of the annulus fibrosus.

As a result of injury or of lifting a heavy weight, part of the nucleus pulposus may be forced through the annulus (Fig. 6.5) and compress a nerve root, particularly in the lower spine between L5 and S1 and L4 and L5 and less commonly in the neck between C5 and 6 (Hook et al. 1960). Lumbar discs are particularly common in those under the age of 40 and may be caused by a fall, or especially lifting heavy weights in a stooping position. As the majority of

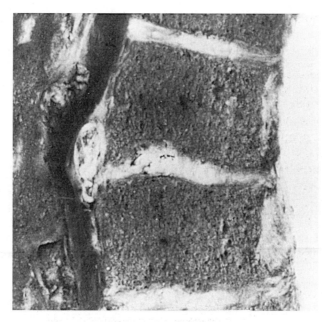

Fig. 6.5. Prolapsed intervertebral disc. Sagittal section of vertebral column, showing ruptured disc protruding beneath the posterior longitudinal ligament. (Reproduced with permission from *Muir's textbook of pathology*, 12th edn. J.R. Anderson (ed), Edward Arnold, London, 1985.)

protrusions are at the levels noted there is no damage to the spinal cord, the effects being those of compression of the roots of the cauda equina. Almost all are due to herniation of the nucleus pulposus, but the spondylolisthesis with disc protrusion may occur between the lowest lumbar vertebra and the sacrum or between the two lowest lumbar vertebrae. The herniations are usually posterolateral, where they project chiefly into the intervertebral foramen to compress only one root, the most common being L4 or L5. When a disc protrudes into the canal the roots which are descending to a lower level are affected: usually only a few are involved but occasionally there is severe damage to most of the lower roots of the cauda equina (Jennett 1956). The cord however is also at risk in the cervical and thoracic regions, particularly if there is a centrally placed disc prolapse. Degeneration of the lumbar discs with osteophyte formation is common at the lumbar level, but prominent bony ridges on the posterior surface of the vertebral bodies are rare compared with those found in the cervical level. In severe cases osteophytes may occlude the intervertebral foramen which contains the important reticular vessels that supply the lumbosacral cord. Herniation may also occur into the body of the vertebrae, an event which by itself is of little importance, particularly as it is seen in some 40% of normal subjects where it is referred to as Schmorl's nodes. However, such herniation is thought to predispose to bulging of the annulus fibrosus and to osteophytosis. Tissue removed at surgery should always be examined histologically when, in most instances, the prolapsed fragments of the disc show mucoid degeneration, the tissue appearing devitalized with only a few normal cells remaining. Sometimes there is evidence of vascularization and macrophages containing haemosiderin may be seen. Less commonly, unexpected lesions such as granulomas and tumours may be found, both of which may simulate prolapse of the nucleus pulposus both clinically and at operation.

Spondylosis Deformans

This is a condition that affects the cervical and lumbar regions of the spine in which there is progressive degeneration of intervertebral discs. The condition is common with radiological evidence of its presence in 50% of people over the age of 50 and 75% over the age of 65 years. (Frykholm 1951; Brain et al. 1952). It is characterized by ossification of the margins of the vertebral bodies in relation to thickening or lipping of the annulus fibrosus. Anterior lipping causes no neurological symptoms in many cases with minor degrees of posterior lipping also being asymptomatic. In some cases, however, bony transverse ridges on the dorsal surface of the cervical vertebrae associated with disc protrusions are the cause of paraparesis or tetraparesis. Osteophytes develop laterally where they may encroach sufficiently on the lateral recess of the spinal canal along the intervertebral foramen to compress nerve roots. The affected nerve roots become thickened and there may be interference with the blood supply of the root entry zones. There is also a risk of cord compression, but the pathogenesis of this myelopathy is complex and involves factors such as interference with the blood supply, trauma and protrusion of disc material. In some cases paraplegia may develop suddenly after a minor degree of flexion or extension of the neck and has occurred after tooth extraction or tonsillectomy. In such cases there is often radiological evidence of previous degeneration of one or more discs, so that it is doubtful whether paraplegia can follow such minor strains unless there is already degeneration of a disc. In contrast, cord compression in middle-aged patients tends to be due not to disc herniation but rather to the backward protrusion of the annulus fibrosus which both at surgery and at post mortem is recognized by transverse bony ridges with which the bulging is associated. In the neck, herniation of the nucleus pulposus occurs either between the 5th and 6th or the 6th and 7th bodies, which are the same sites where chronic degenerations of the type noted above are equally common.

The important fact in the production of myelopathy is congenital narrowing of the cervical spinal canal: the average antero−posterior diameter of the spinal canal in controls was 17 mm and in cases with myelopathy due to cervical spondylosis the average measurement was 14 mm (Payne and Spillane 1957). When the neck is extended the antero−posterior diameter of the spinal canal may be reduced by 2 mm and if there is any posterior movement of one vertebra upon the other the distance is even further reduced. Posteriorly in hyperextension the ligamentum flavum may be infolded and press upon the cord. In addition there may be mechanical compression of the anterior spinal artery and tension on the ligamentum denticulatum prevents the cord from moving backwards. Under these conditions cord compression may occur and may be recognized because a segment is flatter than normal because of compression in its antero−posterior diameter. Histologically, in early lesions there are usually ill-defined areas of spongy degeneration due to distension of myelin sheaths many of which contain swollen axons. These changes are commonly found in the ventral parts of the posterior columns and in the white matter at the point of attachment of the thickened ligamentum denticulatum. The anterior third of the white matter usually remains normal. Frank necrosis may develop and in older lesions cavitation may affect both grey and white matter.

Herniation of thoracic intervertebral discs is uncommon: some are due to trauma whereas others appear to have a more gradual onset. As with other discs they develop as a result of herniation of nucleus pulposus which later becomes fibrosed, calcified and even ossified. Such lesions are said to occur in 2%–3% of all disc protrusions occurring mainly below the level of T6 in patients of middle or later age.

Osteitis Deformans

Paget's disease of the spine is usually accompanied by a degree of kyphosis. Of greater importance, however, in patients who present with paraplegia is the general reduction in the size of the lumen of the spinal canal by prominences that develop on the posterior aspects of the vertebral bodies.

Bony Abnormalities in the Region of the Foramen Magnum

Serious neurological symptoms may result from one of three main bony abnormalities (McRae 1953). First, partial or complete fusion of the atlas with the foramen magnum; second, protrusion of the tip of the odontoid process above Chamberlain's line, which is a line drawn from the back of the hard palate to the posterior margin of the foramen magnum; and third, anomalies either of the odontoid process itself or in its relation to the atlas. In many cases the lesions are developmental, symptoms often beginning in childhood or early adulthood, but they may be precipitated by trauma to either the head or neck. Assimilation or fusion of the atlas with a margin of the foramen magnum is usually only symptomatic when it is combined with other abnormalities such as the odontoid process which is abnormally long, angled backwards or placed unusually high. Under these circumstances the antero–posterior diameter of the spinal canal behind the odontoid process is usually less than 20 mm. Associated features include platybasia or basilar invagination. Basilar invagination or impression although predominantly developmental in origin, may rarely occur as a result of Paget's disease, rickets or osteogenesis imperfecta. Basilar invagination is commonly accompanied by fusion of two or more cervical vertebrae. Because of the malalignment, symptoms may be provoked by movement of the head, the lowest part of the medulla or the first cervical segment being compressed by the prominence formed by the odontoid process and transverse ligaments. Other anomalies include separation of the odontoid process from the atlas either as a result of a developmental abnormality, or trauma. Atlantoaxial dislocation may also occur in which the atlas is displaced forwards in relation to the axis and lower cervical spine and the odontoid process is separated from the anterior arch of the atlas.

Rheumatoid arthritis. When involving the spine, this disease produces a myelopathy by cervical dislocations which may occur between C1 and C2 and less commonly below the level of C2. These are due to destruction of the articular joint surfaces, joint capsules and the ancillary ligaments (Hughes 1977). It is a notable feature of this disease that there is relatively little reactive bone formation and osteophytes that are so characteristic of spondylosis deformans are not a feature of rheumatoid arthritis.

Trauma by Non-mechanical Forces

Lesions of the spinal cord are one of the more serious features of X-irradiation and acute decompression sickness (barotrauma). The cord may also be damaged by lightning, electrical damage and chemotherapy.

X-Irradiation

Radiotherapy is the mainstay of the treatment of malignant tumours of the cord, the ionizing radiation usually being given as a gamma ray beam from radioactive sources or as megavoltage X-ray beams. The dose is usually fractionated, that is the total dose is divided into equal fractions and typical conventional fractionation might be 1.8–2 cGy per day 5 times per week to a total dose of 60 cGy. Any complications resulting from the effects of the ionizing radiation will depend on many factors which include the total dose of the radiation and the number of fractions, the dose per fraction, the total treatment time, the volume irradiated, the elimination of "hot spots" by the use of multiple fields and the use of other treatments such as steroids, radiosensitizers or antineoplastic chemotherapy. The main effect of irradiation on the tumour itself is to produce necrosis: this is particularly true for radiosensitive tumours where large fluid-filled cysts lined with glial scar tissue can be found following treatment. With less radiosensitive tumours extensive central necrosis may occur although peripheral tumour may remain. Tumour radiation may also lead to a change in tumour cytology and typically mutinucleated giant cells with irregular hyperchromatic nuclei are found: the number of mitotic figures is reduced and the effect of irradiation upon the cerebral blood vessels is to induce hyalinization and thrombotic occlusion.

X-irradiation can cause injury to skin and bone and may result in impaired wound healing. Radiation myelopathy (Fogelholm et al. 1974; Godwin-Austen et al. 1975) however, is the most frequent neurological sequela of radiation therapy of which four different clinico-pathological syndromes have been described. Acute transient myelopathy develops a few weeks after spinal irradiation, symptoms usually resolving completely over some 3 to 5 months. The pathogenesis, is not known, but radiation-induced demyelination has been suggested. An uncommon complication is that of acute progressive myelopathy in which paraparesis or quadriparesis develops rapidly. It is thought to be due to arterial occlusion and ischaemic necrosis of the cord. A further uncommon condition is that of lower motor neurone syndrome in which some months following spinal radiation the symptoms and signs of damage to the ventral horn cells develop. The changes are usually symmetrical and are thought to be due to selective damage to the lower motor neurones.

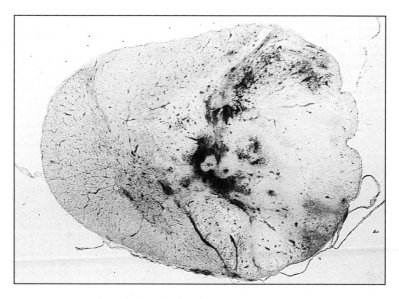

Fig. 6.6. Radionecrosis of cervical cord. The cord is swollen by a focally haemorrhagic necrotic mass of tissue. H & E × 10.

Chronic progressive myelopathy (radionecrosis) is the commonest and most serious of the spinal syndromes caused by radiotherapy (Russell and Rubinstein 1989). The latent period may occur between 6 months and 13 years with a median of 12 to 15 months, the thoracic segments being the most susceptible part of the cord. Examples of this condition have been described following irradiation of extracranial tumours such as nasopharyngeal carcinoma, parotid carcinoma or basal cell carcinoma of the skull and less commonly following irradiation to tumours arising in the mediastinum. This complication is said to occur in 1%–2% of irradiated patients and, as elsewhere in the brain, the lesion is space occupying with all the features of a malignant astrocytoma (Fig. 6.6). The cord is expanded and replaced by focally cystic waxy pale yellow tissue in which there may be petechial haemorrhages. In longstanding cases the affected tissue becomes granular and is apt to crumble. Anatomical definition is blurred but, in the main, grey matter is spared. Histologically the process is characterized by appearances that range from coagulative necrosis (Fig. 6.7A) around which there is no or minimal reactive change to foci of demyelination, loss of axons and infiltration by lipid-containing phagocytes, lymphocytes and plasma cells. The most important change, however, is fibrinoid necrosis and hyalinization of the walls of blood vessels and proliferation of endothelium which may be sufficient to cause an obliterative endarteritis and thrombotic occlusion of small vessels (Fig. 6.7B). Additional features include the formation of telangiectatic vessels, the proliferation of perivascular fibroblasts with the formation in some cases of large amounts of relatively acellular collagen and an associated astrocytosis often with bizarre multinucleated cell formation. In the later stages the segments of cords above and below the lesion are characterized by Wallerian degeneration in ascending and descending fibre tracts respectively.

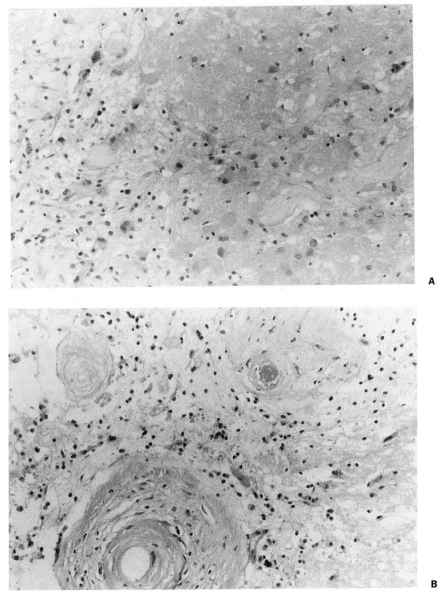

Fig. 6.7. Radionecrosis. **A** There is coagulative necrosis with little in the way of a glial or mesodermal reaction. H & E × 9. **B** Note striking changes in small blood vessels in the form of fibrinoid necrosis and endothelial proliferation. H & E × 130.

The pathogenesis of radionecrosis remains uncertain but vascular change, a direct effect of irradiation on the glia and immunological mechanisms have all been proposed. It is possible, however, that multiple mechanisms operate and that their relative importance varies with the radiation dose, and the interval between exposure and occurrence of damage. There have been many attempts to establish the tolerance level of the spinal cord to radiation. For example, a limit of 33 Gy in 42 days for field sizes less than 10 cm in length has been proposed and generally accepted.

It is sometimes difficult to differentiate effects of radiation from other myelopathies, especially paraneoplastic syndromes and intramedullary metastatic disease. CSF findings are non-specific and myelography is usually normal in radiation-induced myelopathy, but the cord can occasionally be swollen to such a degree that a spinal block is produced. Here CT scanning and more recently MR imaging are helpful.

Chemotherapy

Treatment with antineoplastic agents may be given as a primary treatment, or more commonly as adjunctive therapy, following surgery and/or radiotherapy. The factors that limit the effectiveness of chemotherapy on malignant tumours include drug access by virtue of the blood–brain barrier for agents that are not highly lipid soluble and low sensitivity of most tumours to single-agent chemotherapy. Multiple-agent treatments are commonly used which increases the number of potential drug-induced complications but as a low dose of each individual agent can be used it will reduce the risk of any specific complication arising. The cause of most CNS complications is sensitivity of the normal brain to chemotherapeutic agents, a number of syndromes having been described that include an acute or chronic myelopathy. The neurological side-effects range from the insignificant acute reversible to the dose-limiting debilitating chronic and permanent. In some cases these effects are predictable, varying with the dosage, duration and route of administration. However, other complications are unpredictable and often misinterpreted because of their rarity, idiosyncratic nature or latency. The pathophysiology of these disorders is not known and may differ for each implicated drug. The differential diagnosis should include the important problem of opportunistic infection due to drug-induced immunosuppression. Myelopathies are particularly associated with the antimetabolite drugs methotrexate and cytosine arabinoside and the alkylating agent thiopeta.

Embolism

Blood flow through the spinal cord may be arrested by emboli which according to their size become impacted in arteries, arterioles or capillaries. They may arise as a result of valvular, congenital or ischaemic heart disease and atheroma of the aorta and its large branches. They may also consist of air, nitrogen (hyperbaric and hypobaric as in decompression sickness) and fat.

Hyperbaric Decompression

This is brought about by the reduction of an elevated (hyperbaric) atmospheric pressure to a normal level, an environment that is common to underwater divers and to workers in caissons. Decompression is necessary before ascent to the surface and if carried out slowly according to recommended practice there are no adverse affects. If too rapid, symptoms of caisson disease may appear with damage to bone and inner ear, but particularly to the spinal cord and even result in death.

At any given atmospheric pressure inspired gases dissolve in blood, tissue fluids and fat. Nitrogen is particularly soluble in fat. If the subject then passes too rapidly the dissolved gases come out of solution. Whereas oxygen and carbon dioxide are rapidly reabsorbed, nitrogen tends to form small bubbles which may coalesce. In addition to causing cord damage the "bends" may develop when the bubbles collect around joints and the "chokes" when they develop within the interstititial tissues of the lungs. Bubbles of nitrogen may appear in the bloodstream. At autopsy in patients surviving for only a short time, the brain and spinal cord are intensely congested and there may be haemorrhages. After a longer survival, multiple small infarcts may be seen particularly in the upper levels of the thoracic cord. In the affected segment ischaemic damage is essentially restricted to white matter most commonly in the central portions of each posterior column. Recent histological studies of the spinal cord from professional and amateur divers who died accidentally revealed Marchi positive degeneration in the cords of three professional divers variously affecting the posterolateral and to a lesser extent the anterior columns. Both ascending and descending Wallerian degeneration have been seen in the cord of a 50-year-old amateur diver who survived paraplegia for 4 years after an episode of spinal "bends" (Palmer et al. 1981). The pattern of damage was attributed to multiple infarcts within the cervical blood supply of the cord. The grey matter was normal.

Hypobaric Decompression

This is the reduction of atmospheric pressure from a normal level (sea) to a lower (hypobaric) level as at high altitude or in a hypobaric decompression chamber. If decompression is slow enough there are no adverse effects, but if not there may be symptoms of brain damage and even death. There are only a few reports detailing the neuropathological findings in subjects dying either from exposure to simulated high altitude in decompression chambers or after high altitude flights. Characteristically, there are multiple foci of ischaemic damage accentuated in the grey matter of the cerebral hemispheres, the cerebellum and the brain stem: there is relative sparing of the spinal cord, though in some cases the findings were similar to those described in caisson disease. The lesions have been attributed to a combination of gaseous and fat embolism and circulatory collapse.

Electricity and Lightning

When death is due to electrocution the only abnormality visible in the cord may be hyperaemia, possibly with petechial haemorrhages. If the discharge has been direct through the neuraxis as in death due to lightning, there may be charring or widespread fissuring of its surface.

System Disorders

The so-called degenerative diseases of the nervous system are a diverse group many of which are familial, have a hereditary basis and are characterized by a progressive degeneration of neurones and their processes within anatomically and functionally defined regions or systems, but usually sparing the cerebral cortex. In many there are features of involvement of more than one system, the so-called multiple system atrophies. The current classification is often based on the clinical features which vary both within and between affected families and are due to differences in distribution and extent of the lesions. System disorders that affect the spinal cord include Friedreich's ataxia, hereditary spastic paraplegia (Strumpell), hereditary posterior column ataxia (Biemond) and motor neurone disease.

Friedreich's Ataxia

This rare progressive degenerative disease is the most common of the hereditary ataxias with a prevalence of 1–2 per 100 000 of the population. It is recessively inherited and presents usually before the age of 20 years and is characterized clinically by slowly progressive ataxia, loss of deep sensation, dysarthria, skeletal deformities and cardiac abnormalities. Patients often die of heart disease and there is an association with diabetes mellitus.

At autopsy the most striking macroscopic appearances are those of atrophy of the posterior roots in the lumbosacral region and cauda equina and of the spinal cord and brain stem. Histologically this is due to atrophy of the spinal posterior roots and their associated ganglia (Oppenheimer 1979). This results in prominent degeneration of the posterior columns affecting the gracile more than the cuneate fasciculi, and of the corticospinal and spinocerebellar tracts. In typical cases the spinal cord is small, the changes in the ascending tracts being particularly affected in the upper dorsal and cervical regions while the changes in the descending fibre tracts are more marked in the lower spinal cord (Fig. 6.8). There is variable loss of neurones in Clarke's column. Transneuronal degeneration is seen in the gracile and cuneate nuclei and there is usually marked involvement of the dentate nuclei in the cerebellum, which in turn results in marked atrophy of the superior cerebellar peduncles. In contrast the Purkinje cell complement of the cerebellar hemispheres is usually normal. Variable loss of neurones has also been described in the motor cortex and occasionally there is degeneration of the retina, the optic nerves and tracts, and the lateral geniculate bodies.

There are similarities between Friedreich's ataxia and Marie's hereditary cerebellar ataxia. The two conditions sometimes overlap and there are intermediate forms. Friedreich's ataxia is frequently associated with a chronic progressive myocarditis in which focal coagulative necrosis of the muscle fibres is followed by replacement fibrosis.

Apart from impaired glucose tolerance the only other known association with Friedreich's ataxia is that of increased sensitivity to ionising radiation.

Hereditary Spastic Paraplegia (Strumpell)

This is a slowly progressive disorder characterized by weakness of the legs that develops into a spastic paraparesis. It presents most commonly in adolescent or young adult males: in most cases inheritance is of autosomal dominant type though some also appear to be of an autosomal recessive nature.

The spinal cord may appear normal at autopsy. Histological examination shows degeneration of the lateral corticospinal tracts, particularly in the lower part of the spinal cord. There is also degeneration of the posterior columns, particularly the gracile tracts in the cervical region. The spinocerebellar tracts may also be affected. The pathogenesis is not known, but the nature and distribution of the lesions are strongly suggestive of a distal axonopathy affecting central pathways. It has, therefore, been likened to a prolonged form of the "dying back" process.

Hereditary Posterior Column Ataxia (Biemond)

This is a rare condition with an autosomal dominant mode of inheritance. It is characterized clinically by numbness of the hands and feet that later progresses to total absence of posterior column sensation. The spinal cord is atrophic due to degeneration of the posterior columns and partial degeneration of the posterior nerve roots.

Motor Neurone Disease

This is a progressive, occasionally familial, degenerative disorder of motor neurones with a worldwide distribution that presents clinically with wasting, weakness and eventually paralysis of muscles. It tends to occur in middle and late adult life and is more common in males than females. The disease is usually fatal in 2 to 3 years, but occasionally patients die in less than 12 months while others may survive for 10 years or more. Death is usually due to respiratory failure.

The striking feature clinically is that of loss of motor function with sparing of sensation and sphincter function and cognition. While the name motor neurone disease highlights that the pathological features are within upper and lower motor neurones and is used as a unifying term embracing the historically defined patterns of the disease, there are nevertheless three principal variants that are recognized depending on the distribution of the disease process. Progressive muscular atrophy presents with selectively severe involvement in the cervical region of the spinal cord as a result of which there is fasciculation and then atrophy of the small muscles of the hand. Involvement then spreads to the muscles of the arm and shoulder girdle. The term amyotrophic lateral sclerosis is used when upper motor neurones are affected leading to degeneration of the corticospinal tracts and a spastic paraparesis. Occasionally there is selectively severe damage to the motor nuclei in the lower brain stem, the process then being known as progressive bulbar palsy resulting in progressive wasting and paralysis of the muscles of the tongue, lips, jaw, larynx and pharynx.

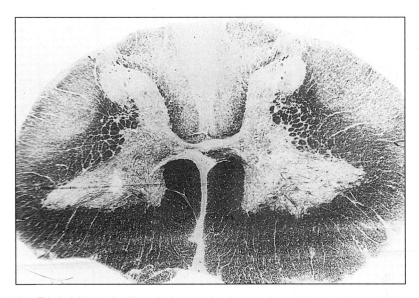

Fig. 6.8. Friedreich's ataxia. There is degeneration in posterior and lateral columns. Weigert-Pal. (Reproduced with permission from J.H. Adams and D.I. Graham, *An introduction to neuropathology*, Churchill Livingstone, Edinburgh, 1988.)

Patients with motor neurone disease usually die as a result of respiratory insufficiency and sometimes of pneumonia. As noted above not all muscle groups are equally affected and the external ocular muscles are usually spared. At autopsy the ventral nerve roots of the spinal cord are shrunken and grey compared with the normal thick white posterior nerve roots. (Brownell et al. 1970; Castaigne et al. 1972).

Transverse sections through the spinal cord show the ventral horns to be smaller than normal and in many instances the lateral columns of the cord are rather grey in colour in contrast to the striking preservation of the white colour of the posterior columns (Fig. 6.9).

The principal histological change is a loss of motor neurones and associated astrocytosis seen most easily in the ventral horns of the cervical and lumbar segments of the spinal cord (Figs. 6.10A and 6.10B) and in the hypoglossal nuclei of the lower brain stem. This is in contrast to the nuclei of the oculomotor, trochlear and abducent nerves which are rarely affected. Within the affected part, it is the larger motor neurones that are principally involved, the smaller and intermediate size cells tending to be preserved. Various changes are seen in the remaining neurones and include neuronophagia and ballooning (ghost cell change) and chromatolysis. Other cells show atrophy and may contain small eosinophilic inclusions (Bunina bodies). Long tract degeneration is usually present (Fig. 6.11) and may extend cranially beyond the cervical region into the brain stem, the cerebral peduncles, internal capsule and hemispheric white matter, all of these changes being the distal manifestation of pyramidal cell disease in the motor cortex. Detailed analysis of the motor cortex is difficult but in severe cases there is some loss of Betz cells. Sensory changes are rare in motor neurone disease and routine microscopy does

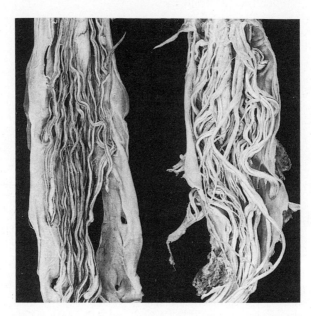

Fig. 6.9. Motor neurone disease. Compared with the normal cauda equina on the right, there is atrophy of ventral nerve roots on the left in a patient with motor neurone disease. (Reproduced with permission from J.H. Adams and D.I. Graham, *An introduction to neuropathology*, Churchill Livingstone, Edinburgh, 1988.)

not reveal obvious changes in sensory or autonomic nerves or the posterior columns. Minor changes, however, can sometimes be shown in the spino-cerebellar tracts and their parent cell bodies in Clarke's column as well as in other sensory pathways.

The pathogenesis of motor neurone disease is not known, there being no good evidence that it is due to a specific viral infection and in particular to chronic poliomyelitis. Intoxication with lead and more so recently by cycad nut poisoning have been considered, the latter possibly being mediated through excitotoxins. The possible exogenous causes of motor neurone disease stem from observation of the Parkinsonism-dementia complex which occurs in Guam which is characterized by diffuse neuronal loss and neurofibrillary tangles in the cortex, the deep grey structures, the substantia nigra and the brain stem. The Guamanian Parkinson's dementia complex associated with Guamanian motor neurone disease appears to be quite different from both idiopathic Parkinsonism associated with dementia and with sporadic motor neurone disease. The principal features are that in addition to the changes of either idiopathic Parkinsonism associated with dementia or sporadic motor neurone disease there is widespread neuronal loss and the formation of neurofibrillary tangles in the brain, brain stem and spinal cord.

The effects of denervation are well seen in muscle comprising collateral reinnervation from healthy subterminal axons, fibre type grouping and group atrophy. A muscle no more than moderately affected should be selected for biopsy.

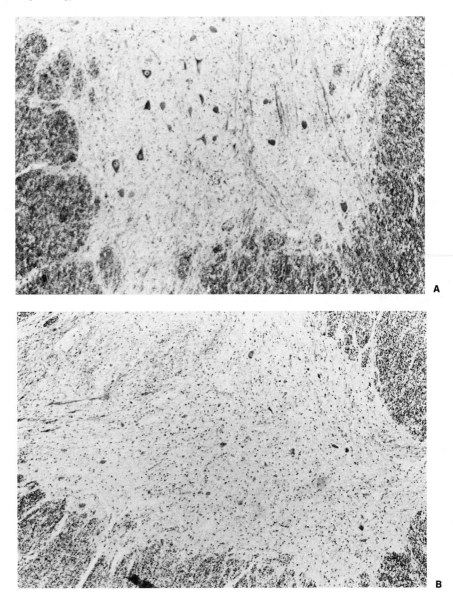

Fig. 6.10. Motor neurone disease. **A** Normal ventral horn; **B** Loss of ventral horn and neurones in case of motor neurone disease. Luxol Fast Blue A and B × 50. (**A** and **B** reproduced with permission from J.H. Adams and D.I. Graham, *An introduction to neuropathology*, Churchill Livingstone, Edinburgh, 1988.)

Werdnig-Hoffmann Disease

This condition, also known as familial spinal muscular atrophy, is caused by degeneration of the lower motor neurone due to autosomal recessive inheritance. It is characterized by delayed motor development, weakness and hypotonia

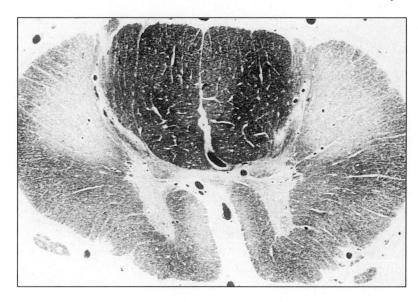

Fig. 6.11. Motor neurone disease. There is degeneration in the lateral, and to a lesser extent in the anterior, columns and preservation of the posterior columns. Heidenhain for myelin. (Reproduced with permission from J.H. Adams and D.I. Graham, *An introduction to neuropathology*, Churchill Livingstone, Edinburgh, 1988.)

that begins at or shortly after birth. It has been one of the causes of the "floppy baby" syndrome. It is rapidly fatal. The earlier the onset, the sooner the child dies. The principal pathological features are those of loss of ventral horn cells, atrophy of the ventral spinal nerve roots and denervation atrophy of muscles. The pyramidal and other long tracts are unaffected.

In addition to the classic and the Werdnig-Hoffman types of motor neurone disease, there is a range of comparatively rare types with onset in later childhood or adolescence. Most are autosomal recessive in nature and do not appear to form a continuum with classic motor neurone disease.

Demyelinating Disorders

By definition these are characterized by the destruction of myelin with the relative preservation of axons. They, therefore, differ from genetic disorders of myelin formation – the leucodystrophies – and from diseases causing breakdown of myelin due to destruction of neurones or their axons – Wallerian degeneration. The disorders in which demyelination is the only pathological process include a spectrum that ranges from acute conditions – acute disseminated (perivenous) encephalomyelitis and acute haemorrhagic leucoencephalopathy – to chronic disorders, the most important of which is multiple (disseminated) sclerosis. Forms intermediate in both clinical and pathological features are not uncommon (Lumsden 1970; Allen 1985; Weller 1985).

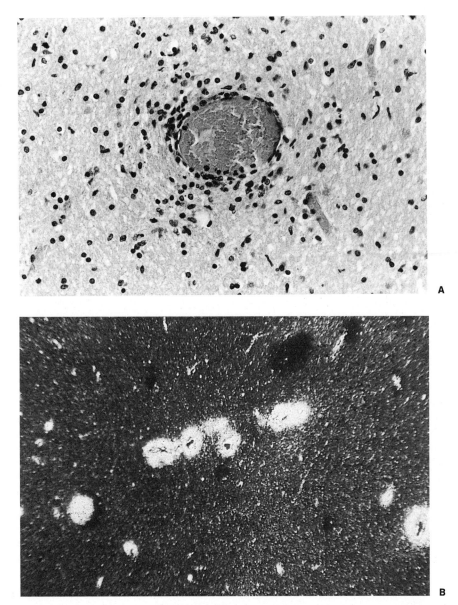

Fig. 6.12. Acute disseminated (perivenous) encephalomyelitis. **A** There is a diffuse inflammatory process in which lymphocytes and some monocytes are seen around a small vessel and in white matter. H & E × 330. **B** There is perivascular demyelination. Heidenhain for myelin × 50. (**A** and **B** reproduced with permission from J.H. Adams and D.I. Graham, *An introduction to neuropathology*, Churchill Livingstone, Edinburgh, 1988.)

Acute Disseminated (Perivenous) Encephalomyelitis

This monophasic and usually self-limiting disease occurs in older children and young adults after measles, mumps, chickenpox or rubella (post-infectious encephalitis). Of rapid onset it develops some 4 to 5 days after the appearance of the rash. Recovery is generally good but the condition is associated with a 10%–20% mortality following measles or chickenpox. There is also an association with upper respiratory tract infections presumed to be viral in nature and with primary vaccination against smallpox (post-vaccinial) encephalitis and antirabies inoculation.

At autopsy the CNS may either appear normal or merely show congestion and oedema. This contrasts with widespread histological changes in the white matter in which there is widespread cuffing of small blood vessels (probably venules) by inflammatory cells (Fig. 6.12A). Initially, the inflammatory infiltrate comprises neutrophil polymorphs but these are replaced by lymphocytes and macrophages. The inflammatory process may extend into the meninges. The most distinctive histological change, however, is that of perivascular demyelination (Fig. 6.12B) within which axon cylinders are preserved in contrast to a total loss and disintegration of myelin sheaths. In the spinal cord especially these lesions may coalesce and with recovery there is an astrocytosis.

The available evidence is that acute disseminated perivenous encephalomyelitis is not infectious in nature but represents a delayed hypersensitivity reaction. The clinical course of the disease, the inability to isolate any virus consistently from the brain, the interval between a virus infection and the onset of the illness and the similarity between the lesion to those seen in experimental allergic encephalomyelitis, all suggest that autoimmune mechanisms may be involved. The exact cause of the immunological reaction has not been established, but it would seem that a humoral reaction to constituents of myelin and a T-lymphocyte reaction to myelin basic protein combine to cause myelin to be the target of the immunological attack. Other possibilities include shared antigens between viruses and oligodendrocytes or that the demyelination is simply a consequence of a "bystander" effect in which myelin becomes damaged as a result of an immunologically mediated attack on viral particles.

Acute Haemorrhagic Leucoencephalitis

This is a relatively uncommon disorder which may occur as a sequel to any one of a number of severe viral infections that may also complicate septic shock, treatment with various drugs, and various other diseases assumed to be hypersensitive reactions, e.g. asthma and acute glomerular nephritis. It has a rapid course and is usually fatal within a few days of onset.

The principal finding at autopsy is that of swelling and multiple petechial haemorrhages, particularly in the white matter. The grey matter of both the cerebral cortex and basal ganglia is often spared, but there may be involvement of the brain stem, cerebellum and spinal cord. The haemorrhagic lesions are often symmetrical and if severe the haemorrhages may become confluent. Histologically the principal abnormalities are those in the walls of small blood vessels in which there is necrosis and exudation of fibrin into and through the vessel walls into the perivascular spaces. Some of the vessels may be occluded by thrombus. In cases of short survival there is perivascular infiltration by neutrophil polymorphs and later by monocytes and lymphocytes. The disease is characterized by perivascular demyelination with associated microglia and macrophages. In some cases, because of the intensity of the vascular reaction, small infarcts develop.

Aetiology is unknown but is thought to be a hyperacute variant of acute disseminated encephalomyelitis and to be caused by the deposition of immune complexes and the activation of complement.

Multiple (Disseminated) Sclerosis

This is the most common of the demyelinating disorders with an incidence that varies with latitude ranging from 30 per 100 000 with a band of high frequency that lies between the 40th and the 60th parallels to less than 10 per 100 000 in lower latitudes. The disease virtually disappears at the equator.

It is more common in women than men and its incidence increases from early adolescence with a peak at the third and fourth decade. The disease in its classic form is characterized by relapses and remissions and some two-thirds of patients ultimately show continuous deterioration. While this is true for the majority there are a small number, however, who have an acute unremitting form of the disease. The initial symptoms and signs vary but include paraesthesiae, limb weakness, ataxia, bladder dysfunction, nystagmus, optic neuritis and, very rarely, psychiatric symptoms.

The pathological features at autopsy vary with the rapidity with which the disease is progressing. For example naked eye examination in cases of *acute active multiple sclerosis* may reveal few abnormalities though when the brain is sliced lesions may appear as areas of yellow granular discoloration in white matter. Histologically, there are sharply defined areas of demyelination within which there are many surviving axons. Stains for lipid show large amounts of the breakdown products of myelin within phagocytes and there is widespread cuffing of vessels by lymphocytes, plasma cells and macrophages. Most of the lympocytes are T-cells and the plasma cells contain IgG. Such cells also define the margins of the plaques. A further feature of acute lesions is that of considerable hypertrophy and hyperplasia of astrocytes. This is in contrast to the oligodendrocytes in the centre of the lesions which are greatly reduced in number: at the margins, however, attempts at remyelination may be seen giving rise to an appearance that has been referred to as shadow plaques. Finally, using silver impregnation techniques and/or immunochemistry for neurofilament proteins, the integrity of the majority of axons can be readily identified.

Again in *chronic multiple sclerosis* there may be little abnormality to be seen post mortem, though as with the ventral aspect of the pons and medulla, it may be possible to see irregular shrunken grey plaques on stripping the meninges from the spinal cord. Plaques of multiple sclerosis may occur anywhere within the CNS, although the optic nerves and chiasma, the periventricular white matter, the brain stem and spinal cord are sites of predilection. Indeed in some patients the optic nerve, brain stem and spinal cord (Fig. 6.13) are severely affected and the brain may contain only a few plaques. Multiple sectioning of the spinal cord reveals plaques to be rather shrunken grey areas

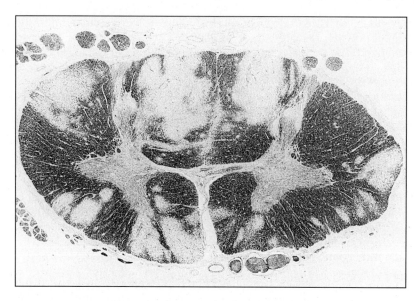

Fig. 6.13. Chronic multiple sclerosis. There are multiple plaques in the spinal cord. Luxol fast blue/cresyl violet. (Reproduced with permission from J.H. Adams and D.I. Graham, *An introduction to neuropathology*, Churchill Livingstone, Edinburgh, 1988.)

of demyelination which are commonly present in the cervical region with a high proportion involving the lateral columns (Oppenheimer 1978). As a result of the plaques, secondary changes may be seen in the form of long tract degeneration.

Histologically the disease is characterized by sharply defined areas of demyelination (Fig. 6.14A) many of which are centred on small venules. If the plaque involves grey matter within the demyelinated area the neurones are preserved, a feature that distinguishes the lesion from infarction. Oligodendrocytes are reduced in number and there is an astrocytosis which in all plaques takes the form of a dense network of fibrillary processes. In chronic active plaques, a few of the associated vessels are cuffed by lymphocytes and macrophages (Fig. 6.14B) and at the margins of the lesion signs of active myelin breakdown are seen in the form of lipid-containing macrophages. Similar cells may be seen in the related meninges and there is preservation of the majority of axons (Fig. 6.14C). In chronic multiple sclerosis the histological appearances differ in that there are very few inflammatory cells. Astrocytes are less prominent although there is a marked gliosis and there are very few macrophages. Again the number of oligodendrocytes is greatly reduced and although many axons are preserved their numbers become reduced over time. The histological appearance in chronic multiple sclerosis, therefore, will vary depending on the activity of the process ranging from chronic active to chronic burnt out plaque formation. Commonly, in longstanding cases there is ultimately Wallerian degeneration in ascending and descending tracts within the spinal cord.

There is a variant of multiple sclerosis (Devic's disease) or neuromyelitis optica in which there is a clinical association of visual failure and signs of

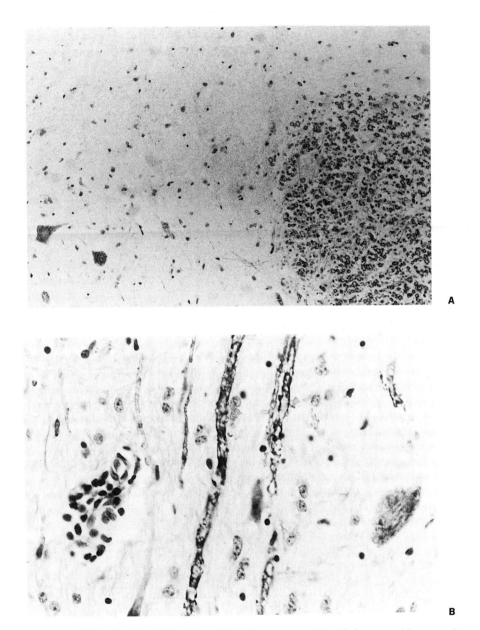

Fig. 6.14. Multiple sclerosis. **A** The edges of the plaque are usually well demarcated because of the complete demyelination. Luxol fast blue/cresyl violet × 130. **B** There is mild perivascular cuffing of vessels by lymphocytes. H & E × 330. **C** There is preservation of axons within the plaques. Palmgren × 130.

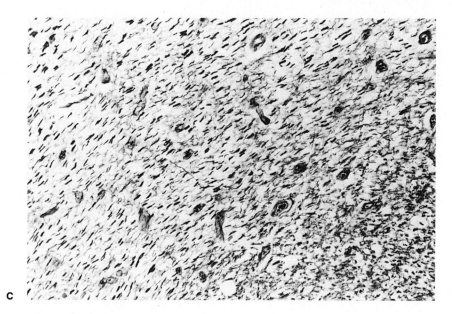

c

Fig. 6.14. (continued)

spinal cord involvement. Apart from the distribution of the plaques, the pathological features are those of the classic form of multiple sclerosis. Fulminating
examples have also been described in which there is necrosis over several
segments of the spinal cord, possibly due to secondary vascular damage.

Following an episode of exacerbation in multiple sclerosis, there may be
partial or complete recovery of neurological function. This may in part be
explained by subsidence of inflammation and swelling in and around the plaque
and by physiological adaptation. Certainly there is little evidence of effective
remyelination probably due to the widespread destruction of oligodendrocytes.
Post-mortem studies have shown that in some cases of clinically mild multiple
sclerosis, there are large numbers of plaques whereas devastating clinical
disease may be associated with a relatively small number. Furthermore, in
as many as 10%–20% of cases in which multiple sclerosis is observed post
mortem, there may be no clinical signs of the disease during life.

The pathogenesis of multiple sclerosis is not known, but epidemiological
studies on individuals migrating from areas of high incidence to areas of low
incidence suggest an environmental factor inter-reacting with genetic factors
may be important. Thus patients born in low latitudes appear to carry the
lower attack rate with them if they move to higher latitudes after the age of 15
years. Conversely, patients migrating after the age of 15 from Northern Europe
to, for example, South Africa and to Israel retain the high risk of their country
of origin; those leaving at a young age seem to be relatively protected. There is
also an increased incidence of multiple sclerosis in the families of patients with
the disease but it is not known whether this is attributable to genetic or
environmental factors or to a combination of both. While these studies might
suggest an infective aetiology, there is no convincing evidence yet for this

theory. Multiple sclerosis has not been transmitted to experimental animals and no viral agent has been consistently isolated from brain tissue, though many studies have demonstrated an increased titre of antibodies – particularly to measles and less consistently to vaccinia, rubella and herpes simplex. The meaning of these increased titres is not clear, as it has not been possible to relate the specific antibodies to the oligoclonal bands of immunoglobulin that are so commonly found in CSF. It is also pertinent to note that the disease does not resemble any known persistent or slow virus infection of the CNS in man or animals. There is considerable evidence for an immune reaction in the pathology of multiple sclerosis. Certainly the presence of lymphocytes and plasma cells in acute plaques is in keeping with such a theory. Recent work has shown that in patients with acute attacks of multiple sclerosis there is a marked decline in the activity of suppressor T-cells in the peripheral blood, the activity rising again after an attack. So multiple sclerosis may, therefore, be a disorder of immune regulation. In support of an autoimmune aetiology, antibodies which together with complement cause demyelination of cultures in neural tissue have been detected in the serum of patients with multiple sclerosis. Such antibodies have also been found in various non-demyelinating diseases. In spite of considerable effort, the antigens under immune attack are not known. One suggestion is that some patients with multiple sclerosis have an increased cell-mediated immunity against myelin basic protein. However, even in diseases such as acute post-infectious encephalomyelitis in which antibodies to myelin basic protein are present in the serum, it is uncertain whether this indicates a primary aetiological factor or a secondary effect of the disease. As with acute disseminated encephalomyelitis it has been suggested that demyelination in multiple sclerosis may be the result of a "bystander" effect. In this way myelin damage would result from the immune attack on a non-myelin antigen.

Metabolic Disorders

It is not intended in this section to cover the primary metabolic diseases which make a considerable contribution to morbidity and mortality in children. Many of these are inherited as autosomal recessive diseases. Although the onset of clinical symptoms may not become apparent until adult life, the majority appear during childhood and frequently in the first few days of life.

For the brain to function normally, it requires that other systems in the body are also functioning normally. In view of this dependence it is perhaps not surprising that secondary metabolic effects on the CNS are an early manifestation of systemic disease. In many instances the clinical features are reversible and there are minimal morphological changes, both occurrences supporting the belief that many of the disorders are attributable to biochemical derangement rather than a structural abnormality. It is only when the metabolic disorder has been profound and prolonged that structural changes occur, thus accounting for the permanent clinical neurological deficits that some of these patients manifest. Such secondary acquired CNS manifestations of systemic disease occur at all ages. However, only a few that affect the spinal cord will be highlighted.

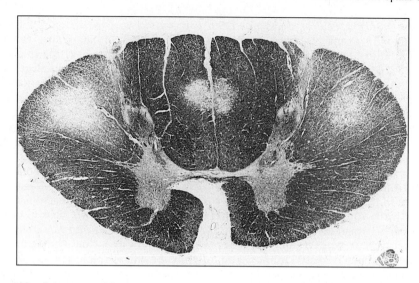

Fig. 6.15. Subacute combined degeneration of the cord. There is focal pallor of myelin staining in the posterior and lateral columns. Luxol fast blue/cresyl violet. (Reproduced with permission from J.H. Adams and D.I. Graham, *An introduction to neuropathology*, Churchill Livingstone, Edinburgh, 1988.)

Subacute Combined Degeneration

Since highly effective purified preparations of vitamin B12 have become available for the treatment of pernicious anaemia this complication is now uncommon. Similar lesions have been found even more rarely in some other chronic diseases, e.g. malabsorption syndromes, leukaemia, diabetes and carcinoma. The administration of vitamin B12 in adequate doses is completely effective in preventing the development of CNS lesions.

Signs and symptoms referable to the spinal cord are usually marked in early features of the disorder. The cord may appear entirely normal externally and on section at autopsy. Histologically however, the disease is characterized by the multifocal development of vacuoles in the white matter of the dorsal and lateral columns (Fig. 6.15), particularly of the lower thoracic region before extending both upwards and downwards. As the vacuolation increases in amount and severity it is accompanied by the breakdown of myelin and some evidence of axonal degeneration. Lipid-containing macrophages are present around small vessels. In untreated cases there is a remarkable absence of astrocytic reaction but with long survival and appropriate treatment, gliosis eventually develops. The symptoms depend on the degree and extent of tract involvement.

Vitamin B12 is required for the normal growth and maintenance of the nervous system. With the exception of vegans, dietary deficiency of the vitamin is uncommon. Other conditions, however, may be associated with the reduced absorption of vitamin B12 and include the absence of the "intrinsic factor" from gastric mucosa that is required for its absorption, infestation by tapeworms and severe gastritis or gastric surgery which removes the region secreting the intrinsic factor. Biochemistry has identified that within the nervous system of mammals there are two vitamin B12 requiring enzymes, namely methionine synthetase and methylmalonyl CoA (co-enzyme A) mutase. There is evidence that methyl donation is the underlying biochemical defect, the peculiar sensitivity of humans as compared to other species in the development of myelin lesions being their higher requirement of myelin basic protein for labile methyl groups. Evidence in support of such a mechanism has been found from various experimental studies that include the study of cage paralysis in primates, intoxication by nitrous oxide and intoxication by cycloleucine.

Acquired Hepatocerebral Encephalopathy

A metabolic encephalopathy invariably accompanies severe liver failure. Cases of massive hepatic necrosis are accompanied by an acute hepatic encephalopathy characterized by rapidly developing coma. On the other hand in cases of liver disease with cirrhosis, particularly when there is porto–systemic shunting, chronic hepatic encephalopathy develops. Both types are potentially reversible so the patients often present an episodic and relapsing course: it may, however, become chronic and progressive. One such manifestation of hepatic disease is the occasional development of myelopathy in which there is symmetrical demyelination of the lateral corticospinal tracts of the cervical cord. There may in addition also be some loss of fibres in the gracile tracts of the dorsal columns. The pattern of the pathology is suggestive of the "dying back" type of neuronal degeneration.

Myelopathy of Diabetes Mellitus

Complications of diabetes in the CNS are usually attributable to cerebrovascular disease. An exception to this generalization is the not uncommon finding of partial demyelination of the posterior columns of the spinal cord. The changes may be so marked that the cord acquires a distinctive shape referred to as "pseudotabes". Demyelination of the lateral columns has been reported as diabetic amyotrophic lateral sclerosis. The pathogenesis of the demyelination is not known: possibilities include primary demyelination, toxic metabolic factors or a microangiopathy due to thickening of the basement membrane and changes in the blood–brain barrier. The loss in the posterior columns is invariably associated with a chronic peripheral neuropathy.

Non-metastatic (Remote) Effects of Carcinoma

Many patients present with deposits of metastatic carcinoma within the brain and fewer with signs of cord compression as a result of deposits in the extradural tissues. Other tumours, particularly carcinoma of the bronchus and lymphoma, may have indirect (remote) effects upon the central or peripheral nervous system either singly or in combination. Indeed up to 6% of patients with carcinoma are said to present neurological syndromes as a manifestation of the non-metastatic effects of carcinoma (Henson and Urich 1982). There is no constant relationship between the course of the neurological disorder and that of the carcinoma, in that they may develop concurrently or the neurological disorder may antedate objective evidence of tumour by several years. Furthermore, the severity of the neurological disease is not related to the size of the tumour.

There are five main categories of disorder that include metabolic and vascular syndromes and those secondary to infections and therapy. Included within the neuromuscular syndromes are a group of conditions that closely simulate motor neurone disease, and an amyotrophic lateral sclerosis-like syndrome. Within the encephalomyelitic syndromes, is the uncommon condition of subacute necrotizing myelopathy, the principal features of which are the presence of lymphocytes and some plasma cells around small vessels within the spinal cord and small aggregates of microglia (Fig. 6.16). Grey matter is affected more than white matter and inflammatory changes are associated with loss of neurones and Wallerian degeneration. Many suggestions have been put forward about the pathogenesis of these neurological syndromes that include toxins, infection, autoimmune processes and both metabolic and endocrine disorders. The presence of inflammatory lesions similar to those seen in virus infections, certainly suggests the possibility that a neurotropic virus is the causal agent. An alternative explanation is that of an antigen–antibody reaction following the discovery of specific circulating antibodies against neural tissue.

Malformations of the Spinal Cord

To be discussed here are syringomyelia and disraphic abnormalities of the cord, the most common form of which is diastematomyelia (Friede 1989).

Syringomyelia

This is an uncommon condition in which a cyst-like space (syrinx) or spaces develop within the spinal cord and contain clear fluid enclosed by neuroglia. The lesion may extend over several centimetres usually lying immediately dorsal to the central canal, though it may extend eccentrically into one or both dorsal horns of the grey matter (Fig. 6.17). Occasionally the cyst communicates with either the fourth ventricle or the central canal. As it enlarges the cord becomes swollen and not infrequently there is an associated Chiari Type 1 malformation. Occasionally, syringomyelia occurs in association with intradural spinal tumours and vascular malformations.

The clinical effects are due principally to destruction of the cord by the enlarging cavity. The first fibres to be affected are the decussating fibres conveying the sensations of heat and pain. This results in dissociated anaesthesia which is a selective insensibility to heat and pain in the region corresponding to the involved segments of the cord. A neuropathic arthritis similar to that seen in tabes is common, but as syringomyelia usually occurs in the cervical region, the joints of the upper limbs are chiefly involved. Trophic lesions also occur in

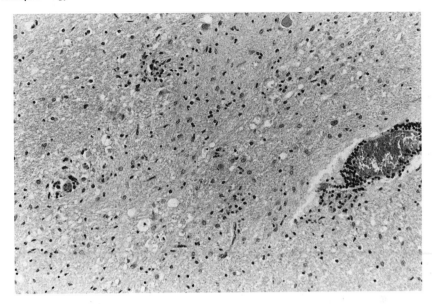

Fig. 6.16. Non-metastatic effects of carcinoma: spinal cord. There is slight perivascular cuffing by lymphocytes, clusters of microglia and an astrocytosis. H & E × 130.

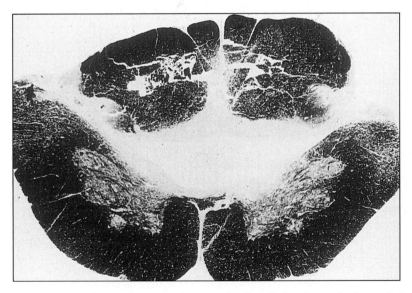

Fig. 6.17. Syringomyelia. There is a cavity extending into both columns in the cervical cord. Weigert-Pal for myelin. (Reproduced with permission from J.H. Adams and D.I. Graham, *An introduction to neuropathology*, Churchill Livingstone, Edinburgh, 1988.)

the skin. If the cavity enlarges it ultimately affects the lateral white columns leading to spastic paraparesis, the ventral grey horns leading to neurogenic atrophy of muscles and the posterior white columns leading to even greater disturbances of sensation.

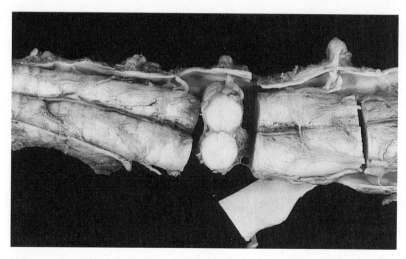

Fig. 6.18. Diastematomyelia. There are two hemicords within a single dural sac and separated by a fibrovascular septum. (Reproduced with permission from J.H. Adams and D.I. Graham, *An introduction to neuropathology*, Churchill Livingstone, Edinburgh, 1988.)

The nature and pathogenesis of syringomyelia remain controversial. However, it is now well accepted that in at least some cases it is caused by CSF being propelled through a valve-like opening between the caudal extremity of the fourth ventricle and the central canal. An alternative view is that syringomyelia is a form of dysraphism in which there has been instability in the lines of junction of the alar and basal laminae with each other. In other words the cavity is a greatly distended central canal.

Diastematomyelia

In this condition the cord is split by either a bony or fibrous septum projecting into the spinal canal. There is a variable degree of separation which in turn determines whether each half of the cord has its own pial and dural sheath or whether these investments are shared (Fig. 6.18). This form of spinal cord dysraphism occurs predominantly in the thoracolumbar spine and is often associated with other anomalies such as spina bifida occulta and the Arnold-Chiari malformation. There is usually a localized kyphoscoliosis at the site of the lesion.

Acknowledgements. My thanks to Mrs. A. Whyte for having typed this manuscript.

References

Allen IV (1985) Demyelinating diseases. In: Adams JH, Corsellis JAN, Duchen LW (eds) Greenfields' neuropathology, 4th edn. Edward Arnold, London, pp 338–384

Brain WR, Northfield D, Wilkinson M (1952) The neurological manifestations of cervical spondylosis. Brain 75:187–225

Brownell B, Oppenheimer DR, Hughes JT (1970) The central nervous system in motor neurone disease. J Neurol Neurosurg Psychiatry 33:338–357

Castaigne P, Lhermitte F, Cambier J, Escourolle R, Le Bigot P (1972) Etude neuropathologique de 61 observations de sclerose laterale amyotrophique: discussions nosologique. Rev Neurol 127:401–414

Duchen LW (1985) General pathology of neurones and neuroglia. In: Adams JH, Corsellis JAN, Duchen LW (eds) Greenfields' neuropathology, 4th edn. Edward Arnold, London, pp 1–52

Esiri MM, Oppenheimer DR (1989) Histology. In: Esiri MM, Oppenheimer DR (eds) Diagnostic neuropathology. Blackwell Scientific, Oxford, pp 46–66

Fink RP, Heimer L (1967) Two methods for selective impregnation of degenerating axons and their synaptic endings in the central nervous system. Brain Res 4:369–374

Fogelholm R, Haltia M, Andersson LC (1974) Radiation myelopathy of cervical spinal cord simulating intramedullary neoplasm. J Neurol Neurosurg Psychiatry 37:1177–1180

Friede RL (1989) Malformations. In: Friede RL (ed) Developmental neuropathology, 2nd edn. Springer-Verlag, Berlin, pp 247–404

Frykholm R (1951) Lower cervical vertebrae and intervertebral discs. Surgical anatomy and pathology. Acta Chirurgica Scand 101:345–359

Godwin-Austen RB, Howel DA, Worthington B (1975) Observations in radiation myelopathy. Brain 98:557–568

Henson RA, Urich H (1982) Cancer and the nervous system. The neurological manifestations of systemic malignant diseases. Blackwell Scientific, Oxford

Hook O, Lidvall H, Astrom KE (1960) Cervical disk protrusions with compression of the spinal cord. Neurology 10:834–841

Hughes JT (1974) Pathology of spinal cord damage in spinal injuries. In: Feiring EH (ed) Brock's injuries of the brain and spinal cord, 5th edn. Springer, New York, pp 668–687

Hughes JT (1977) Spinal cord involvement by C4–C5 vertebral subluxation in rheumatoid arthritis. A description of 2 cases examined at necropsy. Ann Neurol 1:575–582

Hughes JT (1978) Introduction. In: Hughes JT (ed) Pathology of the spinal cord. Lloyd-Duke, London, pp 1–16

Hughes JT (1984) Regeneration in the human spinal cord: a review of the response to injury of the various constituents of the human spinal cord. Paraplegia 22:131–137

Jennett WB (1956) A study of 25 cases of compression of the cauda equina by prolapsed intervertebral disc. J Neurol Neurosurg Psychiatry 19:109–116

Lantos PL (1990a) Cytology of the normal central nervous system. In: Weller RO (ed) Nervous system, muscle and eyes. Systemic pathology, 3rd edn, vol 4. Churchill Livingstone, Edinburgh, pp 3–35

Lantos PL (1990b) Histological and cytological reactions. In: Weller RO (ed) Nervous system, muscle and eyes. Systemic Pathology, 3rd edn, vol 4. Churchill Livingstone, Edinburgh, pp 36–63

Lumsden CE (1970) The neuropathology of multiple sclerosis. In: Vinken PJ, Bruyn GW (eds) Handbook of clinical neurology, vol 9. North-Holland, Amsterdam, pp 296–298

McRae DL (1953) Bony abnormalities in region of foramen magnum: correlation of anatomic and neurologic findings. Acta Radiologica 40:335–355

Nauta WJH, Gygax PA (1954) Silver impregnation of degenerating axons in the central nervous system. A modified technic. Stain Technol 29:91–93

Oppenheimer DR (1978) The cervical cord in multiple sclerosis. Neuropathol Appl Neurobiol 4:151–162

Oppenheimer DR (1979) Brain lesions in Friedreich's ataxia. Can J Neurol Sci 6:173–176

Palmer AC, Calder IM, McCallum RI, Mastaglia FL (1981) Spinal cord degeneration in a case of "recovered" spinal decompression sickness. Br Med J 283:888

Payne EE, Spillane JD (1957) The cervical spine. An anatomo-pathological study of 70 specimens (using a special technique) with particular reference to the problem of cervical spondylosis. Brain 80:571–596

Rossier AB, Foo D, Shillito J, Dyro FR (1985) Post-traumatic cervical syringomyelia. Brain 108:439–461

Russell DS, Rubinstein LJ (1989) Effects of radiation and other forms of energy on intracranial and intraspinal tumours and their surrounding tissues. In: Russell DS, Rubinstein LJ (eds) Pathology of tumours of the nervous system, 5th edn. Edward Arnold, London, pp 871–879

Smith MC (1951) The use of Marchi staining in the later stages of human tract degeneration. J Neurol Neurosurg Psychiatry 14:222–225

Smith MC, Strich SJ, Sharp P (1956) The value of the Marchi method for staining tissue stored in formalin for prolonged periods. J Neurol Neurosurg Psychiatry 19:62–64

Vaughn JE, Pease DC (1970) Electron microscopic studies of Wallerian degeneration in rat optic nerves II. Astrocytes, oligodendrocytes and adventitial cells. J Comp Neurol 140:207–226

Vaughn JE, Hinds PL, Skoff RP (1970) Electron microscopic studies of Wallerian degeneration in rat optic nerves I. The multipotential glia. J Comp Neurol 140:175–206

Weller RO (1985) Pathology of multiple sclerosis. In: Mathews WB, Acheson ED, Batchelor JR, Weller RO (eds) McAlpine's multiple sclerosis. Churchill Livingstone, Edinburgh, pp 301–343

Chapter 7

Embryonic Development of the Spinal Cord and Associated Disorders

M.J. Noronha

Embryology

The three primary germ cell layers – ectoderm, mesoderm and entoderm – are present in the embryonic disc by the end of the second gestational week. At this time, a single sheet of cells (i.e. the midline ectoderm) undergoes a time-specific induction by underlying mesoderm to become the neural plate. During the third week, the ectodermal neural plate enlarges and is further induced by mesoderm and entodermally derived notochord to form a midaxial groove which sinks deeper. Its edges (neural folds) converge and fuse dorsally to form the primitive neural tube. Fusion commences near the midpoint of the embryo and progresses rostrally and caudally and is usually complete by the end of the fourth week. The early formation of the neural tube by primary neurulation is now basically complete.

As the neural tube develops it moves apart from the surface ectoderm. Specific cells at the edges of the neural fold separate away to form the neural crests from which will develop the dorsal root ganglia of the spinal nerves, the sympathetic nervous system and Schwann cells. Simultaneously, mesodermal tissues are organized to form structures which support and surround the neural axis, such as bone, cartilage, connective tissue and meninges.

Developmental neural tube defects may involve multiple germ cell layers i.e. ectoderm and mesoderm resulting in clinical manifestations that can vary from a symptomless occult laminar defect of the lumbar spine detectable only radiologically to a complete spinal rachischis when the spinal cord lies on the dorsal surface of the infant (spina bifida cystica).

The pathogenesis of these defects is not known but the most likely hypothesis is that the neural tube fails to close during embryogenesis. Lack of closure of the posterior neuropore may explain frequently accompanying lumbosacral malformations, but the abnormality may involve the entire length of the spinal cord. An additional feature may be an associated defect of neural induction in mesodermal tissues. It should be noted that "the malformation complex" frequently exhibits so many abnormalities of the nervous system, that it is difficult to base a theory of pathogenesis upon a single primary error of development (Anderson and Carlson 1966).

Primary neurulation of the neural tube is complete between the 26th and 28th day of gestation and is coincidental with the formation of the 28th and

30th somites. The 29th somite corresponds to the 5th sacral vertebra in the adult. The limit of primary neurulation is the last sacral vertebra and secondary neurulation begins caudally beyond this point, resulting in the tail which may have up to 10 coccygeal somites. In man most of the caudal somites disappear. In studying human embryos, the spinal cord segments correspond to the somites level for level. Differential growth of the spinal cord and vertebral canal leads to changes in their relative positions. At birth, the conus medullaris lies opposite the third or fourth lumbar vertebrae and it attains the "adult level" at the lower level of L1 vertebra by about 2 months postnatally (Barson 1970).

During the embryonic period (up to 12 weeks) of intense differentiation, most teratogens are highly effective in producing many serious malformations. Teratogenic agents acting before neural tube closure, which occurs by the end of the fourth week, include radiation, maternal hyperthermia, gestational diabetes mellitus, hypoxia, chemical toxins, drugs and folic acid deficiency (Holmes et al. 1976; Shepard 1982).

Incidence at Birth

Congenital malformations of the CNS consisting principally of spina bifida (cystica), anencephaly and hydrocephalus, comprise a large but diminishing proportion of all congenital malformations. In England and Wales, the occurrence of CNS defects of all types in 1974 was 2452 infants (3.79 per 1000 deliveries) but in 1983 only 917 affected infants (1.45 per 1000 deliveries) were reported. These infants comprised 19.3% falling to 6.6% of all congenital defects reported. The causes of this decline are largely unknown though in part are related to prenatal diagnosis and abortions carried out because of CNS defects. There are large variations in the incidence of CNS defects in different parts of the world. Spina bifida rates per 10000 births have varied from 1.2 in Hong Kong Chinese (Ghosh et al. 1981) to 21.2 in Dublin (Coffey 1983) and 25.0 in North India (Verma 1978).

Spina bifida occulta represents a fusion failure of the posterior vertebral arches unaccompanied by herniation of meninges or neural tissue. Spina bifida cystica is a term used to designate collectively meningocele and myelomeningocele (Fig. 7.1).

Spina Bifida Cystica

This common malformation together with anencephaly occurs in approximately 3 per 1000 live births. Anencephaly is incompatible with life and accounts for about half the cases in this group, while the majority of the myelomeningocele infants are born alive. The lesion may vary from a small parchment-like membrane on the baby's back without any neurological deficit present, to a large myelomeningocele occupying several segments and causing complex loss of neurological function affecting the lower limbs and sphincters.

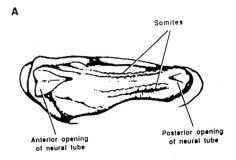

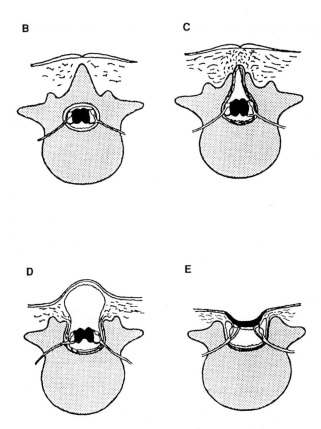

Fig. 7.1. **A** Embryo at day 23 with amnion removed to show the somites on each side of the neural tube, which is closed except in the head and lumbar regions. **B–E** Cross-sections of neonatal lumbar vertebrae to show spinal cord (black) and meninges: **B** Normal; **C** Spina bifida occulta; **D** Meningocele; **E** Severe spina bifida with unclosed neural tube (myelomeningocele).

A myelomeningocele occurring in the cervical region is usually small, has a narrow neck and seldom contains important nervous tissue. In the thoracic region, small lesions without evidence of neurological deficit sometimes occur though at other times the lesions are large with a considerable loss of neurological function below the level of the lesion. Over 80% of myelomeningoceles involve the lumbar or sacral regions, possibly because the lower end of the neural tube is the last part to close during development.

The lesions can be classified as follows:

1. *Meningocele*. There is a defect of the vertebral arches with herniation of the membranes of the spinal cord to form a sac usually with good skin cover. There are no neural elements in the sac.

2. *Myelomeningocele*. The spinal cord or nerve roots are displaced through the spina bifida defect. The dura mater lines the sac for only part of the way, being replaced by arachnoid up to the point where the spinal cord or cauda equina lie on a free surface forming the fundus of the sac wall, while the ectodermal skin reaches only to the base of the sac. In its most severe form with complete failure of the neural tube to close, the spinal cord lies on the dorsal surface of the infant.

3. *Hydrocephalus*. Myelomeningocele is associated with hydrocephalus in 73% of patients. The incidence rises to 90% when the myelomeningocele is situated in the thoracolumbar region (Lorber 1961). Although hydrocephalus was thought to be present at birth in only 25% of babies, with modern imaging techniques the abnormality is almost invariably present in the newborn. It is important to differentiate between hydrocephalus without an accompanying myelomeningocele and progressive forms of hydrocephalus which require surgical intervention. Hydrocephalus is almost invariably associated with a developmental abnormality of the hind brain consisting of downward displacement of the cerebellar tonsils and medulla into the upper cervical canal (Arnold-Chiari type II malformation).

Aqueductal stenosis may be associated with the Arnold-Chiari malformation in 40%–75% of cases (Peach 1965a; Stein and Schut 1979). Abnormalities of cranial nerves and cervical cord may also complicate the Arnold-Chiari malformation resulting in dysphagia, bradycardia, poor head control and upper extremity weakness (Park et al. 1983). Upper airways obstruction due to vocal cord abductor paralysis and central apnoea occur in a small number of children but these features carry a high mortality (Hays et al. 1989). The appearance of microgyria has been described in 55%–95% of cases (Ingraham et al. 1944; Peach 1965b). This finding probably reflects a true cortical dysgenesis and may be important because of a potential relationship to intellectual deficits or the occurrence of epileptic seizures (Bartholesky et al. 1985).

Antenatal Diagnosis and Prevention

The presence of abnormally high alpha-fetoprotein levels in the amniotic fluid suggests myelomeningocele. Alpha-fetoprotein probably leaks into the amniotic fluid from an open neural tube defect. Hence in closed lesions, alpha-fetoprotein levels are not elevated. Maternal serum alpha-fetoprotein levels are also elevated during pregnancy *after* the first trimester. In open neural tube lesions, the optimal time of screening suggested for measuring alpha-fetoprotein levels is at 14 to 16 weeks in the amniotic fluid and at 16 to 18 weeks of gestation in the maternal serum. The detection rate for open neural tube defects using serum screening is approximately 80% with a low false-positive rate (Report of UK Collaborative Study 1977). Ultrasonography of the fetus can usually detect or confirm the extent of the neural tube defect as well as the presence of hydrocephalus.

True prevention of myelodysplasia may be possible by periconceptual vitamin supplementation, based on the observation that there is a higher risk of neural tube defects in the poorer socioeconomic classes and that in a group of women giving birth to an infant with this disorder, the mean blood levels of folate, ascorbic acid and riboflavin were lower than in controls (Smithells et al. 1981).

Management and Prognosis

Management is directed towards the preservation of function and the recognition and management of treatable complications. It will usually require the involvement of many specialists. Treatment includes the prevention of infection, surgical reduction and covering of the myelomeningocele, control of hydrocephalus, management of urinary bladder and bowel problems, and the treatment of paralysis and deformities of the lower limbs.

Four adverse conditions were identified by Lorber (1971) as contraindications to surgical treatment: (1) a high level of paraplegia, (2) hydrocephalus apparent at birth (head circumference 2 cm above the 90th centile), (3) gross kyphosis and (4) major malformations in other systems. Presence of any of these criteria tends to result in a poor prognosis in that the child will survive, grossly physically handicapped and often with mental impairment as well. The decision for vigorous treatment of the most severely affected infants with myelomeningocele is beset by medical and moral considerations. Each child must be assessed individually in the context of advances in technology and medical care and with full consultation with the parents. Counselling is essential so that parents understand the nature and severity of the deformities, the extensive surgical and rehabilitative measures that will be needed, and the child's potential for intellectual and physical development.

More than 70% of treated infants were alive at 6 years of age, whereas more than 80% of untreated infants were dead at 3 months (Smith and Smith 1973; Stark and Drummond 1973). Children born with myelomeningocele may live for months or years if they receive supportive care only. All decisions regarding treatment should be directed towards the best interests of the infant, including the child's contentment and comfort (Zachary 1973).

Initial Management

Paediatricians and surgeons experienced with dealing with problems of spina bifida, should be involved with the baby's care preferably from the first hours or day after birth. Closure of the open defect, relief of intracranial hypertension, and evaluation of urinary and skeletal problems are important from the start.

The extent of the spinal defect, the degree of paralysis and sensory impairment in the lower limbs, and the presence of any sphincter disturbances are identified. When the lesion is below L2, the cauda equina bears the brunt of the damage resulting in varying degrees of a flaccid, areflexic paraparesis and sensory deficits distal from dermatomes L3 or L4. Sphincter and bladder involvement results in dribbling incontinence of urine, poor tone in the anal sphincter and rectal prolapse may occur. If the lesion is located at the thoracolumbar level or higher, anal tone is usually normal, the urinary bladder hypertonic and the paraparesis may sometimes show features of upper motor neurone involvement due to an isolated segment of functioning spinal cord below the level of the meningocele (Stark and Baker 1967). In lesions affecting the sacral spinal cord, the nerve supply to the lower limbs is usually normal but the nerve supply to the sphincters and pelvic floor muscles is impaired so that the child will have a normal gait but urinary and faecal incontinence will occur. Saddle anaesthesia involving dermatomes of S3 to S5 may also be present.

Assessment of the functional level of the lesion allows reasonable estimates of potential future capacities. Thus most patients with lesions below S1 ultimately are able to walk unaided, whereas those with lesions above L2 are wheelchair dependent for at least the major portion of their activities. Patients with intermediate lesions will exhibit similar degrees of wheelchair dependency or will be primarily ambulatory with calipers and crutches. Most important, deterioration to a lower level of ambulatory function readily occurs in the absence of careful management.

Closure of the myelomeningocele should be done as early as possible to prevent the risk of infection and subsequent deterioration in neurological function. If primary closure is not possible due to the large cutaneous area involved or the severity of other risk factors, epithelialization must be encouraged and surgery to cover the defect can be performed later. Cranial ultrasonography should be performed early to determine the presence of hydrocephalus. Hydrocephalus may be present even though the baby's head is not enlarged (Lorber 1961). A shunting procedure, usually a ventriculo–peritoneal shunt, will alleviate the pressure problems due to the hydrocephalus.

Later Complications

Bladder dysfunction and urinary incontinence occur in the majority of patients. Interruption of the sacral nerve roots and fibre connections between the brain stem and sacral cord is the cause of the dysfunction. Normal bladder function occurs in only 10% of these children (Eckstein and Chir 1972; Rink and Mitchell 1984). Prevention of bladder infection involves clean intermittent catheterization to maintain low residual volumes and the administration of prophylactic antibacterial drugs (Charney et al. 1982; Eckstein and Molyneux 1982). Vesicoureteral reflux often develops in the second or third year of life and may necessitate reimplantation of ureters into the bladder.

Bowel function is impaired in half of these children. Welch and Wiston (1987) reported that 45% of children studied aged over 2.6 years had acceptable bowel control for age, but the remaining group had no apparent voluntary control. Chronic constipation was a problem for about half the children with myelomeningocele.

Deformities of the lower limbs do not occur if the limbs are totally denervated and flaccid or if the lower limbs are essentially normal (sacral lesions). The majority of patients will have partial paralysis depending on the level of spinal involvement with only certain groups of muscles being affected. Orthopaedic defects may be severe and necessitate early intervention. Hip subluxation is usually treated with splinting or plaster casting. Sensory deficits in the lower limbs may enhance the likelihood of pressure sores. Physiotherapy may help to preserve the full range of movement in the joints and prevent the onset of contractures.

Epilepsy occurs in over 20% of children with myelomeningocele (Bartholesky et al. 1985). Important antecedent factors include infections, malformations of the brain, perinatal problems and possibly the trauma of the shunt procedures. These features together with the presence of severe hydrocephalus at birth, uncontrolled hydrocephalus in infancy and CNS infections are additional important risk factors for the presence of mental retardation.

Late neurological features may relate to underlying tethering of the spinal cord, hydromyelia, uncontrolled hydrocephalus, the Arnold-Chiari malformation associated with brain stem or cervical cord abnormalities, and previously unrecognized malformations of the brain. Fractures of long bones of the lower extremities are not uncommon because of disuse osteoporosis. Obesity may be the result of, and a cause of, inactivity (Asher and Olsen 1983).

In addition to the medical complications seen in the child, myelomeningocele causes major psychological and social stresses on both the child and the family. The family must face the daily burden of care which often requires a great commitment of time and energy. Family members may never achieve equilibrium as they may be at different stages of the grieving process which is associated with having a child with a major defect thereby making communications, understanding and support between them difficult. The child may develop manipulative and demanding behaviour or may demonstrate regression and withdrawal in response to the stresses of frequent hospitalizations, painful or embarrassing procedures and a realization that he is different to his peers. Learning disabilities may lead to poor school performance, poor self-esteem, loss of interest in school and a downward spiral of failure (Liptak et al. 1988).

Problems of Teenage and Adult Spina Bifida Patients

While the clinical follow-up arrangements for spina bifida patients present no great difficulties in the paediatric age groups, the problems become enormous when these children outgrow their paediatric facilities. Adult facilities for these multi-handicapped patients are lacking and the involvement of various specialists is essential in the management of the differing aspects of their problems. Provision of training schemes is important as a significant number can ultimately be employed and become independent socially and financially. The question of sexual potency and ability to reproduce may cause considerable concern to the teenager with spina bifida (Dorner 1977). Medical and rehabilitative problems often persist into adult life (Hinderer et al. 1988).

Spina Bifida Occulta

The term "spina bifida occulta" is applied to cases in which fusion defects of the vertebral column occur without protrusion of intraspinal contents on to the surface of the body. The condition is common and occurs in at least 5% of the population, but it is usually asymptomatic. Several abnormalities may be found in association with spina bifida occulta. However, the Arnold-Chiari malformation and hydrocephalus are not associated with it. The accompanying conditions include: dermal sinus tract and dermoid cyst, short or tight filum terminale, diastematomyelia, anterior meningocele, a neuroenteric cyst and distortion of spinal cord or spinal nerve roots by fibrous bands and adhesions or subcutaneous lipoma (lipomeningocele). The mechanism of injury to the underlying spinal cord appears most likely to be due to ischaemia whether the spinal cord is anchored by lipoma, short or tight filum terminale, fibrous bands or by diastematomyelia (Yamada et al. 1981).

Symptoms of occult spinal dysraphism may be absent, minimal or severe, depending on the degree of neural involvement. The patient may present with static or a slowly progressive weakness or sensory loss in the legs or feet, foot deformities, or problems with their gait. Bowel and bladder disturbances such as incontinence, repeated urinary infections or enuresis may also be the presenting complaint. Less commonly, scoliosis, back stiffness or pain in the back of the leg may be a feature (Anderson 1975; Till 1975; Hendrick et al. 1983).

Common findings are shortened heel cords, high arches or equinovarus deformities of the feet, asymmetry in size or girth of feet and legs, diminished tendon reflexes, trophic ulcers on the feet and decreased rectal sphincter tone. Rarely, presentation is with bacterial meningitis in those children with an unrecognized dermal sinus extending to the dura.

The diagnosis and management of these disorders have been greatly facilitated by real time ultrasound examination and MRI techniques (Bale et al. 1986; Brumberg et al. 1988). CT myelography with the contrast medium injected into the cisterna magna may be helpful if MRI is not available. Surgery is indicated in symptomatic patients; prophylactic intervention is becoming more common due to technical advances and a desire to prevent the development of complications (McLone and Nadich 1986).

Dermoid Cyst and Dermal Sinus Tract

The tract consists of a stalk of firm connective tissue surrounding a lumen lined by dermis. A cutaneous opening or dimple in the midline at the back may exude a purulent discharge. The stalk may extend to the dura or, more commonly, pierce the dura and attach to the conus medullaris or, if higher, to the spinal cord itself. In a minority, a bulbous dermoid cyst, in continuity with the stalk may intrude between the roots of the cauda equina and into the spinal cord. Infection and recurrent meningitis are ever-complicating factors and can be prevented by the early recognition of the significance of cutaneous dimples and sinuses and excision of the tract and dermoid cyst (Fig. 7.2).

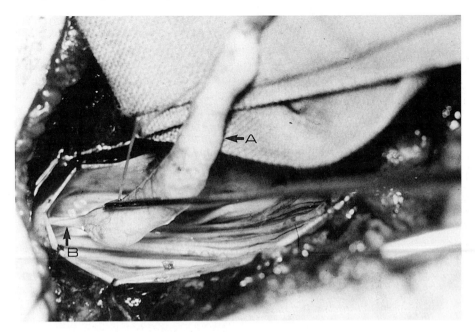

Fig. 7.2. The dermal sinus tract has been excised (A) and is attached to the cauda equina (B).

Short or Tight Filum Terminale or Adhesions

A tethered cord is the most frequent finding associated with spina bifida occulta. It may occur alone or may be associated with any of the other anomalies. The conus medullaris is abnormally low and is tethered by one or more forms of intradural abnormalities such as a short and thickened filum terminale, fibrous bands and adhesions, or a totally intradural lipoma. These features are a result of disturbances in the closure of the neural folds and occur early in embryonic development, approximately between 20 and 30 days of gestation (Marin-Padilla 1985).

Typical symptoms and signs may be absent in infancy but progressive motor or sensory deficit in the lower limbs, foot deformities and gait disturbance may present later. Disturbance of bowel or bladder control occurs in about 20% of patients. Release of the tethered cord in the asymptomatic patient usually prevents the onset of complications and may arrest or reverse neurological features once they have occurred (Hoffman 1985).

Diastematomyelia

A midline septum which may be bony, cartilaginous or fibrous, divides the spinal cord longitudinally into two, usually unequal portions. The septum is anchored to the ventral dura mater on the posterior aspect of the vertebral bodies and may be attached posteriorly to the vertebral arch or dura mater. There is usually an overlying cutaneous abnormality characterized by a patch of hypertrichosis (Fig. 7.3) often with a naevus in the underlying skin. Less frequently a meningocele, a spinal scoliosis or an irregular prominent spinous process may be present at the level of the lesion (Guthkelch 1974). Another common presentation is a unilaterally weak, deformed and hypoplastic lower leg and foot, and neurological signs consisting of an absent ankle jerk and extensor plantar response. Sensory impairment in the area of supply of the lower lumbar and/or sacral roots may be found (James and Lassman 1960).

Treatment consists of removal of the septum prophylactically. Any existing neurological deficit remains unchanged but if the child is managed expectantly, the majority develop evidence of progressive spinal cord dysfunction (Guthkelch 1974).

Lipomeningocele

A subcutaneous lipoma in the lumbosacral region is usually present. The fibro-fatty tissue extends deeply and is attached to the filum terminale and to the dorsum of a low conus medullaris or to the roots of the cauda equina (James and Lassman 1981). Hoffman (1985) stresses that the majority of these children are normal at birth but that the incidence of disability increases with age because the spinal cord is tethered by fat to the overlying skin as well as being tethered to the bottom of the dural sac. He suggests that early surgical treatment to untether the spinal cord and reconstitute the dural sac, will result in the majority of these children retaining normal neurological function.

Sacral Agenesis (Caudal Regression Syndrome)

Rarely, the coccyx and sacrum fail to develop as may the sacral and lumbosacral segments of the spinal cord. There are often accompanying genitourinary abnormalities (Welch and Alterman 1984). The extent of neurological features is similar to that of myelomeningocele, ranging from minimal deficit to equinovarus deformities of the feet or more extensive sensory and motor deficits of the lower limbs. Most patients have a neurogenic bladder and bowel impairment. Maternal diabetes mellitus is associated in 16% of cases (Passarge and Leuz 1966).

Spinal Cord Injury

Spinal cord injury during delivery results from excessive traction or rotation of the spine. Traction is the more important cause in breech deliveries and

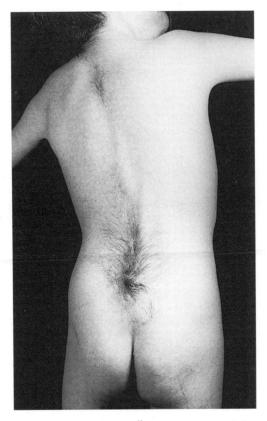

Fig. 7.3. Hairy patch overlying a diastematomyelia.

accounts for the majority of cases, whilst torsion in cephalic deliveries accounts for the minority of cases. In the newborn, the bony vertebral canal is almost entirely cartilaginous and very elastic whilst the dura is somewhat less elastic. The spinal cord is anchored above by the medulla and the roots of the brachial plexus and below by the cauda equina and filum terminale. Excessive longitudinal traction, as may occur in a vaginal breech delivery, results in rupture of the dura and spinal cord at the site which is most mobile i.e. the lower cervical and upper thoracic cord. With extreme rotational movements, as with forceps rotation in difficult cephalic deliveries, the site of particular cord mobility and most frequent rupture is in the upper cervical cord (Towbin 1969; Volpe 1987).

The clinical syndromes of spinal cord injury in the newborn are principally threefold (Koch and Eng 1979; Volpe 1987):

1. Stillbirth or rapid neonatal death secondary to respiratory failure: these children generally have an upper cervical section syndrome usually related to cephalic delivery with hyperextension of the neck. Neurological features are characterized by a flaccid tetraplegia with areflexia, lack of spontaneous respiration and pin-prick sensory level up to the neck. Facial and extraocular movements are spared.

2. Long-term survivors who present with a flaccid paraparesis in the neo-natal period but who proceed to develop a spastic paraparesis in the ensuing months: varying degrees of upper limb involvement, a sensory level in the upper trunk, diaphragmatic breathing and a Horner's syndrome may also be present. The lesion is at the cervicothoracic cord level and is generally associated with breech deliveries.

3. Children with subtle neurological signs of spasticity who are often con-fused with cerebral palsy: they have partial cord injuries and occasional vas-cular accidents to the brain.

Clinical evaluation of spinal cord birth injury is difficult in the early phases. Associated cerebral hypoxic-ischaemic lesions and brachial plexus injury can often combine to make differentiation impossible. Clinical suspicion is often triggered by a history of a difficult breech or forceps extraction. The diagnosis initially is often confused with spinal muscular atrophy, respiratory distress syndrome or cerebral palsy. Radiological investigations play an important role in making the diagnosis. Plain X-ray films of the cervical spine are usually normal. Ultrasound examination of the spinal canal and CT myelography are important procedures in identifying the presence and extent of damage to the spinal cord and nerve roots (Babyn et al. 1988).

Rarely, spinal cord injury in the neonatal period occurs in association with vascular occlusion, observed with umbilical artery catheterization or acci-dental injection of air in a peripheral vein (Aziz and Robertson 1973; Brown and Phibbs 1988; Willis et al. 1981). Congenital spinal cord haemangioblastoma has been described as a cause of spinal cord section syndrome in the newborn.

Hypoxic-Ischaemic Spinal Cord Injury Following Perinatal Asphyxia

Following acute perinatal asphyxia prominent clinical signs of neurological disturbance are dominated by the cerebral signs of depressed mental status and seizures. The accompanying features of diminished movements, reduced tone and depressed tendon reflexes are usually presumed also to reflect cerebral dysfunction. The potential contribution of a spinal cord disturbance in the causation of these abnormal neuromuscular signs following asphyxia has received little attention. Sladky and Rorke (1986) have reported the neuropath-ological features of hypoxic-ischaemic spinal cord injury in asphyxiated babies. Ischaemic necrosis of the ventral grey matter of the spinal cord was observed and the authors postulated that this represented the watershed hypoperfusion territory between the radial branches of the single anterior spinal artery and the paired dorsal spinal arteries.

Clancy et al. (1989) reported in acutely asphyxiated infants that there was good qualitative correlation between clinical cerebral signs and the extent of cerebral lesions. Infants described as lethargic and without seizures, displayed less severe cerebral lesions than those with frank coma and seizures at post mortem. Also, the most inactive, flaccid and areflexic babies had obvious spinal cord grey matter necrosis. Survivors showed changes of acute denerva-tion on electromyographic examinations indicating recent ischaemic injury of the anterior horn cells.

Table 7.1. CSF findings in childhood

Cell Count

RBC: First 14 days of life	up to $675 \times 10^6/l$
Later	$0-2 \times 10^6/l$
Leucocytes: Newborns/preterm	up to $20 \times 10^6/l$
First year of life	up to $10 \times 10^6/l$
After 1 year	up to $5 \times 10^6/l$

Protein (Lumbar fluid)

Preterm	up to $3.0\,g/l$
Term baby	$1.5-2.0\,g/l$
At 1 month	$0.7\,g/l$
6 months and later	up to $0.4\,g/l$

Glucose

CSF glucose should be 50% or more of blood glucose
Low CSF glucose ($<1.0\,mmol/l$) in infant strongly suggests
meningitis but may also occur if the baby is hypoglycaemic

Pressure

Newborns	$50-80\,mm$ water
Infants	$40-150\,mm$ water
Children	$70-200\,mm$ water

Volume

Infants	$40-60\,ml$
Young children	$60-100\,ml$
Older children	$80-120\,ml$
Adults	$100-160\,ml$

CSF Findings in Childhood

The normal ranges are given in Table 7.1. When bloody CSF is obtained then the ratio of red cells to white cells should be calculated and this is compared with the ratio in the peripheral blood at that time: in uninfected CSF this is usually 500:1 or more. In clinical practice, any polymorphonuclear leucocyte count higher than $20/mm^3$ in newborns or preterm infants should be regarded as suspicious of meningitis. The CSF protein levels are raised in meningitis and markedly raised levels have often been associated with a poor prognosis and a high incidence of post-meningitic hydrocephalus. CSF glucose estimations must be done with simultaneous measurement of blood glucose, as CSF glucose should be 50% or more of blood glucose levels.

References

Anderson FM (1975) Occult spinal dysraphism: a series of 73 cases. Pediatrics 55:826–835

Anderson H, Carlson C-A (1966) The surgical management of myelomeningocele with a preliminary report of 31 cases. Acta Paediatr Scand 55:626–635

Asher M, Olsen J (1983) Factors affecting the ambulatory status of patients with spina bifida cystica. J Bone Joint Surg 65A:350–356

Aziz EM, Robertson AF (1973) Paraplegia: a complication of umbilical artery catheterisation. J Pediatr 82:1051–1052

Babyn PS, Chaung SH, Daneman A, Davidson GS (1988) Sonographic evaluation of spinal cord birth trauma with pathologic correlation. AJNR 9:765–768

Bale JF, Bell WE, Dunn V, Afiffi AK, Menezes A (1986) Magnetic resonance imaging of the spine in children. Arch Neurol 43:1253–1256

Barson AJ (1970) The vertebral level of termination of the spinal cord during normal and abnormal development. J Anat 106:489–497

Bartholesky LE, Haller J, Scott RM, Wojick C (1985) Seizures in children with meningomyelocele. Am J Dis Child 139:400–402

Brown MS, Phibbs RH (1988) Spinal cord injury in newborns from use of umbilical artery catheters. J Perinatol 8:105–110

Brumberg JA, Latchaur RE, Kanal E, Burke DL, Albright I (1988) Magnetic resonance imaging of spinal dysraphism. Radiol Clin North Am 26:181–205

Charney EB, Kalichman MA, Snyder H (1982) Multiple benefits of clean intermittent catheterisation for children with myelomeningocele. Z Kinderchir 37:145–147

Clancy RR, Sladky JT, Rorke LB (1989) Hypoxic-ischaemic spinal cord injury following perinatal asphyxia. Ann Neurol 25:185–189

Coffey VP (1983) Neural tube defects in Dublin: 1953–54, 1961–82. Ir Med J 76:411–413

Dorner S (1977) Problems of teenagers. Physiotherapy 63:190–192

Eckstein HB, Chir M (1972) Myelomeningocele. Postgrad Med J 48:496–500

Eckstein HB, Molyneux A (1982) Intermittent catheterisation of the bladder for neuropathic incontinence. Z Kinderchir 37:143–144

Ghosh A, Woo JSK, Poon IM, Ho-Kei M (1981) Neural tube defects in Hong Kong Chinese. Lancet 2:468–469

Guthkelch AN (1974) Diastematomyelia with median septum. Brain 97:729–742

Hays RM, Jordan RA, McLaughlin JF, Nickel RE, Fisher LD (1989) Central ventilatory dysfunction in myelodysplasia: an independent determinant of survival. Dev Med Child Neurol 31:366–370

Hendrick EB, Hoffman HJ, Humphreys RP (1983) The tethered spinal cord. Clin Neurosurg 30:457–463

Hinderer S, Hinderer K, Dunne K, Shurtleff D (1988) Medical and functional status of adults with spina bifida. Dev Med Child Neurol (suppl 57) 30:28

Hoffman HJ (1985) The tethered spinal cord. In: Holzman RWN, Stein BM (eds) The tethered spinal cord. Thieme Shalton Inc, New York, pp 91–98

Holmes LB, Driscoll SG, Atkins L (1976) Etiological heterogeneity of neural tube defects. N Engl J Med 294:365–369

Ingraham FD, Swan H, Hamlin H (1944) Spina bifida and cranium bifidum. Harvard University Press, Cambridge

James CCM, Lassman LP (1960) Spinal dysraphism: an orthopaedic syndrome in children accompanying occult forms. Arch Dis Child 35:315–327

James CCM, Lassman LP (1981) Spina bifida occulta: orthopaedic, radiological and neurosurgical aspects. Academic Press, London

Koch B, Eng G (1979) Neonatal spinal cord injury. Arch Phys Med Rehabil 60:378–381

Liptak GS, Bloss JW, Briskin H, Campbell JE, Herbert EB, Revell GM (1988) The management of children with spinal dysraphism. J Child Neurol 3:3–20

Lorber J (1961) Systematic ventriculographic studies in infants born with meningomyelocele and encephalocele: the incidence and development of hydrocephalus. Arch Dis Child 36:381–389

Lorber J (1971) Results of treatment of myelomeningocele: an analysis of 524 unselected cases with special reference to possible selection for treatment. Dev Med Child Neurol 13:279–303

Marin-Padilla M (1985) The tethered cord syndrome. In: Holtzman RWN, Stein BM (eds) The tethered spinal cord. Thieme Shalton Inc, New York, pp 3–13

McLone DG, Nadich TP (1986) Laser resection of fifty spinal lipomas. Neurosurgery 18:611–615

Park TS, Hoffman HJ, Hendrick EB, Humphries RP (1983) Experience of surgical decompression of the Arnold-Chiari malformation in young infants with myelomeningocele. Neurosurgery 13:147–152

Passarge E, Leutz W (1966) Syndrome of caudal regression in infants of diabetic mothers. Pediatrics 37:672–675

Peach B (1965a) Arnold-Chiari malformation: morphogenesis. Arch Neurol 12:527–535

Peach B (1965b) Arnold-Chiari malformation. Anatomic features of 20 cases. Arch Neurol 12:613–621

Report of UK collaborative study on alpha-fetoprotein in relation to neural-tube defects (1977) Maternal serum alpha-fetoprotein measurement in antenatal screening for anencephalopathy and spina bifida in early pregnancy. Lancet 1:1323–1332

Rink RC, Mitchell ME (1984) Surgical correction of urinary incontinence. J Pediatr Surg 19:637–641

Shepard TH (1982) Detection of human teratogenic agents. J Pediatr 101:810–815

Sladky JT, Rorke LB (1986) Perinatal hypoxic/ischemic spinal cord injury. Pediatr Path 6:87–101

Smith GK, Smith ED (1973) Selection for treatment in spina bifida cystica. Br Med J 4:189–197

Smithells RW, Shepard S, Schorah CJ, et al. (1981) Apparent prevention of neural tube defects by periconceptual vitamin supplementation. Arch Dis Child 56:911–918

Stark GD, Baker GCW (1967) The neurological involvement of the lower limbs in myelomeningocele Dev Med Child Neurol 9:732–744

Stark GD, Drummond M (1973) Results of selective early operation in myelomeningocele. Arch Dis Child 48:676–683

Stein SC, Schut L (1979) Hydrocephalus in myelomeningocele. Child's Brain 4:413–419

Till K (1975) Paediatric neurosurgery for paediatricians and neurosurgeons. Blackwell Scientific, Oxford

Towbin A (1969) Latent spinal cord and brain stem injury in newborn infants. Dev Med Child Neurol 11:54–68

Verma IC (1978) High frequency of neural tube defects in North India. Lancet 1:879–880

Volpe JJ (1987) Neurology of the newborn, 2nd edn. Saunders, Philadelphia

Welch JP, Alterman K (1984) The syndrome of caudal dysplasia: a review including etiologic considerations and evidence of heterogeneity. Pediatr Path 2:313–327

Welch K, Wiston KR (1987) Spina bifida. In: Vinken PJ, Bruyn GW, Klawans HL (eds) Handbook of clinical neurology, vol 50, revised series 6. Elsevier, Amsterdam, pp 477–508

Willis J, Duncan C, Gottschalk S (1981) Paraplegia due to peripheral venous air embolism in a neonate: a case report. Pediatrics 67:472–473

Yamada S, Zinke DE, Sanders D (1981) Pathophysiology of "tethered cord syndrome". J Neurosurg 54:494–503

Zachary RB (1973) Severely malformed children. Br Med J 2:482 (letter)

Chapter 8

Imaging of the Spine and Spinal Cord

J.S. Lapointe

Introduction

Between 1896, when Roentgen discovered X-rays, and 1975, when spinal computed tomography (CT) became available thanks to improvements to Hounsfield's 1971 invention, the spinal cord had to be studied by indirect means. Plain film radiography, and linear and complex motion tomography were used to image the bony spine. The outline of the spinal cord was first seen with pneumomyelography, after Dandy outlined the medulla with air in 1919 but a safe opaque contrast medium for myelography was only introduced in 1940. This iophendylate (Pantopaque) was replaced by non-ionic water-soluble metrizamide (Amipaque) in 1973. Spinal angiography, since its introduction by Djindjian in 1963, has had a limited role in the investigation of vascular lesions of the spinal cord.

After 1975, perfected CT body scanners made axial images of the spinal cord possible. With the aid of intrathecal contrast, better visualization of the contour of the cord and its position within the spinal canal was achieved. Following improved resolution of the CT scans in the 1980s, cysts, haemorrhages, and tumours within the substance of the cord could be detected without intrathecal contrast and without or with intravenous contrast enhancement (Ruggiero et al. 1981). At the same time, rapid progress in the image quality of magnetic resonance studies was being made and the first clinical units became available at the beginning of the 1980s. This new and expensive technology, whose first images were produced by Lauterbur in 1973, will be the imaging modality of choice in the 1990s for diseases affecting the spinal cord, as it is the first method which consistently outlines the substance of the cord in any plane and the effect of the surrounding tissues on it. Recent advances have increased the resolution in MRI of the cord to the point that grey and white matter differentiation is possible.

Imaging Tools

In this period of concern over health care costs, it is important for the physician ordering examinations to understand what information each type of examination is likely to yield, and to tailor these requests to the patient's neurological status. The availability of the technology should not be the only determining factor in the choice of examination. The degree of radiological expertise available and the familiarity with the conditions being studied are also very important. If the patient is to be transferred to a more specialized centre for management, it is often advisable to have that centre's neuro-radiologists perform the examinations, to reduce unnecessary duplication and to increase diagnostic yield. While the following is not all-inclusive, its aim is to elucidate what place these examinations have in the overall investigation.

Plain Films

Plain film radiography (Banna 1985) is available in all radiology depart-ments and is the first radiographic examination performed when trauma to the spine has been sustained. Obtained supine, often on a trauma board, with the neck in a brace or collar, the examination consists mainly of AP and cross-table lateral films. In an uncooperative patient, it may be difficult to obtain a good open-mouth view to see the base of the odontoid. When the patient has a short neck or wide shoulders, a swimmer's view will delineate the cervicothoracic junction. Oblique views of the cervical spine may not be routinely obtained in trauma. Satisfactory information may be gained by angling the X-ray tube without moving the patient, resulting in a somewhat distorted view of the oblique cervical spine. Another method is to obtain oblique views of the cervical spine by doing oblique scout views (digital radio-graph) by CT. These add only a few seconds to a CT examination of the head. Alignment of pedicles and shingling or imbrication of the laminae can be easily ascertained by either method, attesting to the normal alignment of the vertebral bodies and obviating the need for spinal precautions in the multi-traumatized patient (Fig. 8.1A and B).

The size of the intervertebral foramina and the integrity of the pedicles and laminae are assessed on routine oblique views of the cervical spine, while oblique views of the lumbar spine help to assess the pars interarticularis and the apophyseal joints. Flexion and extension views are performed if abnormal mobility of the spine, usually at the cervical level but occasionally at the lumbar level, is suspected. Ligamentous injury of the cervical spine can easily be missed on the initial supine study. These flexion and extension views should always be performed with the patient's cooperation and in a sitting or standing position, when the patient's condition permits. Supine flexion and extension films done passively may give the physician a false sense of security and not demonstrate the presence of ligamentous injury. Spinal precautions should be maintained as long as instability is still suspected.

Tomography

Tomography is of two types, linear and complex motion, and is equipment dependent. The second type better delineates bony detail and is used to study complex congenital anomalies of the spine such as segmentation anomalies and scoliosis. It is also used to study fractures of the spine, where CT scanning is

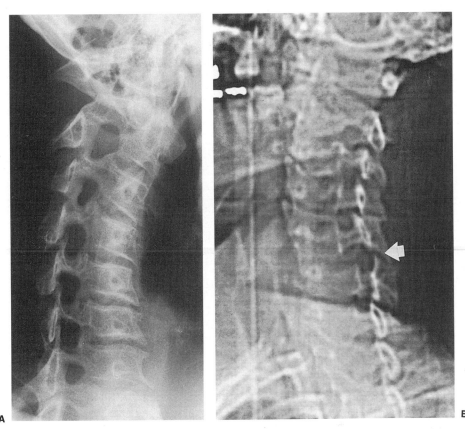

A   B

Fig. 8.1. A Oblique view of the cervical spine showing normal imbrication (shingling) of the cervical laminae. **B** Oblique digital radiography (scout view) showing a facet look at C5–6: loss of shingling of the laminae, disrupted alignment of the round pedicles and of the posterior margin of the vertebral bodies.

not available. As many cases of trauma occur in young people, CT scanning is preferred because the dose of radiation is much less with CT scanning than with tomography, and the examination can be performed more quickly and with better resolution, and with less manipulation of the injured spine (Donovan-Post 1984).

Myelography

This consists of injection of a iodinated contrast medium into the subarachnoid space and gravitation of this contrast to various segments of the spinal canal under fluoroscopic control. Myelography helps to determine the presence of blocks due to intradural, extradural, and intramedullary lesions, as well as to outline the position, size and shape of the spinal cord and nerve roots. While it was the investigation of choice for 40 years to determine the presence of disc herniation and tumour, it has largely been replaced by CT scanning and MR

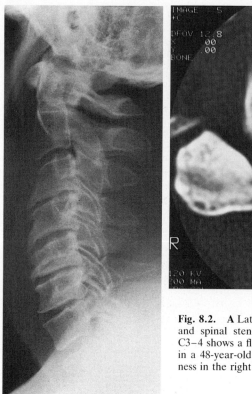
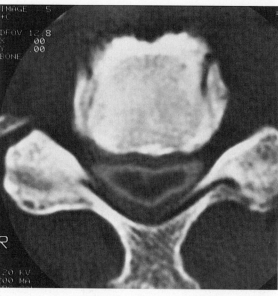

B

Fig. 8.2. **A** Lateral cervical spine shows severe spondylosis and spinal stenosis. **B** Postmyelogram axial CT scan at C3–4 shows a flattened spinal cord consistent with atrophy in a 48-year-old man complaining of neck pain and weakness in the right arm.

A

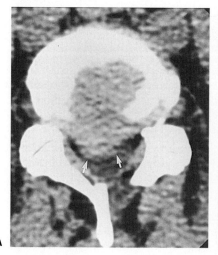
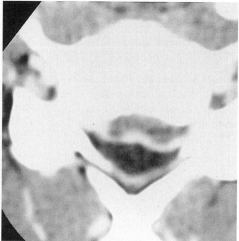

A   **B**

Fig. 8.3. **A** Axial CT scan showing a large central lumbar disc herniation at L5–S1 in a 40-year-old woman with back pain. **B** Axial CT scan with intravenous contrast enhancement showing a large central and left sided C4–5 disc herniation in a 36-year-old man with left arm weakness.

imaging. It is still used in many centres that do not have ready access to these two latter technologies, and the introduction of improved non-ionic, water-soluble contrast media such as iohexol (Omnipaque) and iopamidol (Isovue) has greatly decreased the amount of side-effects of this procedure. The incidence of post lumbar puncture headache in many centres has been further decreased by the use of 25 and 26 gauge spinal needles (Vézina et al. 1989). Myelography is currently used in conjunction with computed tomography when CT scanning or MRI (either non-enhanced or intravenously enhanced) have not resolved the clinical dilemma. It is particularly useful in delineating subtle mass effect on root sleeves due to disc herniation, as well as subtle epidural spread of tumour, and also for demonstrating cord atrophy due to spondylosis presenting as cervical myelopathy (Shapiro 1984) (Fig. 8.2A and B).

CT Scanning

This has been widely used since the early 1980s to study disc herniations and spinal stenosis. CT scanning of the virgin lumbar spine requires no intravenous contrast as the presence of fat in and around the spinal canal helps define disc margins, root sleeves, thecal sac, and epidural veins and outlines the relationship of these soft tissue structures to the bony canal, intervertebral foramina, and apophyseal joints. Intravenous contrast is used to outline the epidural venous plexus and in some instances to help differentiate between recurrent disc herniation and post surgical scarring (Figs. 8.3A and B, 8.4A and B). In the cervical spine, the convex configuration of the end plate makes visualization of the margin of the disc more difficult; intravenous contrast, by highlighting the vertebral venous plexus, which is closely apposed to the posterior margin of the vertebral body and disc, is used routinely to detect subtle indentation on the dural sac and nerve roots. Neoplasms such as neurofibromas, meningiomas, and intramedullary tumours may also be enhanced with intravenous contrast, improving their delineation (Fig. 8.5) (Newton and Potts 1983).

MR Imaging

This is the newest addition to imaging techniques. The lack of radiation is viewed as an advantage over CT scanning by both physicians and patients. Contraindications to its use are many and include the presence of ferromagnetic metals such as certain cerebral aneurysm clips and metallic orbital foreign bodies, which may be displaced by the pull of the magnet, and the presence of pacemakers which may malfunction. The current configuration of the scanner and its relatively small aperture makes scanning large patients, claustrophobic patients, and certain severely ill patients difficult or impossible. Patient co-operation is important as motion degrades the quality of the images. Sagittal and coronal imaging of the spinal canal is easily obtained, contrary to CT. While the cord can be seen on one image from the foramen magnum to the conus, surface coils over areas of interest have improved resolution and focus attention on specific areas of the cord. Paramagnetic contrast agents such as gadolinium DTPA enhance lesions in a similar fashion as CT intravenous

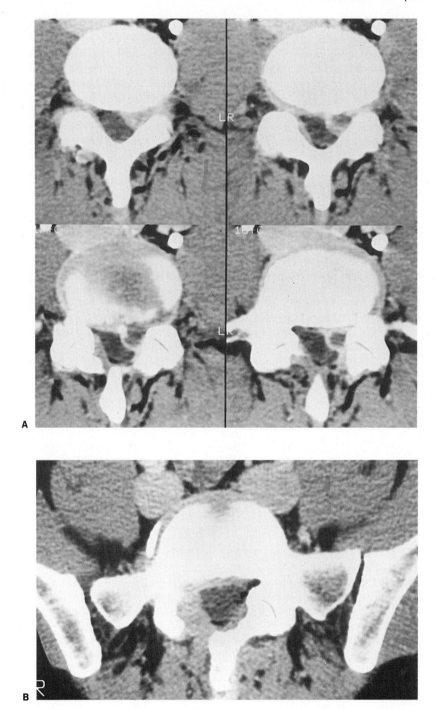

Fig. 8.4. A Axial CT scan with intravenous contrast enhancement showing a recurrent left sided L4–5 disc herniation in a 45-year-old man with left L5 root symptoms. **B** Axial CT scan with intravenous contrast showing enhancing scar along the right side of the dural sac, at the site of previous L5–S1 laminectomy in a 46-year-old man complaining of recurrent right leg pain.

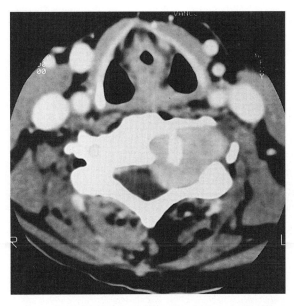

Fig. 8.5. Axial CT scan of the cervical spine, with intravenous contrast, showing an enhancing dumb-bell schwannoma of the left C2–3 foramen in a 69-year-old woman with left shoulder pain and weakness for six months and a prior history of breast carcinoma.

contrast, increasing lesion conspicuity. MRI is rapidly replacing myelography, especially when an intramedullary lesion is suspected. Cysts, syrinxes, and intramedullary masses and cerebellar tonsillar herniation are readily demonstrated (Figs. 8.6, 8.7) and physiological processes such as myelination and CSF flow can be studied (Norman 1987).

Spinal Angiography

This examination is used when myelography, CT scan, or MRI have suggested the presence of an arteriovenous malformation, a dural fistula or a vascular tumour. It is time-consuming and tedious and results in a large amount of radiation to the patient. To outline the vascular supply of the spinal cord, selective injections in all the intercostal and lumbar arteries are necessary, with additional injections of vertebral arteries, thyrocervical trunks, costocervical trunks, and internal iliac arteries sometimes necessary. This often means 25 to 50 separate vessels must be studied at one or more sittings. Digital subtraction angiography, when available, speeds the examination as well as decreases the radiation dose and the volume of iodinated contrast material. Embolization, surgery, or a combination of both can then be planned. This type of examination should be limited to specialized centres (Thron 1988) (Fig. 8.8A and B).

Nuclear Medicine Bone Scans

These are useful to pinpoint early metastatic disease not evident on plain film, and may help localize benign bone lesions such as osteoid osteoma which is a

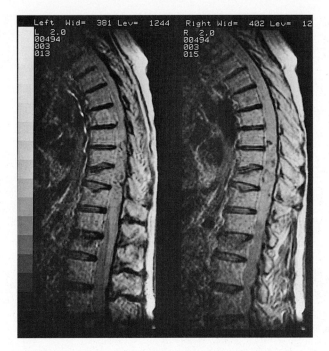

Fig. 8.6. Sagittal MRI of the thoracic cord showing mixed density changes of an astrocytoma in a 73-year-old woman with multiple compression fractures.

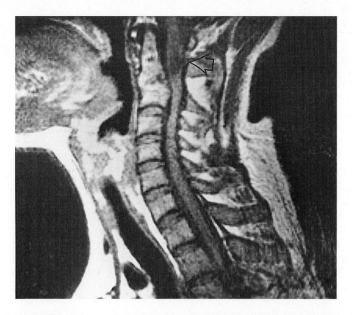

Fig. 8.7. Sagittal MRI of the cervical spine showing a high cervical cord syrinx in a 31-year-old man who suffered an injury to C2 and C3 ten years ago with persistent mild quadriparesis and recent increasing left limb weakness.

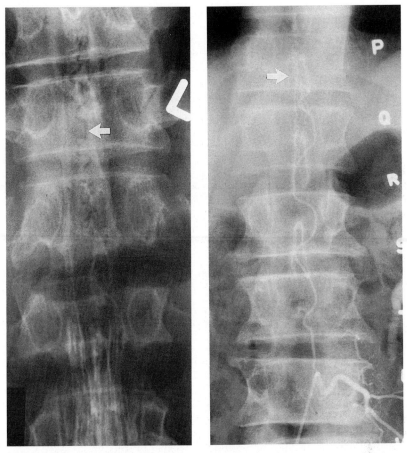

Fig. 8.8. **A** Myelogram and **B** spinal angiogram showing the abnormal vessels of a dural fistula of the conus medullaris in a 52-year-old man complaining of progressive lower limb weakness with sphincter difficulties.

common source of bone pain in young people and which occasionally presents in the spine. Gallium scans and tagged leucocyte scans may pinpoint vertebral infection in the absence of plain film bony changes. Further studies by CT or MRI may then be warranted.

Ultrasound

This can be used as readily in the neonatal spine as it is in the neonatal brain. It is particularly useful in patients with dysraphic states of the lower lumbar spine suspected because of a skin covered lumbosacral mass and can be performed without radiation or sedation. Lipomyelomeningocele, teratoma, and status post repair of myelomeningocele can be evaluated. Absence of cord motion on real-time scanning indicates cord tethering and the need for further evaluation. In the adult, ultrasound of the spine is an intraoperative tool used to localize intramedullary cysts for shunting, intramedullary masses for removal, and to minimize the myelotomy and thus reduce postoperative sensory changes, to assess the spinal canal for adequate decompression of spinal stenosis, and to rule out the presence of subarachnoid cysts (Pasto et al. 1984). It is also used to determine the adequacy of decompression of spinal fractures and normal realignment of structures and to localize foreign bodies such as bone fragments or bullet fragments intraoperatively (Naidich and Quencer 1987).

Current Concepts

A review of the entire spectrum of conditions studied with these available tools is outside the scope of this monograph. The enclosed references will yield more specific detail to the interested reader. A summary of current practices and new knowledge of common conditions follows. It is hoped that the reader will be able to extrapolate from these examples useful and practical information concerning the investigations of conditions affecting the spine and spinal cord.

Anatomy – Normal vs. Abnormal

Evaluation of the alignment of the vertebral bodies, the pedicles, the spinous processes, the apophyseal joints and the laminae, symmetry of the soft tissues including the discs and ligaments and the integrity of the bone and its density can and should be determined.

The appearance of the various bony structures evolves during growth, but following closure of the epiphyses, a fairly uniform configuration is attained. Familiarity with the spine in childhood helps to recognize developmental abnormalities, such as limbus vertebra, hypoplastic disc, transitional vertebra, tropism of the apophyseal joints, and prevents erroneous diagnoses.

Plain films depict the bones well, but CT scan with its greater sensitivity to calcium illustrates subtle bony alterations to better advantage. Cross-sectional imaging may make it easier to understand the compressive or obstructive effects of certain types of lesions on the dural sac and the exiting nerve roots, for example, nerve roots exiting through a narrowed intervertebral foramen or the extraspinal extension of tumour or infection.

MRI, because of its ability to image more subtle changes in tissue density than CT, has improved our understanding of the changes affecting the ageing spine in health and disease. Alterations in vertebral bone marrow and in the intervertebral disc are now better understood and can be distinguished from disease. Distinction of grey and white matter columns in the cord has been achieved (Czervionke et al. 1988; Carvlin et al. 1989; Curtin et al. 1989).

Until the advent of MRI, the spinal cord, intrathecal nerves, and the cerebellar tonsils could only be accurately depicted with intrathecal contrast during myelography or CT. Concurrently, improved real-time ultrasound scanning led to visualization of the lumbar spine and its contents in the neonate, but abnormalities were usually confirmed by invasive studies prior to surgery.

The cerebellar tonsils and the conus medullaris are now easily visible on MRI and their normal position has been determined in vivo. Tonsillar ectopia (Chiari I) takes many forms and is deemed to be present when the tip of the rounded or pointed tonsils are found 5 mm below the level of the foramen magnum, measured by a line drawn from the caudal cortex of the basion to the opisthion (Barkovich et al. 1986). Similarly, the position of the normal conus is at the adult level in the first few months of life. The normal range of the tip of the conus extends from T12 to L3 (Wilson and Prince 1989).

Tethering of the conus is no longer a condition found mainly in childhood and adolescence, but is being increasingly recognized in middle-aged adults. In children with lumbosacral dimples or hair patches, without or with a subcutaneous lipoma, cord tethering can be easily diagnosed on CT scan and MRI or by ultrasound in neonates. Adults often have no cutaneous abnormality and present with an abnormal gait or difficulty in urination, which in males can mimic prostatic hypertrophy. Myelography, intrathecally enhanced CT or MRI will show the thickened filum terminale, usually associated with a lipoma (72%) and a conus below L2 (84%). An associated cavitary lesion or myelomalacia was recognized in 9 of 20 patients on MRI in one series (Merx et al. 1989; Raghavan et al. 1989).

A better understanding of complex anomalies of the spine including segmentation anomalies, tethering, diastematomyelia and syringomyelia associated with meningomyelocele usually require combined investigations to elucidate all facets of the process so that adequate treatment may be instituted.

Trauma

Plain films are the mainstay of the investigation of spinal trauma as they are readily obtained and measures to stabilize the spine may be instituted rapidly. Spinal trauma is often associated with multiple head, chest, or abdomen injuries which require more immediate attention. It is rarely necessary to obtain detailed information on the spine once the level of injury has been recognized, on an emergency basis, as experience has shown that immediate decompression of spinal fractures does not alter the prognosis for recovery, the maximum deficit having been caused at the time of injury. It is necessary to determine the extent of the injury before the patient is mobilized, especially in those patients who have suffered fractures with little or no neurological deficit to prevent the occurrence of secondary injury. In many instances, the plain film findings underestimate the extent of the bony injuries. CT scanning in particular and, where not available, tomography should be used (Figs. 8.9A and B, 8.10A and B).

Spinal Stability vs. Instability

One of the main questions regarding a spinal fracture is determining its stability (Dunsker et al. 1986) i.e., will motion with resulting change in position of the various elements of the spine further compromise the spinal cord? Fractures affecting both the vertebral body and neural arch are always unstable. When in doubt, a useful system is to divide the spine into three columns, the first centred on the interlaminar line, the second on the posterior margin of the vertebral body, and the third on its anterior margin. The integrity of the bones and ligaments is considered along each of these lines. If the injury has disrupted ligaments and/or bones of two of the three columns, the spine is considered acutely unstable and appropriate management precautions should be taken (Denis 1983). A more chronic instability may occur if only one column, usually the posterior one, is damaged.

Intraspinal Haemorrhage

Haemorrhage has to be sizable before it can be detected on non-contrast spinal CT in an epidural, subdural, subarachnoid or intramedullary location. MRI has rarely been used in acute spinal trauma because of the difficulties in obtaining an adequate examination. Once the patient is stabilized, however, it may prove quite useful for prognosis and management. Any deterioration of spinal function following spinal trauma warrants thorough investigation. Early diagnosis and treatment may reverse the deterioration and maintain function. Early MRI results suggest that recovery is insignificant with intramedullary haematoma and good with contusion or oedema (Naseem et al. 1986; Kadoya et al. 1987; Kulkarni et al. 1987).

Post-traumatic Syrinx (Fig. 8.7)

A progressive neurological deficit whether subacute or chronic warrants detailed investigation. The most common lesion is the development of post-traumatic syringomyelia which can progress in a cranial or caudal direction (Aubin et al. 1987). Cranial extension of the syrinx results in an ascending neurological deficit. MRI is particularly useful in delineating the extent of these cysts, believed by some authors to represent dilatation of the central canal secondary to obstruction or compression of the cord and subarachnoid space. The absence of haemosiderin as a marker of previous haemorrhage does not support the theory of a syrinx starting from a cord haematoma (Norman 1987).

Water-soluble intrathecal contrast medium, followed by a 6 to 24 hour or 48 hour delayed CT scan of the spine, was used in the past to delineate these syrinxes. While it was useful prior to the advent of MRI, it is no longer the study of choice because the timing of contrast accumulation within the cord varies from patient to patient, making diagnosis more difficult, and the extent of the cyst is not accurately shown.

CSF flow dynamics is currently an area of intense MRI study. Shunting of the syrinx into the subarachnoid space or into the peritoneum is used to arrest progression of the deficit. Syrinxes exhibiting flow are thought more likely to be undergoing active expansion (water-hammer effect) and the patient should benefit from shunting, while cysts with non-pulsatile fluid are believed to be at little risk of expansion (Sherman et al. 1986; Castillo et al. 1987). The most caudal position possible for the shunt is preferred to assist in decompression and to minimize new deficits.

Fractures (Figs. 8.9A and B, 8.10A and B)

The types of spinal fractures are too numerous to detail here and the reader is referred to the works of Rogers (1982) or Banna (1985) for easy reading. The following points warrant special attention:

1. Patients can survive craniovertebral dislocation; alignment of the tip of the clivus with the tip of the odontoid should always be ascertained on the lateral view of the skull or cervical spine to avoid missing this injury (Woodring et al. 1981; Lee et al. 1987).

2. Fractures of the base of the odontoid can be missed if undisplaced. Its cortical outline should be easily followed on the lateral and open-mouth view. In an uncooperative patient with an inadequate open-mouth view, a Caldwell view of the skull often shows the C2 vertebra well.

3. To view the cervicothoracic junction, a frequent site of fracture dislocation, it may be necessary to obtain the oblique views discussed previously before resorting to tomography (Fig. 8.1).

4. Burst fractures frequently result in serious neurological injury. They can mimic a simple compression fracture on the lateral view if the integrity of the

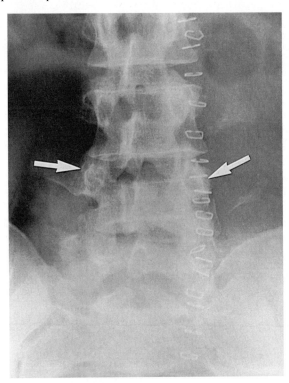

A

Fig. 8.9. **A** Plain film of the lumbar spine obtained portably after an emergency laparotomy on a 20-year-old man who sustained multiple injuries in a motor vehicle accident. The left L3 and L4 transverse processes are avulsed, the pedicles of L4 are splayed, and the body of L4 is decreased in height. **B** The axial CT scan shows a burst fracture of L4 with marked narrowing of the spinal canal by retropulsed bone fragments.

Fig. 8.9. (continued)

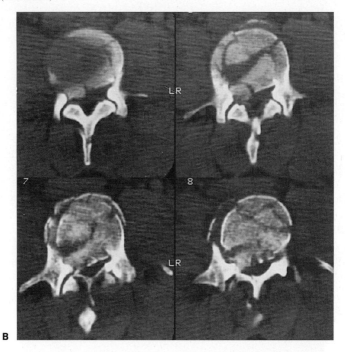

posterior margin of the vertebral body is not properly assessed and if the intraspinal position of the fragment of bone originating from the posterior superior aspect of the vertebral body is not recognized. CT scan frequently shows more extensive fractures than originally demonstrated on plain films (Atlas et al. 1986; Kim et al. 1988).

5. Injuries in a purely axial plane, such as the so-called seat belt fracture and ligamentous disruption without or with subluxation, are difficult or impossible to see on axial images alone. Reformatted sagittal or coronal images will give adequate information provided the patient has not moved between slices which have been obtained at small intervals, usually 3 or 5mm. This technique is useful when a short segment of spine is being studied. Not only the level of injury but also usually at least one-half of the vertebral body above and below the fracture should be imaged.

6. It is not uncommon for the patient to suffer injury at more than one vertebral level, sometimes quite distant from the first. Only a high index of suspicion will lead to its early recognition and investigation (Gehweiler et al. 1980).

Degenerative Disc Disease and Spinal Stenosis (Fig. 8.11)

Back and neck pain are very common complaints. Pain radiating to an extremity, especially when localized in a neuroanatomical distribution, helps to pinpoint the source of the symptom. A neurological deficit need not be present.

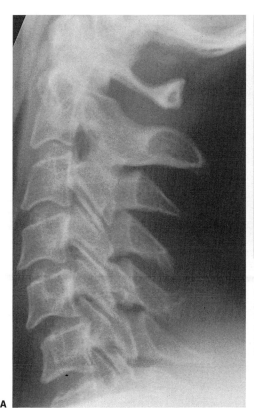

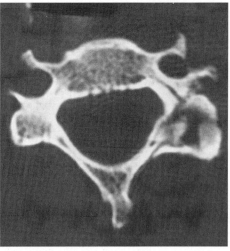

B

A

Fig. 8.10. **A** The lateral cervical spine shows subluxation of C5 on C6 without distortion of the interlaminar line. **B** The axial CT scan shows a unilateral fracture involving the left C5 pedicle, lamina and articular pillar in a 40-year-old woman who sustained a fall.

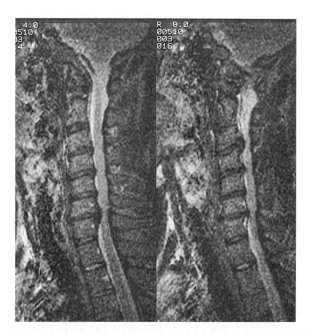

Fig. 8.11. Sagittal MRI of the cervical spine showing spondylosis maximum at C6–7, with cord compression in a 40-year-old man with hyper-reflexia.

In the past, investigation by myelography was reserved for presumed surgical candidates. When the myelogram was normal the patient was sometimes sent to a psychiatrist for treatment of functional pain. Even after apparently successful surgery, a large number of patients suffered from persistent or recurrent symptoms. This has been termed the "failed back syndrome".

Degenerative Disc Disease

CT and MRI have shown that degenerative disc disease is very prevalent, especially after age 45. In one series, asymptomatic cervical cord impingement (by disc) was found in 26% of patients over 64 years of age on MRI (Teresi et al. 1987). The progressive changes in the intervertebral disc with ageing have been documented with MRI and pathological correlation obtained, from the neonatal period to adulthood (Pech and Haughton 1985; Ho et al. 1988; Yu et al. 1988a,b,c; Yu et al. 1989). Types of tears of the annulus fibrosis have been characterized on MR (Yu et al. 1988b) and the radial tear may be responsible for the bulging annulus. Transverse tears, resulting in rupture of Sharpey's fibres at the periphery of the annulus near the ring apophysis, may account for the focal herniation (Yu et al. 1988a,b,c; Bonneville et al. 1989).

Not all disc bulges (defined as a concentric extension of disc material with an intact but often thin annulus), or disc herniations (diagnosed when a disruption of the annulus is associated with focal disc extrusion), are symptomatic (Norman 1987). Free fragments, often called sequestered discs, herniate through the lateral part of the posterior longitudinal ligament because its midportion is much thicker than its lateral aspects. This lateral herniation is more likely to result in symptoms because the exiting nerve roots are impinged upon by the free fragment. Myelography is not always capable of distinguishing herniation from bulge, especially when the defect is central. MRI and CT are of similar sensitivity and specificity in the diagnosis of herniation (Brown et al. 1988; Hedberg et al. 1988; Masaryk et al. 1988) (Fig. 8.3).

CT and MRI both demonstrate types of disc herniation not visible on myelography. The far lateral or extreme lateral disc herniation is the type that compresses the exiting nerve root in the intervertebral foramen and slightly lateral to it, distal to the nerve root sleeve. Often an overlooked entity and a cause for failed back syndrome, it is more commonly found at higher disc levels than routine disc herniations, with about one-half seen at L2–3 and L3–4 and only one-third or so at L4–5. Migratory (free) fragments are found in half the cases and typically there is no intraspinal herniation (Osborn et al. 1988). A routine laminectomy will not disclose this type of herniation and a facetectomy or foraminotomy may be necessary to remove the fragments.

Institutions with large volumes of spinal MRI are noticing an apparent increased incidence of thoracic disc herniations (Ross et al. 1987a). As in other parts of the spine, not all are symptomatic, but the small diameter of the subarachnoid space surrounding the cord increases the potential for harm. Some of these herniations have mimicked spinal multiple sclerosis. Prior to MRI, thoracic disc herniation was diagnosed with myelography. In the absence of a block, supine AP and cross-table lateral films of the thoracic region were obtained and subtle indentations on the dural sac sought. A postmyelogram CT scan of the suspicious area may be obtained to determine whether the herniation is central or lateral. If the patient has symptoms localized to a specific dermatome, an intravenously enhanced CT scan with thin slices (1.5–3 mm) may disclose the herniation, in a similar fashion to herniated cervical discs.

The above types of disc herniation have been termed neurogenic and represent the well known disc herniations. Recently, vertebrogenic symptoms, consisting of local and referred pain and autonomic reflex dysfunction, mainly sympathetic, have been ascribed to lumbar disc extrusion anterior to the pedicles. Twenty-nine per cent of patients in one series had this anterior type of disc herniation (Jinkins et al. 1989). Further studies will determine the place of this type of herniation in the diagnosis of back pain.

Spondylosis and Diffuse Idiopathic Skeletal Hyperostosis

Spinal pathology causing pain or neurological dysfunction is not limited to disc disease. Spondylosis, the formation of osteophytes at the margins of the vertebral bodies due to loss of resilience of the discs and increased stress on Sharpey's fibres, can impinge on the dural sac or nerve roots. Extensive ossification of the anterior longitudinal ligament, with preservation of the disc height, has been termed diffuse idiopathic skeletal hyperostosis (DISH). While this entity was thought benign, affecting only the mobility of the spine, a 50% incidence of associated ossification of the posterior longitudinal ligament (OPLL) has been documented (Resnick et al. 1978). OPLL can contribute to spinal stenosis and lead to severe myelopathy. Its current treatment consists of unroofing of the spinal canal, either anteriorly or posteriorly, to relieve the stenosis.

Spinal Stenosis

Spinal stenosis, or narrowing of the spinal canal, can be congenital (due to short pedicles and/or laminae) (Fig. 8.2), acquired (due to overgrowth of the articular facets without or with arthrosis, thickening of the laminae or ligamentum flavum), or a combination of these factors (Rosa et al. 1986; Postacchini 1988). It is commonly focal, affecting only short segments of the spinal canal, and is recognized on axial images (on CT or MRI) as distortion of the dural sac from its rounded shape to a triangular shape. Normally the dural sac tapers gradually the more caudally the scans progress, maintaining its rounded shape. Assessment of adequate surgical decompression is aided in some centres by intraoperative ultrasound; lateral decompression has been achieved when the dural sac has a normal configuration. Effects of chronic cervical cord compression seen as increased intensity on MRI are thought to be proportional to the severity of the myelopathy and the degree of spinal stenosis. The presence of these changes suggests a less favourable response to medical or surgical therapy (Takahashi et al. 1989).

Post Surgical Scarring

(See Fig. 8.4B.) The formation of excessive scar following surgery is a cause of recurrent symptoms. Re-exploration is difficult or impossible and can exac-

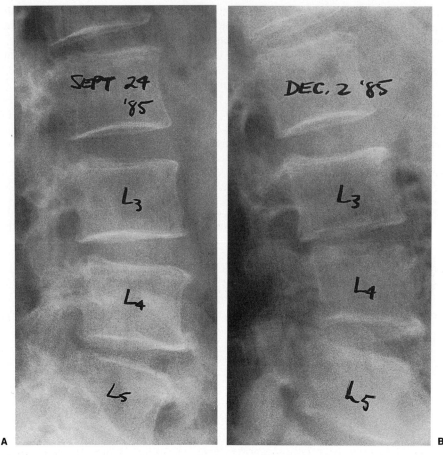

Fig. 8.12. A and **B** Lateral lumbar spine views showing discitis as progressive disc space narrowing of L3–4, with demineralization of the adjoining end plates, following L3 to L5 laminectomy for spinal stenosis in a 65-year-old man.

erbate symptoms. It has always been a difficult diagnostic problem, because retained or recurrent disc herniation can coexist with scar.

On intravenously enhanced CT, scar enhances while herniated disc rarely does (Teplick and Haskin 1984; Braun et al. 1985; Yang et al. 1986; Sotiropoulos et al. 1989). The degree of enhancement is variable however and is dependent on the amount of iodine (total grams) used and the timing of the scans. The amount of scar present will also vary and the evolution of scar enhancement on CT is still being determined. A large amount of contrast, such as 300 ml of Conray 60%, representing 84 g of iodine, infused rapidly while scans are being obtained yields the best results. The use of a similar amount of iodine with the safer non-ionic materials remains costly.

On MRI, epidural scar is of variable intensity. Its irregular configuration and extension is an important feature in differentiating it from recurrent disc herniation (Bundschuh et al. 1988a; Hochhauser et al. 1988). The mechanism and time course of enhancement of epidural fibrosis with gadolinium-DTPA has been studied. As in CT, herniated disc does not enhance, while epidural fibrosis surrounding herniated disc does. In the unoperated spine, epidural fibrosis occurs as an attempt at healing around a herniation, and it must be distinguished from the epidural venous plexus (Ross et al. 1989a,b).

Infection and Inflammation

Infection (Figs. 8.12A and B, 8.13A and B)

Discitis and vertebral osteomyelitis, whether bacterial or tuberculous, though infrequent in developed countries, may be insidious in onset and difficult to recognize and to treat (Burke and Brant-Zawadzki 1985; Kopecky et al. 1985). Disc space narrowing, irregularity and sclerosis of vertebral end plates followed by more pronounced bone destruction and demineralization are its signs on plain films, tomography, CT and MRI. Paravertebral spread of infection and epidural or subdural extension may be recognized with intravenously enhanced CT scan, intrathecally enhanced CT scan, and MRI without or with gadolinium-DTPA. Myelography is rarely needed. The examination most likely to produce the best information in the cooperative patient is MRI; intravenously enhanced CT is the next choice. Subtle changes in the disc and bone marrow on MRI may pinpoint the infection before it is visible by other imaging modalities. Tuberculous spondylitis may spare the discs and mimic metastatic disease (Smith et al. 1989; Thrush and Enzmann 1989).

Arachnoiditis

This inflammatory process results in adhesion of the pia-arachnoid to the cord or, more commonly, lumbar nerve roots and it may be associated with spinal cord atrophy (Donaldson and Gibson 1982). In the late stages, fibrosis involves the dura, leptomeninges, and nerve roots. On myelography, CT, or MRI, the nerve roots are clumped together and move poorly in the decreased sub-arachnoid space. The margins of the dural sac are irregular, with amputation of the nerve root sleeves. Complete obstruction may occur (Ross et al. 1987b). Iophendylate (Pantopaque, Ethiodan, Myodil), used for myelography until the late 1970s when safe water-soluble compounds became widely available, is known to have caused arachnoiditis, especially if blood was present in the CSF. It is absorbed at the rate of 1 ml per year and evidence of previous oil myelography is still present in many patients. This retained oily contrast has the MRI characteristics of fat (Braun et al. 1986). It is often loculated and may have caused small arachnoid cysts at the points of adhesion, which may further compromise root sleeves.

Rheumatoid Arthritis

Rheumatoid arthritis is another condition which has greatly benefited from the advent of MRI as pannus can now be readily discerned and its effect on the

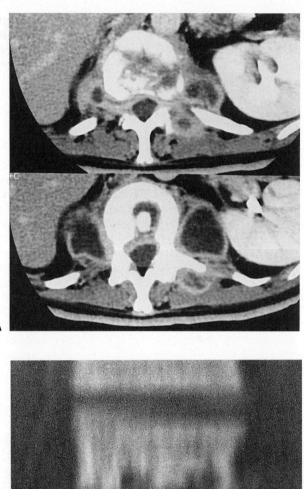

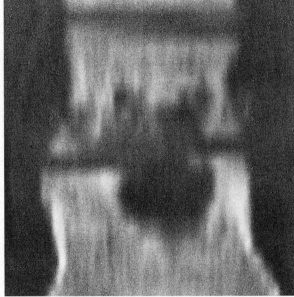

Fig. 8.13. A Axial CT scans with intravenous contrast enhancement, showing bilateral psoas abscesses with T12–L1 tuberculous discitis in a 37-year-old man presenting with low back pain, gradual weight loss, and recent fevers and chills. **B** Coronal reformatted image showing the bone destruction of the end plates.

thecal sac observed. Abnormal mobility due to ligamentous laxity or disruption is best assessed with flexion and extension views. Plain films, tomography, and CT scans show the bone changes to best advantage.

Synovial hypertrophy, joint effusion, and cartilage thinning are better appreciated on MRI (Beltran et al. 1987). Sagittal MRI of the cervicomedullary junction in one group of 15 patients showed that those with a cervicomedullary angle of less than 135 degrees had brain stem compression, cervical myelopathy or C2 radicular pain, and all were neurologically abnormal. Purely bone changes such as apophyseal joint disease, cystic changes of the C1–2 facets, erosion of the spinous processes and the basiodental interval were better studied by other methods than MRI (Bundschuh et al. 1988a,b; Petterson et al. 1988).

Stainless steel fixation wires used to reduce C1–2 instability may result in poor MR images. For this reason, surgeons are urged to use titanium wires or alloys which do not interfere with the MRI signals. Fixation will not only immobilize the spine and reduce cord compression, but pannus may regress as a consequence, further reducing cord impingement (Mirvis et al. 1988; Larsson et al. 1989a).

Neoplasms

The management of spinal tumours has been altered as a result of improved imaging and surgical techniques (Jeanmart 1986) (Figs. 8.5, 8.6, 8.14A and B, 8.15). Removal of many of these tumours is feasible, the effect of radiation therapy and the follow-up of the consequence of longstanding compressive lesions is now possible. Myelomalacia, atrophy and small intramedullary cysts may be found at the site of compression. Some believe that syringomyelia, which develops months to years after removal of the mass, has its origin in these areas of abnormal tissue (Castillo et al. 1987). Early detection of such syrinxes and their treatment may prevent progression and result in maintenance of neurological function. Clinical deterioration can also be due to tumour recurrence which can be detected and in some cases removed, with preservation or restoration of function.

Myelography is traditionally used to confirm the level of spinal block often caused by epidural spread of metastatic tumour, the most common type of spinal neoplasm. Intradural masses can be sharply demarcated and the extent of intramedullary expansion visualized. Contrast administered via a lumbar puncture can be supplemented by further water-soluble contrast injected at the C1–2 level. The entire length of the subarachnoid space is thus evaluated and the level and number of spinal segments involved determined, to limit the number of decompressive laminectomies or to define radiation portals.

CT scanning following a myelogram sometimes discloses an incomplete block where the myelogram suggested it was complete. This is because very small amounts of contrast passing beyond the block can be detected by CT. A C1–2 puncture can be averted in these patients when the limits and the character of the mass have been satisfactorily shown on CT.

Intravenously enhanced CT can be used to localize the solid component of an intramedullary mass, or extraspinal extension of an intradural extramedullary tumour. Epidural and paravertebral masses, especially when asso-

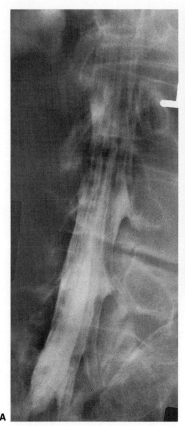

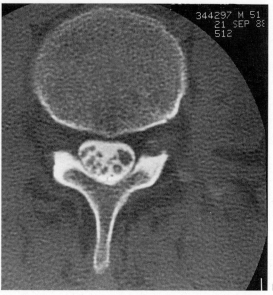

Fig. 8.14. A Oblique view of a lumbar myelogram. **B** axial image of the postmyelogram CT scan showing thickened nodular nerve roots consistent with metastatic subarachnoid seeding in a 51-year-old man presenting with weakness and pain in his legs, who had an adenoid cystic carcinoma of his larynx removed one year ago.

ciated with bone destruction, are also well shown (Lapointe et al. 1986; Shapiro et al. 1986).

Spinal angiography is performed when the presence of a haemangioblastoma is suspected in isolation or associated with Von Hippel-Lindau disease. Single or multiple tumours may be intramedullary or extramedullary. A cyst may be associated with the tumour nodule, as in cerebellar haemangioblastoma, and be responsible for most of the symptoms including an ascending deficit due to cephalad progression of the "syrinx" (Rebner and Gebarski 1985).

MRI delineates intramedullary masses very well and provides more information than other imaging modalities (DiChiro et al. 1985; Carsin et al. 1987). Ependymomas and astrocytomas comprise 90% of all intramedullary tumours. Of these, 30%–50% have one or more cysts adjacent to the solid portion. These cysts, of variable size, can be proximal and/or distal to the solid component. Enhancement with gadolinium DTPA demarcates the tumour nodule to best advantage (Sze et al. 1988a,b; Valk 1988; Parizel et al. 1989). Evidence of prior haemorrhage within a tumour is seen on MRI as well as peritumoural oedema. Calcification, rare in spinal tumours and found most commonly in schwannoma and meningioma, is not easily detected on MRI. CT scan is the most sensitive method for the detection of calcium.

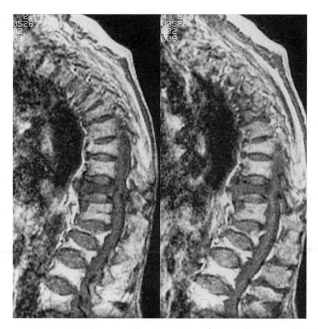

Fig. 8.15. Sagittal MRI of the thoracic spine showing breast carcinoma metastasis in T10 and T11 replacing normal bone marrow, with cord compression at T10 and severe compression fractures of T12 and L1, with normal marrow, in a 78-year-old woman with urinary symptoms.

Leptomeningeal metastatic disease may be subtle. On myelography or on intrathecally enhanced CT, small tumour nodules along the margins of the dural sac, irregularity and/or nodularity of cord or nerve roots, are considered diagnostic (Fig. 8.14A and B). Early experience with MRI was discouraging, but new imaging sequences and the use of gadolinium DTPA have greatly increased the diagnostic yield (Smoker et al. 1987; Krol et al. 1988; Sze et al. 1988a,b; Carmody et al. 1989).

Ultrasound of spinal tumours is utilized intraoperatively to localize the solid component within an expanded cord. Small cysts may be detected which were not apparent on MRI (Goy et al. 1986).

Multiple Sclerosis

Multiple sclerosis (MS) remains a diagnostic dilemma. While only 15%–20% of patients present with purely spinal symptoms, investigation of the patient for silent cerebral plaques has proved useful and an aid to diagnosis (Edwards et al. 1986). Spinal plaques are only very rarely visible on CT scan obtained with a double dose delay technique (scan obtained 45 minutes after injection of 84 g of iodine), the technique most commonly used to demonstrate cerebral plaques. MRI consistently shows intracranial plaques better than CT. In the event of a normal cerebral MRI study, a spinal study should be performed, as plaques may be demonstrated in the cord. The MS plaques are seen as high signal intensity and with the improved resolution of grey and white matter of the cord, it may be possible to correlate the clinical findings with the actual spinal tracts involved, similar to what is possible in the brain, bearing in mind that the appearance of cerebral lesions wax and wane with time and that the location of cerebral plaques does not always correlate with symptoms and/or signs. Gadolinium DTPA may prove useful to study the activity of the plaques (Larsson 1989b). These MRI studies have disclosed the presence of un-recognized herniated thoracic discs in some patients presumed to have MS. No doubt a large number of asymptomatic disc herniations will also be discovered.

Myelography was traditionally used in suspected spinal MS to rule out compressive lesions such as disc herniation or foramen magnum meningioma. Dural arteriovenous fistulas (Fig. 8.8) are another mimic of spinal MS, increas-ingly diagnosed since the use of water-soluble contrast for myelography became widespread in the late 1970s. Presenting as paraparesis, paresthesias, sphincter disturbance, sensory deficits or muscle atrophy, usually in middle age, the effects of these arteriovenous shunts can be arrested or reversed with surgery and/or embolization. Congestion of the spinal cord and resulting hypoxia caused by interference with normal venous drainage by the arteriovenous shunt is believed responsible for the symptoms. Myelography, and in some cases MRI, discloses the presence of tortuous draining veins, usually on the dorsal aspect of the cord. Only spinal angiography will accurately outline the vascular supply of the dural nidus, originating from one or more radicular branches of a segmental artery. Spinal angiography should not be carried out when tortuous and moderately dilated vessels on the dorsal aspect of the thoracolumbar enlargement are found incidentally, and in the absence of suggestive symptoms or signs of a fistula, as these "varices" may be a normal finding (N'Diaye et al. 1984; Thron 1988).

Conclusion

Development of CT in the 1970s resulted in the first cross-sectional images of the brain. Development of MRI in the 1980s has furthered the evaluation of the spinal cord and its adjoining structures. Resolution of spinal cord cross-sectional anatomy is approaching that of brain. MRI has improved our understanding of CSF flow dynamics. By revealing the temporal alterations in multiple sclerosis, it is helping to elucidate the pathophysiology of this disorder and to discern the effects of various therapies.

Improved knowledge of spinal anatomy, pathology, and physiology is largely responsible for the favourable outcome of many of these patients who are now treated more aggressively than in the past.

References

Atlas SW, Regenbogen V, Rogers LF, Kim KS (1986) Radiographic characteristics of burst fractures of the spine. AJNR 7:675–682; AJR 147:575–582

Aubin ML, Balériaux D, Cosnard G, et al. (1987) MRI in syringomyelia of congenital, infectious traumatic or idiopathic origin. A study of 142 cases. J Neuroradiol 14:313–336

Banna M (1985) Clinical radiology of the spine and spinal cord. Aspen Systems Corp, Rockville, Maryland

Barkovich AJ, Wippold FJ, Sherman JL, Citrin CM (1986) Significance of cerebellar tonsillar position on MRI. AJNR 7:795–799

Beltran J, Caudill JL, Herman LA, et al. (1987) Rheumatoid arthritis: MR imaging manifestations. Radiology 165:153–157

Bonneville JF, Runge M, Cattin F, Potelon P, Tang Y-S (1989) Extraforaminal lumbar disc herniations: CT demonstration of Sharpey's fibers avulsion. Neuroradiology 31:71–74

Braun IF, Hoffman Jr JC, David PC, Landman JA, Tindall GT (1985) Contrast enhancement in CT differentiation between recurrent disk herniation and postoperative scar: prospective study. AJNR 6:607–612; AJR 145:785–790

Braun IF, Malko JA, Davis PC, Hoffman Jr JF, Jacobs LH (1986) The behavior of pantopaque on MR: in vivo and in vitro analyses. AJNR 7:997–1001

Brown BM, Schwartz RH, Frank E, Blank NK (1988) Preoperative evaluation of cervical radiculopathy and myelopathy by surface-coil MR imaging. AJNR 9:859–866; AJR 151:1205–1212

Bundschuh CV, Modic MT, Ross JS, Masaryk TJ, Bohlman H (1988a) Epidural fibrosis and recurrent disc herniation in the lumbar spine. MR imaging assessment. AJNR 9:169–178; AJR 150:923–932

Bundschuh C, Modic MT, Kearney F, Morris R, Deal C (1988b) Rheumatoid arthritis of the cervical spine: surface coil MR imaging. AJNR 9:565–571; AJR 151:181–187

Burke DR, Brant-Zawadzki M (1985) CT of pyogenic spine infection. Neuroradiology 27:131–137

Carmody RF, Yang PJ, Seeley GW, Seeger JF, Unger EC, Johnson JE (1989) Spinal cord compression due to metastatic disease: diagnosis with MR imaging versus myelography. Radiology 173:225–229

Carsin M, Gandon Y, Rolland Y, Simon J (1987) MRI of the spinal cord: intramedullary tumors. J Neuroradiol 14:337–349

Carvlin MJ, Asato R, Hackney DB, Kassab E, Joseph PM (1989) High-resolution MR of the spinal cord in humans and rats. AJNR 10:13–17

Castillo M, Quencer RM, Green BA, Montalvo BM (1987) Syringomyelia as a consequence of compressive extramedullary lesions: postoperative clinical and radiological manifestations. AJNR 8:973–978; AJR 150:391–396

Curtin AJ, Chakeres DW, Bulas R, Boesel CP, Finneran M, Flint E (1989) MR imaging artifacts of the axial internal anatomy of the cervical spinal cord. AJNR 10:19–26

Czervionke LF, Daniels DL, Ho PSP, et al. (1988) The MR appearance of gray and white matter in the cervical spinal cord. AJNR 9:557–562

Denis F (1983) The three column spine and its significance in the classification of acute thoracolumbar injuries. Spine 8:817–831

DiChiro G, Doppman JL, Dwyer AJ, et al. (1985) Tumors and arteriovenous malformations of the spinal cord: assessment using MR. Radiology 156:689–697

Donaldson I, Gibson R (1982) Spinal cord atrophy associated with arachnoiditis as demonstrated by computed tomography. Neuroradiology 24:101–105

Donovan-Post JM (1984) Computed tomography of spinal trauma. In: Donovan-Post JM (ed) Computed tomography of the spine. Williams and Wilkins, Baltimore, London, pp 765–808

Dunsker SB, Schmidek HH, Frymoyer J, Kahn E (eds) (1986) The unstable spine (thoracic, lumbar and sacral regions). Grune and Stratton, Orlando, New York

Edwards MK, Farlow MR, Stevens JC (1986) Cranial MR in spinal cord MS: diagnosing patients with isolated spinal cord symptoms. AJNR 7:1003–1005

Gehweiler Jr JA, Osborne RL, Becker RF (1980) The radiology of vertebral trauma. Saunders, Philadelphia

Goy AM, Pinto RS, Raghavendra BN, Epstein FJ, Kricheff II (1986) Intramedullary spinal cord tumors: MR imaging, with emphasis on associated cysts. Radiology 161:381–386

Hedberg MC, Drayer BP, Flom RA, Hodak JA, Bird CR (1988) Gradient echo (GRASS) MR imaging in cervical radiculopathy. AJNR 9:145–151; AJR 150:683–689

Ho PSP, Yu S, Sether LA, Wagner M, Ho K-C, Haughton VM (1988) Progressive and regressive changes in the nucleus pulposus. Part I. The neonate. Radiology 169:87–92

Hochhauser L, Kieffer SA, Cacayorin ED, Petro GR, Teller WF (1988) Recurrent postdiskectomy low back pain. MR-surgical correlation. AJNR 9:769–774; AJR 151:755–760

Jeanmart L (ed) (1986) Radiology of the spine. Tumors. Springer-Verlag, Berlin, Heidelberg, New York, Tokyo

Jinkins JR, Whittemore AR, Bradley WG (1989) The anatomic basis of vertebrogenic pain and the autonomic syndrome associated with lumbar disk extrusion. AJNR 10:219–231; AJR 152:1277–1289

Kadoya S, Nakamura T, Kobayashi S, Yamamoto I (1987) Magnetic resonance imaging of acute spinal cord injury. Neuroradiology 29:252–255

Kim KS, Chen HH, Russell EJ, Rogers LF (1988–89) Flexion teardrop fracture of the cervical spine: radiographic characteristics. AJNR 9:1221–1228; AJR 152:319–326

Kopecky KK, Gilmor RL, Scott JA, Edwards MK (1985) Pitfalls of computed tomography in diagnosis of discitis. Neuroradiology 27:57–66

Krol G, Sze G, Malkin M, Walker R (1988) MR of cranial and spinal meningeal carcinomatosis. Comparison with CT and myelography. AJNR 9:709–714; AJR 151:583–588

Kulkarni MV, McArdle CB, Kopanicky D, et al. (1987) Acute spinal cord injury: MR imaging at 1.5T. Radiology 164:837–843

Lapointe JS, Graeb DA, Nugent RA, Robertson WD (1986) Value of intravenous contrast enhancement in CT evaluation of intraspinal tumors. AJR 146(1):103–107

Larsson EM, Holtås S, Zygmunt S (1989a) Pre and postoperative MR imaging of the craniocervical junction in rheumatoid arthritis. AJNR 10:89–94

Larsson EM, Holtås S, Nilsson O (1989b) GD-DTPA-enhanced MR of suspected spinal multiple sclerosis. AJNR 10:1071–1076

Lee C, Woodring JH, Goldstein SJ, Daniel TL, Young AB, Tibbs PA (1987) Evaluation of traumatic atlanto-occipital dislocation. AJNR 8:19–26

Masaryk TJ, Ross JS, Modic MT, Boumphrey F, Bohlman H, Wilber G (1988) High resolution MR imaging of sequestered lumbar intervertebral disks. AJNR 9:351–358; AJR 150:1155–1162

Merx JL, Bakker-Niezen SH, Thijssen HOM, Walder HAD (1989) The tethered spinal cord syndrome: a correlation of radiological features and peroperative findings in 30 patients. Neuroradiology 31:63–70

Mirvis SE, Geisler F, Joslyn JN, Zrebeet H (1988) Use of titanium wire in cervical spine fixation as a means to reduce MR artifacts. AJNR 9:1229–1231

Naidich TP, Quencer RM (eds) (1987) Clinical neurosonography: ultrasound of the central nervous system. Springer-Verlag, Berlin, Heidelberg, New York, London, Paris, Tokyo

Naseem M, Zachariah SB, Stone J, Russell E (1986) Cervicomedullary hematoma: diagnosis by MR. AJNR 7:1096–1098

N'Diaye M, Chiras J, Meder JF, Barth MO, Koussa A, Bories J (1984) Water soluble myelography for the study of dural arteriovenous fistulae of the spine draining into the spinal venous system. J Neuroradiol 11:327–339

Newton TH, Potts DG (1983) Computed tomography of the spine and spinal cord. Modern neuroradiology vol 1. Clavadel Press, San Anselmo, CA

Norman D (1987) The spine. In: Brant-Zawadzki M, Norman D (eds) Magnetic resonance imaging of the central nervous system. Raven Press, New York, pp 289–328

Osborn AG, Hood RS, Sherry RG, Smoker WRK, Harnsberger HR (1988) CT/MR spectrum of far lateral and anterior lumbosacral disk herniations. AJNR 9:775–778

Parizel PM, Balériaux D, Rodesch G, et al. (1989) GD-DTPA-enhanced MR imaging of spinal tumors. AJNR 10:249–258; AJR 152:1087–2096

Pasto ME, Rifkin MD, Rubenstein JB, Northrup BE, Colter JM, Goldberg BB (1984) Real-time-ultrasonography of the spinal cord: intraoperative and postoperative imaging. Neuroradiology 26:183–187

Pech P, Haughton VM (1985) Lumbar intervertebral disk: correlative MR and anatomic study. Radiology 156:699–701

Pettersson H, Larsson EM, Holtås S, et al. (1988) MR imaging of the cervical spine in rheumatoid arthritis. AJNR 9:573–577

Postacchini F (1988) Lumbar spinal stenosis. Springer-Verlag, Wien, New York

Raghavan N, Barkovich AJ, Edwards M, Norman D (1989) MR imaging in the tethered spinal cord syndrome. AJNR 10:27–36

Rebner M, Gebarski SS (1985) Magnetic resonance imaging of spinal cord hemangioblastoma. AJNR 6:287–289

Resnick D, Guerra J, Robinson C, Vint V (1978) Association of diffuse idiopathic skeletal hyperostosis (DISH) and calcification and ossification of the posterior longitudinal ligament. AJR 131(6):1049–1053

Rogers LF (1982) Radiology of skeletal trauma, vol 1. Churchill Livingstone, New York, pp 273–338

Rosa M, Capellini C, Canevari MA, Prosetti D, Schiavoni S (1986) CT in low back and sciatic pain due to lumbar canal osseous changes. Neuroradiology 28:237–240

Ross JS, Perez-Reyes N, Masaryk TJ, Bohlman H, Modic MT (1987a) Thoracic disk herniation: MR imaging. Radiology 165:511–515

Ross JS, Masaryk TJ, Modic MT, et al. (1987b) MR imaging of lumbar arachnoiditis. AJNR 8:885–892; AJR 149:1025–1032

Ross JS, Delamarter R, Hueftle MG, et al. (1989a) Gadolinium-DTPA-enhanced MR imaging of the postoperative lumbar spine: time course and mechanism of enhancement. AJNR 10:37–46; AJR 152:825–834

Ross JS, Modic MT, Masaryk TJ, Carter J, Marcus RE, Bohlman H (1989b) Assessment of extradural degenerative disease with Gd-DTPA-enhanced MR imaging: correlation with surgical and pathologic findings. AJNR 10:1243–1249; AJR 154:151–158

Ruggiero R, Capece W, Del Vecchio E, Palmieri A, Ambrosio A, Calabro A (1981) High resolution CT spinal scanning with ACTA 0200 FS. Neuroradiology 22:23–25

Shapiro M, Kier EL, Reed D, et al. (1986) Intravenous contrast enhanced CT alternative to myelography in neoplasms involving spinal canal (ASNR abstract). AJNR 7:549

Shapiro R (1984) Myelography, 4th edn. Year Book Medical Publishers, Chicago

Sherman JL, Barkovich AJ, Citrin CM (1986) The MR appearance of syringomyelia; new observations. AJNR 7:985–995

Smith AS, Weinstein MA, Mizushima A, et al. (1989) MR imaging characteristics of tuberculous spondylitis vs. vertebral osteomyelitis. AJNR 10:619–625; AJR 153:399–405

Smoker WR, Godersky JC, Knutzon RK, Keyes WD, Norman D, Bergman W (1987) The role of MR imaging in evaluating metastatic spinal disease. AJNR 8:901–908; AJR 149:1241–1248

Sotiropoulos S, Chafetz NI, Lang P, et al. (1989) Differentiation between postoperative scar and recurrent disk herniation: prospective comparison of MR, CT and contrast enhanced CT. AJNR 10:639–643

Sze G, Krol G, Zimmerman RD, Deck MDF (1988a) Intramedullary disease of the spine: diagnosis using gadolinium DTPA-enhanced MR imaging. AJNR 9:847–858; AJR 151:1193–1204

Sze G, Abramson A, Krol G, et al. (1988b) Gadolinium-DTPA in the evaluation of intradural extramedullary disease. AJNR 9:153–163; AJR 150:911–921

Takahashi M, Yamashita Y, Sakamoto Y, Kojima R (1989) Chronic cervical cord compression: clinical significance of increased signal intensity of MR images. Radiology 173:219–224

Teplick JG, Haskin ME (1984) Intravenous contrast enhanced CT of postop lumbar spine: improved identification of recurrent disk herniation, scar, arachnoiditis and diskitis. AJNR 5:373–383; AJR 143:845–856

Teresi LM, Lufkin RB, Reicher MA, et al. (1987) Asymptomatic degenerative disk disease and spondylosis of the cervical spine: MR imaging. Radiology 164:83–88

Thron AK (1988) Vascular anatomy of the spinal cord. Springer-Verlag, Wien

Thrush A, Enzmann DR (1989) MR of infectious spondylitis (ASNR abstract). AJNR 10:880

Valk J (1988) GD-DTPA in MR of spinal lesions. AJNR 9:345–350; AJR 150:1163–1168

Vézina JL, Fontaine S, Laperrière J (1989) Outpatient myelography with fine needle technique: an appraisal. AJNR 10:615–617; AJR 153:383–385

Wilson DA, Prince JR (1989) MR imaging of the location of the normal conus medullaris throughout childhood. AJNR 10:259–262

Woodring JH, Selke AC, Duff DE (1981) Traumatic atlantooccipital dislocation: two cases with survival. AJNR 2:251–254

Yang PJ, Seeger JF, Dzioba RB, et al. (1986) High dose IV contrast in CT scanning of the postoperative lumbar spine. AJNR 7:703–707

Yu S, Haughton VM, Ho PSP, Sether LA, Wagner M, Ho K-C (1988a) Progressive and regressive changes in the nucleus pulposus. Part II. The adult. Radiology 169:93–98

Yu S, Sether LA, Ho PSP, Wagner M, Haughton V (1988b) Tears of the annulus fibrosus: correlation between MR and pathologic findings in cadavers. AJNR 9:367–370

Yu S, Haughton VM, Sether LA, Wagner M (1988c) Annulus fibrosus in bulging intervertebral disks. Radiology 169:761–763

Yu S, Haughton VM, Lynch KL, Ho KC, Sether LA (1989) Fibrous structure in the intervertebral disk: correlation of MR appearance with anatomic sections. AJNR 10:1105–1110

Chapter 9

Neurophysiological Investigation of the Spinal Cord

M.S. Schwartz and M. Swash

The spinal cord is a long structure that extends from the post-cervical segment, located just caudal to the foramen magnum, to the conus medullaris which, in adults, is located at about the L1 vertebral level. The spinal nerve roots leave the cord by passing slightly caudally to reach the appropriate intervertebral foramina on each side, the ventral and dorsal nerve roots fusing just distal to the posterior root ganglion to form mixed motor and sensory roots. These nerve roots form major branching plexuses in the cervical and lumbosacral regions in which the peripheral nerves innervating the limbs are formed but, in the thoracic region, the mixed nerve roots remain separate and form intercostal nerves. Thus the segmental organization of the human spinal cord reflects the underlying metameric differentiation of body segments in other species.

The spinal cord itself consists of symmetrical, central grey matter, containing anterior horn cells, cells of the autonomic nervous system, sensory neurones and interneurones, surrounded by descending and ascending white matter tracts. Only a few of these grey and white matter structures are directly accessible to neurophysiological investigation (Table 9.1). Other methods can be used to assess the functional state of some of these structures. For example, H reflex excitability studies and F response frequency measurements are an index of anterior horn cell excitability in patients with spasticity due to corticospinal tract disease.

Neurophysiological studies of spinal cord function are especially useful in assessing the extent or level of certain diseases, e.g. in the assessment of the distribution of neurogenic change in patients with motor neurone disease. They are also used to monitor spinal cord function in patients undergoing cord or spinal surgery, especially during operative correction of scoliosis in order to try

Table 9.1. Spinal cord structures accessible to neurophysiological investigation

Posterior columns } Spinocerebellar tracts }	Somatosensory evoked potentials (SEPs) from nerve stimulation
Corticospinal tracts	Magnetic or electrical stimulation of spinal cord or motor cortex
Anterior horn cells	Needle electromyography
Sensory nerve roots	H reflex latency and SEP studies, dermatomal SEP's
Motor nerve roots	F response studies, magnetic, electrical and direct needle electrode stimulation techniques
Spinothalamic tracts	Thermal threshold determinations

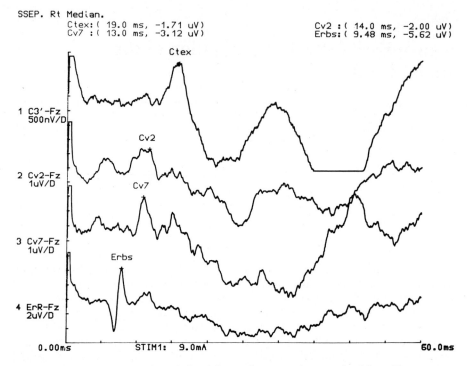

SSEP. Rt Median.
      Ctex:(19.0 ms, −1.71 uV)   Cv2 :(14.0 ms, −2.00 uV)
      Cv7 :(13.0 ms, −3.12 uV)   Erbs:(9.48 ms, −5.62 uV)

Fig. 9.1. SEP from stimulation of the right median nerve in normal subject. The responses recorded at Erb's point, at the levels of the C7 and C2 spinous processes, and at the cortex, are marked on the tracing and the electrode placements are described to the left of the tracing. In addition, the latencies from the stimulus to the waveforms are indicated at the top of the figure.

to prevent the development of paraplegia as a complication of surgery. In addition, neurophysiological assessment has been used in evaluating patients with suspected multiple sclerosis, since clinically silent lesions may be detected by appropriate investigations.

Neurophysiological Techniques Used in Assessment of Spinal Cord Diseases

Somatosensory Evoked Potentials (SEPs)

The SEP can be recorded from the brachial plexus, spinal cord and sensory cortex (Matthews et al. 1974). Although potentials cannot be recorded from the lumbar plexus, the ascending sensory volley in the spinal cord can be recorded in the spinal cord from the conus medullaris to the cervicomedullary junction. The response is obtained by electrical stimulation of mixed peripheral nerves. In the upper limbs the median nerve (Jones 1977) is commonly used, but the ulnar or radial nerve may also be used. In the lower limbs the posterior

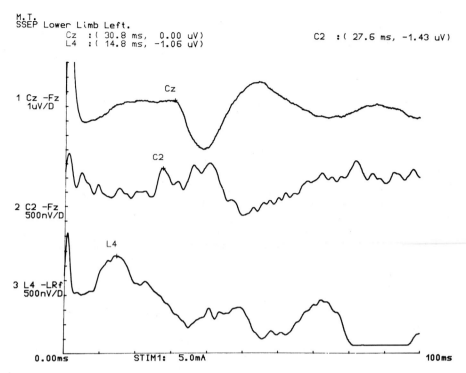

Fig. 9.2. SEP from stimulation of the left deep peroneal nerve in normal subject. Responses have been recorded from the L4 and C2 vertebral levels, and from the cortex at Cz. The latencies of these waveforms from the stimulation point are noted at the top of the figure.

tibial and common peroneal nerves are preferred (Katifi and Sedgwick 1986). Digital averaging is necessary to identify the afferent volley and generated potentials at all recording sites (Dawson 1954; Chiappa 1983).

In upper limb studies (Fig. 9.1) potentials are recorded at Erb's point in the brachial plexus, from the cervical cord at C7 and C2 vertebral levels, and from the cerebral cortex using an active electrode applied to the scalp overlying the primary sensory cortex. In studies of SEPs from the leg (Fig. 9.2), recordings are made from the cord at the L4 vertebral level representing the conus medullaris. Additional recordings can be made from more rostral cord levels, and identical electrode placements at the cervical region and scalp are used, as in upper limb studies.

Recordings made from stimulation of a mixed peripheral nerve include potentials arising from muscle afferents as well as cutaneous afferents (Burke et al. 1981). Dermatomal stimulation, on the other hand, although it produces smaller potentials, involves cutaneous afferents only, and this stimulation technique may have particular application when it is important precisely to delineate involvement of particular afferent nerve roots in a disease process (Sedgwick and Katifi 1987).

The SEP consists of several components. The potential recorded at the brachial plexus is called N9 (signifying a negative peak with a latency of about

9 ms), that at C7 is called N11, that at C2 is called N13 and that at the cortex is called N19. In lower limb studies, the potential recorded at L1 is called the LP component (signifying lumbar potential of latency varying with stature) and the cortical potential is called N37. The latencies of all these potentials are measured, by convention, to their peaks rather than to their often ill-defined onsets. The sites of origin of these potentials, in terms of cellular and white matter structures, are controversial. The N11 potential has been ascribed to the root entry zone, and N13 to the dorsal horns or dorsal columns (Kimura 1989).

Corticospinal Tract Conduction Studies

Percutaneous electrical or magnetically-induced stimulation of the central cortex produces a contralateral muscle twitch that is topographically related to the site of stimulation of the motor cortex. The cortex is activated at lower threshold during slight muscular attraction and by anodal stimulation (Merton and Morton 1980a,b; Rothwell et al. 1987). Using this technique the central motor conduction time (CMCT), representing conduction time from motor cortex to cervical region, can be measured (Cowan et al. 1984). This CMCT has usually been assessed in recordings from upper limb muscles (biceps brachii or first dorsal interosseous muscles) but similar measurements can be made from recordings of quadriceps femoris or tibialis anterior muscles in the lower limb, and if stimulation of the lower part of the spinal cord is utilized in experiments involving recordings from leg or sacral muscles, motor conduction velocity in the fast descending motor pathways in the spinal cord can be estimated directly, from the latency difference and the interstimulus distance (Snooks and Swash 1985; Berger and Shahani 1989).

Transcranial electrical stimulation of the motor cortex or spinal cord requires very high voltage pulses (2 kV with a delay time of 10 ms) and, because it is uncomfortable, has been superseded by magnetic stimulation. A brief, high-current electrical pulse in a coil of wire induces a rapid change in magnetic flux perpendicular to the plane of the coil that, in turn, induces an electric field perpendicular to the magnetic flux sufficiently powerful to stimulate motor cortex and spinal cord (Barker et al. 1985). Since electric current does not flow through scalp skin this technique is relatively painless, and attention to the design of the cord used and to current parameters in the coil, allows focal stimulation of motor areas in the cortex to be achieved (Ammassian et al. 1989).

Needle Electromyography (EMG)

Recordings of electrical activity in muscle, at rest and during voluntary activation, allow conclusions regarding the integrity of anterior horn cells and their motor axons that innervate the motor unit territories of muscle fibres in skeletal muscles. Various techniques are available. *Concentric needle EMG* is useful as an overall measure of neurogenic or myopathic change in muscle (Swash and Schwartz 1988). In neurogenic disorders fibrillation, positive sharp waves and fasciculation potentials may be recorded in resting muscle and the motor unit action potentials recorded during voluntary contraction are characteristically polyphasic and of increased amplitude. *Single fibre EMG* employs a special electrode with a small (25 µm diameter) leading off surface; this is useful in quantifying neurogenic change by measuring the fibre density (an index of packing density of muscle fibres innervated by a single motor unit) (Stalberg and Thiele 1975), and the neuromuscular jitter (an index of safety factor for neuromuscular transmission) (Stalberg et al. 1975). *Macro EMG* is a method for measuring the size of motor units in chronic partial denervation (Stalberg 1982). In concentric needle and single fibre EMG recordings sequential measurements of firing rate regularity and variability are a somewhat neglected aspect of the assessment of patients with upper motor neurone and anterior horn cell disorders.

Motor Root Stimulation

Although it is possible to stimulate motor roots with a monopolar needle electrode inserted through the paraspinal muscles immediately lateral to the spinous process, stimulation of motor nerve roots is more easily accomplished by magnetic induction (Mills and Murray 1986). The latency to a muscle of interest in the limb must be compared to the normal values obtained in the same laboratory, and to that to the same muscle in the opposite limb, since limb length is an important variable.

H Reflex Studies

The H (H = Hoffmann) reflex consists of a monosynaptic reflex response obtained in soleus muscle after stimulation of the medial popliteal (tibial) and, less reliably, in the forearm flexors after median nerve stimulation. In infants H reflexes can be obtained in the appropriate muscles after stimulation of most of the accessible mixed nerves. H reflex studies are useful in clinical practice in assessment of proximal lesions in the C7 and S1/S2 roots, particularly since both the afferent and the efferent components are involved in the response. H reflex studies are also used to measure the excitability of the anterior horn cell pool, e.g. in patients with spasticity (Angell and Hoffmann 1963). A double stimulation method has been used to produce an H reflex excitability curve for quantification.

F Responses

The F (F = foot) response is a late response recorded from a muscle after stimulation of its nerve (Kimura 1983). It represents the electrically evoked excitation of anterior horn cells induced by the retrogradely conducted impulse from the point of stimulation of the nerve; thus no synapse is involved in this response, although there is a short central delay (1 ms) between arrival of the stimulus and the response of the anterior horn cell. The latency represents conduction from the stimulus point to the spinal cord and back again to the muscle from which the response is recorded. F wave responses can thus be used to assess proximal motor conduction, and as a measure of the excitability of anterior horn cells (Fisher 1983).

Poly EMG

This technique has been used in gait analysis, in order to assess the timing and extent of the contraction of different muscles during the gait cycle in patients with neurological disorders. It can also be applied to posturographic and kinaesiological studies of upper limbs. Multiple amplifying channels are used to record from different agonist and antagonist muscles acting around one or more joints in the two legs, and foot switches and goniometers integrated into the recording system are used to time the activity of muscles in relation to the gait cycle, and to limb movement. Large amounts of data are generated and computer analysis is frequently used. This methodology is particularly useful in rehabilitation, in orthotics and in orthopaedic and sports medicine settings (Dimitrijevic 1986).

Applications of Clinical Neurophysiological Investigations

The choice of neurophysiological investigation in spinal cord diseases is dependent on the tracts or cell groups commonly involved in certain diseases. Conversely, in planning investigation of individual patients investigations are used to confirm the clinical impression of involvement of certain tracts or cell groups, to assess the extent of this involvement, and to consider the possibility of subclinical involvement of the spinal cord in patients presenting with visual failure or other lesions in whom multiple sclerosis is suspected. In addition, neurophysiological methods can be used to determine the segmental distribution or level of involvement of the spinal cord by disease.

Multiple Sclerosis

Involvement of the spinal cord is common in multiple sclerosis (MS). The cervical cord is particularly frequently involved, with demyelination in the dorsal columns and corticospinal tracts (Oppenheimer 1978). Evoked potentials, in general, have been studied particularly comprehensively in relation to the diagnosis of MS. These tests are especially useful in this disorder since they are capable of detecting subclinical abnormalities and thus can be used to establish the presence of a second lesion in patients presenting with clinical syndromes suggestive but not diagnostic of the disease. Evoked potentials, including visual, brain stem auditory responses, somatosensory responses and blink reflexes, reveal subclinical abnormalities in 20%–40% of suspected or possible cases of MS depending on the test used (Chiappa 1980; Kimura 1985). The yield of abnormality is greater with visual and somatosensory evoked responses than with brain stem auditory or blink responses (Kimura 1985).

Somatosensory responses are abnormal in about 75% of all patients with suspected MS, including definite, probable and possible cases, and in about 50% of patients without sensory symptoms or signs. Lower limb responses yield a slightly greater proportion of abnormal results than upper limb responses

(Chiappa and Ropper 1982). About 30% of abnormal responses are unilateral. Of patients with sensory symptoms or signs 75% have abnormal somatosensory evoked potentials (Chiappa 1983). In patients with clinically definite MS Baumhefner et al. (1990) found that SEPs from median nerve stimulation were abnormal in 89% of cases and that MRI revealed abnormalities in 97% of cases. Despite these data Matthews et al. (1982) found that SEP studies were of diagnostic value in only 3 of 84 patients with definite or suspected MS; in this series visual evoked responses were more consistently abnormal. Abnormalities in SEPs are more likely in the presence of corticospinal tract signs in the stimulated limb (Aminoff 1984). Most of the abnormalities in SEP latencies are found in potentials derived from structures located caudal to the cervicomedullary junction; thus, delays or absence of the N11 and N13 potentials are common in upper limb studies whereas abnormalities in N19 alone are rare (Chiappa 1983). In normal subjects cortical responses can be recorded after stimulation of the median nerve at frequencies up to 110 Hz, but in patients with MS the cortical responses may fail to follow the stimulus at rates greater than 40 Hz (Sclabassi et al. 1974).

Central motor conduction time (CMCT), derived from magnetic or electrical stimulation of the brain and cervical cord, is often abnormal in patients with MS. In upper limb studies, increased CMCT time is more likely when there are pyramidal signs in the arm, but abnormal CMCT is found in up to 20% of patients with MS in whom there are no abnormal signs in the arms, a yield similar to that found with visual evoked response studies. If strength is normal there is a 50% chance of abnormal CMCT (Hess et al. 1989). In the legs, abnormal CMCT correlates with the presence of signs of corticospinal tract involvement, especially extensor plantar responses, and with the Kurtzke disability scale (Ingram et al. 1988). In addition, motor conduction in the spinal cord, between the C8 and T12 levels, is also sometimes slowed, even to as low a figure as 24 m/s (Snooks and Swash 1985).

F response studies also show abnormalities in MS. The F wave amplitude is increased, the F/M amplitude ratio is increased, and the percentage of F responses is increased in patients with spasticity, weakness or other upper motor neurone signs. These abnormalities also correlated with abnormalities in CMCT (Smith et al. 1989). Needle EMG is generally not helpful in the diagnosis of MS but motor units firing in brief runs may be recorded in patients with myokymia. In addition, the neuromuscular jitter may be increased in single fibre EMG recordings (Weir et al. 1979) and decremental responses have been noted to repetitive stimulation (Eisen et al. 1978), observations indicating lower motor neurone involvement, presumably relating to central myelin damage on the lower motor neurone proximal to the Redlich-Obersteiner zone.

Temperature changes may have marked effects on clinical disability in patients with MS (Uhthoff 1889; Matthews et al. 1985), but inducing an increase in central body temperature does not produce changes in evoked potentials that are specific for multiple sclerosis.

Cord Compression and Spinal Trauma

Neurophysiological investigations in extrinsic compression syndromes may be useful in establishing the level and extent of the lesion. The clinical approach will depend on whether or not there is a root lesion at the level of the cord compression; if this is the case EMG and F wave studies are valuable in characterizing the distribution of abnormality within and at the upper level of the lesion. SEP studies are also informative both in recognizing the level of the lesion, and in demonstrating conduction block in the cord from stimulation in the lower limbs. Central motor conduction studies may also be useful, especially in cervical spondylosis (Masur et al. 1989).

Disturbances in a root distribution at the level of cord compression, for example by disc herniation, neurofibroma, metastasis or meningioma, can be recognized by the features of chronic partial denervation found by concentric needle EMG studies in the muscles innervated by the root or roots involved; this investigation is especially useful in the cervical and lumbosacral segments. In high cervical compression wasting of the hands may occur, probably due to venous engorgement in the lower cervical segments; this is accompanied by EMG changes with increased fibre density in the small hand muscles, remote from the level of compression (Stark et al. 1981). F wave studies are more useful and reproducible in the L5/S1 roots than in the upper limbs. In root lesions F wave studies may show delayed F responses, increased chronodispersion of the responses, or absence of the F responses (Panayiotopoulos 1979; Tang et al. 1988). Somatosensory responses in patients with cervical cord compression can be used to identify the level of the lesion. In lesions at C8/T1 level the SEP response from median nerve stimulation is normal, but the responses from ulnar stimulation are attenuated or absent, indicating the location of the disturbance of input to the cord (Stöhr et al. 1982). In lesions affecting C6/C7 segments there is attenuation or loss of N13 after median nerve stimulation (Stöhr et al. 1982). In lesions rostral to C6 the responses obtained at C7 from median or ulnar stimulation are normal in configuration and latency, but those obtained at C2 are absent, distorted or of low amplitude with abnormal dispersion. In general, in patients with radiculopathies the SEPs are almost always abnormal, but in patients with myelopathy the results of SEP studies are less reliable (Ganes 1980). Lower limb SEP studies, from the posterior tibial nerve, can be used in evaluating cauda equina root lesions (see Chapter 17), and cord lesions above this level. The location of any disruption of the transmitted wave in the posterior columns can be assessed by appropriately placed recording electrodes. The selectivity of SEPs in localizing a lesion on the afferent side can be increased by using dermatomal stimulation (Katifi and Sedgwick 1986).

Comparison of SEP and central motor conduction studies in patients with cervical myelopathies due to spondylosis or trauma have been made by Thompson et al. (1987) and by Masur et al. (1989). The latter group studied 19 patients with cervical spondylosis and stenosis presenting with cervical radiculopathy. The 4 patients with long tract signs all had abnormalities both in SEP and central motor conduction studies. In the remaining 15 patients, 13 had abnormalities in central motor conduction and 12 had SEP abnormalities after stimulation of the tibial nerves. Thompson et al. (1987) studied 6 patients, of whom 3 had cervical cord trauma, and 3 had myelopathies due to cervical spondylosis. All 6 patients had abnormalities of central motor conduction, consistent with the clinical features of myelopathy, but only 2 had abnormal SEP responses. Abbruzzese et al. (1988) found increased latency in motor responses recorded in the biceps, thenar or tibialis anterior muscles after cervical stimulation in 40% of patients with radiculopathy or myeloradiculopathy due to cervical spondylosis. Changes in motor conduction were found even when SEPs were normal, but not the converse.

Intrinsic Cord Lesions

The neurophysiological abnormalities found in patients with intrinsic cord lesions, e.g. spinal infarction, intrinsic cord tumours, syringomyelia and demyelination, will depend on the location and extent of the lesion and on the distribution of abnormality within the ascending and descending tracts, the central grey matter, and the ventral and dorsal spinal roots. Thus *infarction* in the territory of the anterior spinal artery would be expected to cause abnormal motor conduction and normal SEPs because of the sparing of the dorsal horns and posterior columns. The use of neurophysiological investigation of the spinal cord in patients with *multiple sclerosis* is discussed above. *Intrinsic cord tumours* are rare, and neurophysiological investigations have not been systematically evaluated in diagnosis of these lesions (Colon et al. 1988; Kaplan et al. 1988). In *tabes dorsalis* H reflexes are absent, and SEPs from median nerve stimulation are normal (Donofrio and Walker 1988).

Arteriovenous malformations of the spinal cord may produce neurological disability from haemorrhage, infarction or increased venous pressure on the cord remote from the lesion itself. Electrophysiological changes occur, consisting of neurogenic changes on EMG in 77%, abnormal tibial nerve SEPs in 88% and slight slowing of motor conduction in some nerves related to the lesion due to loss of fast-conducting axons and reduced motor action potential amplitude. Sural sensory nerve action potentials are normal (Armon and Daube 1989). In 4 of the 24 patients in this series there were EMG changes at a distance from the arteriovenous malformation (AVM), probably due to increased venous pressure in the cord. The patchily distributed neurophysiological abnormalities found depend on the location of the AVM, its arterial supply and the duration of symptoms (Armon and Daube 1989).

In *syringomyelia* there is damage to the central parts of the cervical spinal cord, medulla and, less frequently, to the upper thoracic cord, caused by an expanding, centrally located cystic cavity. This results in denervation of muscles in the root distribution of the affected cord segments, or cranial nerves. This chronic partial denervation is accompanied by EMG changes which show a constant pattern in the arms, with the C8/T1 segment most affected, C7 segment less severely involved and C6 segment least affected. Double discharges may occur. The complex motor unit potentials in the affected muscles, especially small hand muscles, are usually stable although some may show increased neuromuscular jitter in single fibre EMG studies (Schwartz et al. 1980). SEP responses in syringomyelia show a reduced amplitude or absence of cervical potentials reflecting segmental involvement in the disease, and in some cases there is slowed central sensory conduction of the SEP response due to damage to the ascending sensory pathways, or to rostral cord compression due to tonsillar herniation at the foramen magnum (Anderson et al. 1986). Sensory nerve action potentials and peripheral motor and sensory nerve conduction studies are normal (Fincham and Cape 1968).

Table 9.2. Spinal cord diseases and neurophysiological investigations

	SEP	Cortical/spinal stimulation	EMG	F waves	H reflexes
Demyelinating disease (multiple sclerosis)	3	3	0	1	+/−
Cord compression (disc and extrinsic tumours)	2	2	2	2	1
Spinal trauma	3	3	1	0	0
Degenerative disorders					
Motor neurone disease	+/−	1	3	0	0
Friedreich's ataxia	3	0	+/−	0	0
Subacute combined degeneration (B12-deficiency)	3	0	1	0	0
Hereditary ataxias	2	0	1	0	0
Syringomyelia	+/−	?	3	1	0
Intrinsic cord neoplasms	1	?	1	0	0
Vascular lesions	1	?	0	0	0
Infections					
AIDS (HIV infection)	1	?	2	1	0
HTLV-1 associated myelopathy	2	?	0	0	0
H zoster myelitis	0	0	2	0	0
Poliomyelitis and post-polio syndrome	0	0	3	0	0
Decompression sickness	3	?	0	0	0

Degenerative Disorders

In degenerative disorders affecting the spinal cord the distribution of neuro-physiological abnormality will be related to the specificity of involvement of individual components of the spinal cord grey and white matter, and to the presence or absence of associated involvement of the lower motor and sensory neurones (Table 9.2).

Motor Neurone Disease

In this disease of the motor system there is degeneration both of the upper and lower motor neurone, with loss of fibres in the crossed and uncrossed corticospinal tracts, involvement of the spinocerebellar neurones and tracts (Swash et al. 1988; Williams et al. 1990) and loss of anterior horn cells, with degeneration of motor axons in the peripheral nervous system.

The principal neurophysiological investigation in patients with suspected motor neurone disease is EMG. There are features of widespread denervation and reinnervation, even in muscles that are clinically unaffected. Thus, fibrillations, positive sharp waves and fasciculations can be recorded, and the motor unit action potentials recorded by conventional or single fibre needle EMG are polyphasic, and of increased amplitude and duration. With single fibre EMG velocity may be slightly slowed but sensory conduction studies and SEPs are normal. Repetitive nerve stimulation (Bernstein and Antel 1981) reveals a decremental response to 2 Hz stimulation in some patients, a feature associated with a rapidly progressive course (Stalberg et al. 1975; Swash and Schwartz 1982; Schwartz and Swash 1982; Swash and Schwartz 1988). The generator site of fasciculation potentials in motor neurone disease has for long been controversial (Denny-Brown and Pennybacker 1938; Conradi et al. 1982). Janko et al. (1989) have shown that the more complex fasciculation potentials are more unstable, and that the repetition rate was fastest in the most stable potentials. Current evidence suggests that fasciculation potentials arise proximally in the damaged innervation of motor units, although Roth (1984) thought that most fasciculations arose from generator sites in the distal motor innervation.

F response frequency is decreased in motor neurone disease in parallel with the decrease in M wave amplitude, reflecting loss of functioning anterior horn cells; the frequency of identical responses is increased, however, due to the increased excitability of the anterior horn cell pool associated with damage to the corticospinal tracts (Peiogolu-Harmoussi et al. 1989).

Corticospinal involvement can be assessed by magnetic or electrical cortical motor stimulation and, if this is combined with stimulation of the descending motor pathways in the spinal cord, at C7/T1 and T12/L1 vertebral levels, using the electrical stimulator, the yield of abnormality is increased since recordings can then be made from leg muscles (Ingram and Swash 1987; Berardelli et al. 1987; Schriefer et al. 1989; Eisen et al. 1990). The increase in central motor conduction time, or absence of responses, can be correlated both with weakness and with signs of upper motor neurone disturbance. Motor conduction velocity in the spinal cord was inversely correlated with the presence of extensor plantar responses in the patients studied by Ingram and Swash (1987). Both the lower and upper motor neurone abnormalities may be strikingly asymmetrical.

Friedreich's Ataxia

This is an autosomal recessive disorder, inherited from a genetic locus on the short arm of chromosome 9, that is characterized by degeneration of spinocerebellar tracts, corticospinal tracts and posterior columns. Sensory nerve action potentials are small or absent (McLeod 1971). EMG shows mild neurogenic changes in distal muscles but motor nerve conduction is normal (McLeod 1971). In the peripheral nerve there is marked loss of large myelinated axons, with preservation of unmyelinated nerve fibres. SEP studies (Pedersen and Trojaborg 1981; Vanasse et al. 1988) are always abnormal. In half the patients no SEP responses can be recorded from scalp or spine. In those in whom SEP responses can be recorded all the central components are delayed, and central sensory conduction time is prolonged. Central motor conduction studies, using magnetic stimulation of the motor cortex and electrical stimulation of the cervical motor roots, recording from hand muscles, showed increased central motor conduction time in 10 of 11 patients with Friedreich's ataxia (Claus et al. 1988).

Other Hereditary Ataxias

The principal types of hereditary ataxia of unknown causation are an early-onset cerebellar ataxia with retained tendon reflexes, and a late-onset degenerative cerebellar disease. In other clinical syndromes, the biochemical lesion is understood (Harding 1984). In about half the patients in both the early- and late-onset groups studied by Claus et al. (1988) central motor conduction time was increased. SEP studies show increased central conduction in the brain stem to cortex segment in many patients with hereditary ataxic syndromes (Pedersen and Trojaborg 1981; Vanasse et al. 1988) and abnormalities are generally more severe in longstanding or advanced cases.

Vitamin B12 Deficiency

In the peripheral nervous system vitamin B12 deficiency causes a mild peripheral neuropathy, and in the central nervous system, myelopathy, optic atrophy and dementia are the major features. The myelopathy is characterized by combined degeneration of corticospinal tracts and posterior columns, resulting in the clinical features of an ataxic paraparesis with marked impairment of position and vibration sense, mainly affecting the legs. The peripheral neuropathy is accompanied by slight slowing of motor and sensory nerve conduction in some patients (Mayer 1965), with small or absent sensory nerve action potentials (Fine et al. 1990). EMG shows distal fibrillations and neurogenic potentials (Fine et al. 1990). SEP studies have shown more abnormal responses and more markedly slowed central conduction from stimulation of peroneal nerves than from stimulation of median nerves (Tomado et al. 1988; Fine et al. 1990). Zegers de Beyl et al. (1988) found that slowing of central sensory conduction was more marked in the posterior columns (N11–P14 segment) than in the lemniscal-thalamocortical pathway. These abnormalities in SEP responses improve during treatment with vitamin B12 supplementation.

Infections

Several neurotropic virus infections involve the spinal cord, producing characteristic clinical syndromes (Table 9.2). Neurophysiological investigations are useful in diagnosis and management in several of these.

AIDS Myelopathy

HIV infection may cause a spinal cord disorder characterized by a vacuolar myelopathy presenting with ataxia, spastic paraparesis and sphincter disturbances, and occurring in up to 30% of patients with AIDS (Petito et al. 1988). Vacuolation occurs in the lateral and posterior columns in the thoracic cord. SEP studies have been reported. All 23 patients with this syndrome reported by Helweg-Larsen et al. (1988) showed delayed cortical SEPs following tibial nerve stimulation, the delay occurring in the central components of the cortical SEP.

HTLV-1 Associated Myelopathy

This disorder consists of a chronic, progressive myelopathy of adult onset, occurring in many parts of the world, but especially well recognized in Caribbean and Japanese people. Central manifestations are occasionally noted and CSF abnormalities include a raised CSF protein, a mild increase in lymphocyte content, and raised titres of HTLV-1 antibodies. Spastic paraparesis dominates the clinical picture, but mild distal abnormalities and sphincter dysfunction also develop. In Japanese patients the SEP responses from the arms are normal but after tibial nerve stimulation abnormalities consisting of slowed conduction rostral to T12 are noted, indicating abnormalities in the thoracic cord (Kakigi et al. 1988). The visual evoked responses were abnormal in 2 of 15 cases, and the brain stem auditory evoked potentials in 5 of 16 cases, all of whom had deafness or hearing disturbance (Kakigi et al. 1988). In Jamaican cases (Cruikshank et al. 1989; Gout et al. 1989) the SEP responses from the upper limbs are usually abnormal, in addition to the changes found after stimulation of tibial nerves. Cruikshank et al. (1989) found that visual evoked responses were abnormal in 10 of 19 patients, and that brain stem auditory evoked potentials were abnormal in 4 of 16 cases. Central motor conduction in four Japanese patients showed increased latencies from cortical stimulation, and motor responses of small amplitude (Ugawa et al. 1988).

Herpes Zoster Myelitis

Herpes zoster infection may be followed by segmental motor weakness in the affected radicular distribution, or by encephalomyelitis, Guillain-Barré syndrome, cerebral vasculitis or leucoencephalitis and by post-herpetic neuralgia. EMG assessment of patients with segmental weakness reveals neurogenic changes, including fibrillations, positive sharp waves, fasciculations and high amplitude polyphasic motor unit action potentials in muscles innervated by the affected root and, sometimes, in muscles at a distance from this region (Gardner-Thorpe et al. 1976). Sphincter involvement may occur (Jellinek and Tulloch 1976). Neurophysiological studies in patients with post-herpetic myelopathy have not been evaluated. Nurmikko and Bowsher (1990) have suggested that there are both peripheral and central components to post-herpetic neuralgia.

Poliomyelitis and Post-polio Syndrome

Anterior poliomyelitis is an acute disorder in which there is viral invasion and destruction of anterior horn cells and motor neurones in the cranial motor nuclei, leading to the rapid onset of lower motor neurone paralysis in the distribution of the affected motoneuronal nuclei. EMG features of denervation, especially fibrillation potentials, appear about three weeks after the onset and when recovery begins polyphasic motor unit action potentials of increasing amplitude can be recorded, consistent with reinnervation. Fibrillation potentials can be recorded in affected muscles for many years afterwards in the absence of change in muscular strength. In some patients, several decades after the acute infection, increasing fatiguability develops, a syndrome termed post-polio syndrome (Halstead and Rossi 1985; Cashman et al. 1987). These symptoms develop in muscles initially paralysed during the acute phase of the disease and may be sufficient to cause increasing disability. This late complication can be distinguished from motor neurone disease by the restricted distribution of the new symptoms, and by the absence of upper motor neurone signs. EMG studies show increased jitter and blocking when single fibre EMG techniques are used, probably due to degeneration of the terminal arborization of enlarged reinnervated motor units due to age effects on the surviving motoneuronal pool (Weichers and Hubbell 1981).

Decompression Sickness

Rapid decompression after equilibration during a dive carries the risk of gas bubble formation in the vascular system, and perhaps also in the tissues, that in the nervous system may lead to myelin degeneration in the brain and spinal cord. The latter is a site of special vulnerability to decompression sickness (Type 2 or neurological bend) with consequent spasticity and sensory disturbance. Somatosensory evoked potential studies have been used in the early stages of the illness to document involvement of the spinal cord, in studies with stimulation of the tibial nerves, but there is usually rapid recovery that parallels clinical improvement. Early-detected abnormalities in SEP in divers with Type 2 bends do not predict the neurological outcome (James 1988; Smith and Trojaborg 1988).

Monitoring of Spinal Cord Functions During Spinal Surgery

Because there is a small risk of paraplegia complicating spinal surgery, especially during correction of scoliosis and during laminectomy for cervical and thoracic spondylosis or other myelopathies, neurophysiological methods have been developed to monitor spinal cord function. These consist of three measures, somatosensory evoked responses, electromyography and cortical motor responses. These assess proprioceptive and cutaneous afferents in the spinocerebellar tracts and dorsal columns (Jacobson and Tew 1987), anterior horn cell and root function (Harper et al. 1988) and corticospinal tract function (Boyd et al. 1986) respectively. Only the last technique directly assesses the descending motor tracts.

Somatosensory evoked potentials do not assess motor pathways and in 11 of 351 patients operated for correction of scoliosis in Harper et al.'s (1988) series motor deficit occurred without change on the SEP. In 7 patients the SEP amplitude changed during the operation; in 2 of these the SEP change did not improve and paraplegia developed; in 3 the SEP improved after surgery was halted and there was no permanent neurological disability. Thus SEP monitoring was clinically useful in only 1% of patients. False negative changes in

SEP have been noted by others (Lesser et al. 1986). SEP changes without neurological deficit have also been reported (Chatrian et al. 1988) and this technique is therefore not a reliable predictor of outcome.

During surgery, SEPs must be monitored both rostral and caudal to the level of pathology, using Kirschner wire electrodes placed adjacent to the spinous processes, or needle electrodes placed in the interspinous ligament close to the dura. Stimuli applied to tibial or median nerves are used as appropriate. The deeper levels of anaesthesia result in changes in the SEPs but, generally, a reduction in amplitude of greater than 50%, or an increase in latency greater than 2 ms are significant changes warranting pause in surgery, or even measures to awaken the patient to test motor function in the legs (Lesser et al. 1985).

Stimulation of the motor cortex can be used in the anaesthetized, paralysed patient to assess corticospinal tract function by recording the evoked spinal cord potential, reflecting corticospinal tract function, with epidural electrodes (Levy et al. 1984; Boyd et al. 1986). Kitagawa et al. (1989) used this method in 20 patients undergoing upper cervical spine surgery. In 5 patients transient attenuation of the response did not signify clinical impairment; in 1 patient the response disappeared and there was complete postoperative quadriplegia and in 2 patients initially small responses improved during tumour removal with excellent postoperative recovery.

References

Abbruzzese G, Dall'agata D, Morena M, et al. (1988) Electrical stimulation of the motor tracts in cervical spondylosis. J Neurol Neurosurg Psychiatry 51:796–802

Aminoff MJ (1984) The clinical role of somatosensory evoked potential studies: a critical appraisal. Muscle Nerve 7:345–354

Ammassian VE, Gracco RQ, Maccabee PJ (1989) Focal stimulation of human cerebral cortex with the magnetic coil: a comparison with electrical stimulation. Electroencephalogr Clin Neurophysiol 74:401–416

Anderson NE, Frith RW, Synek VM (1986) Somatosensory evoked potentials in syringomyelia. J Neurol Neurosurg Psychiatry 49:1407–1410

Angell RW, Hoffmann WW (1963) The H reflex in normal, spastic and rigid subjects. Arch Neurol 9:591–596

Armon C, Daube JR (1989) Electrophysiological signs of arteriovenous malformations of the spinal cord. J Neurol Neurosurg Psychiatry 52:1176–1181

Barker AT, Jalinous R, Freeston IL (1985) Non-invasive magnetic stimulation of human motor cortex. Lancet 2:1106–1107

Baumhefner RW, Tourtellotte WW, Syndulko K, et al. (1990) Quantitative multiple sclerosis plaque assessment with magnetic resonance imaging. Arch Neurol 47:19–26

Berardelli A, Inghilleri M, Formisano R, et al. (1987) Stimulation of motor tracts in motor neuron disease. J Neurol Neurosurg Psychiatry 50:732–737

Berger AR, Shahani BT (1989) Electrophysiologic evaluation of spinal cord motor conduction. Muscle Nerve 12:976–980

Bernstein LP, Antel JP (1981) Motor neuron disease: decremental responses to repetitive nerve stimulation. Neurology 31:202–204

Boyd SG, Rothwell JC, Cowan JM, et al. (1986) A method of monitoring function in corticospinal pathways during scoliosis surgery with a note on motor conduction velocities. J Neurol Neurosurg Psychiatry 49:251–257

Burke D, Skuse NF, Lethlean AK (1981) Cutaneous and muscle afferent components of the cerebral potential evoked by electrical stimulation of human peripheral nerves. Electroencephalogr Clin Neurophysiol 51:579–588

Cashman VR, Maselli, R, Wollman RL, et al. (1987) Late denervation in patients with antecedent paralytic poliomyelitis. N Engl J Med 317:7–12

Chatrian GE, Burger MS, Wirch AL (1988) Discrepancy between intra-operative SSEP's and post-operative function. J Neurosurg 69:450–454

Chiappa K (1980) Pattern-shift visual, brain stem auditory and short-latency somatosensory evoked potentials in multiple sclerosis. Neurology 30:110–123

Chiappa KH (1983) Evoked potentials in clinical medicine. Raven, New York, pp 1–340

Chiappa KH, Ropper AH (1982) Evoked potentials in clinical medicine 2. N Engl J Med 306:1205–1211

Claus D. Harding AE. Hess CW, et al. (1988) Central motor conduction in degenerative ataxic disorders: a magnetic stimulation study. J Neurol Neurosurg Psychiatry 51:790–795

Colon EJ, Rottevell JJ, Stegeman DF, et al. (1988) Abnormal EMG and SSEP in a young child with an ependymoma. Clin Neurol Neurosurg 90:249–252

Conradi S, Grimby L, Lundemo G (1982) Pathophysiology of fasciculations in ALS as studied by electromyography of single motor units. Muscle Nerve 5:202–208

Cowan JMA, Dick JPR, Day BL, et al. (1984) Abnormalities in central motor pathway conduction in multiple sclerosis. Lancet 2:304–307

Cruikshank JK, Rudge P, Dalgliesh AG, et al. (1989) Tropical spastic paraparesis and human T cell lymphotropic virus Type 1 in the United Kingdom. Brain 112:1057–1090

Dawson GD (1954) A summation technique for the detection of small evoked potentials. Electroencephalogr Clin Neurophysiol 6:65–84

Denny-Brown D, Pennybacker JB (1938) Fibrillation and fasciculation in voluntary muscle. Brain 61:311–332

Dimitrijevic MR (1986) Neurocontrol of the upper motor neuron and progressive neuromuscular diseases. In: Dimitrijevic MR, Kakulas BA, Vrbová G (eds) Recent achievements in restorative neurology. 2. Progressive neuromuscular diseases. Karger, Basel, pp 39–52

Donofrio PD, Walker FO (1988) Tabes dorsalis: electrodiagnostic features. J Neurol Neurosurg Psychiatry 51:1087–1089

Eisen A, Yufe R, Trop D, et al. (1978) Reduced neuromuscular transmission safety factor in multiple sclerosis. Neurology 28:598–602

Eisen A, Shtybel W, Murphy K, et al. (1990) Cortical magnetic stimulation in amyotrophic lateral sclerosis. Muscle Nerve 13:146–151

Fincham RW, Cape CA (1968) Sensory nerve conduction in syringomyelia. Neurology 18:200–201

Fine EJ, Soria E, Paroski MW, et al. (1990) The neurophysiological profile of vitamin B12 deficiency. Muscle Nerve 13:158–164

Fisher MA (1983) F response analysis of motor disorders of central origin. J Neurol Sci 62:13–22.

Ganes T (1980) Somatosensory conduction times and peripheral cervical and cortical evoked potentials in patients with cervical spondylosis. J Neurol Neurosurg Psychiatry 43:683–689

Gardner-Thorpe C, Foster JB, Barwick DD (1976) Unusual manifestations of Herpes zoster. J Neurol Sci 28:427–447

Gout O, Gessain A, Bolgert F, et al. (1989) Chronic myelopathies associated with human T lymphotropic virus Type 1. Arch Neurol 46:255–260

Halstead LS, Rossi CD (1985) New problems in old polio patients: results of a survey of 539 polio survivors. Orthopedics 8:845–853

Harding AE (1984) The hereditary ataxias and related disorders. Churchill Livingstone, Edinburgh

Harper CM, Daube JR, Litchey WJ, et al. (1988) Lumbar radiculopathy after a spinal fusion for scoliosis. Muscle Nerve 11:386–391

Helweg-Larsen S, Jakobsen J, Borsen F, et al. (1988) Myelopathy in AIDS: a clinical, neuroradiological and electrophysiological study of 23 Danish patients. Acta Neurol Scand 77:64–73

Hess CW, Mills KR, Murray NMF, et al. (1989) Magnetic brain stimulation: central motor conduction studies in multiple sclerosis. Ann Neurol 22:744–752

Ingram DA, Swash M (1987) Central motor conduction is abnormal in motor neuron disease. J Neurol Neurosurg Psychiatry 50:159–166

Ingram DA, Thompson AJ, Swash M (1988) Central motor conduction in multiple sclerosis: evaluation of abnormalities revealed by transcutaneous magnetic stimulation of the brain. J Neurol Neurosurg Psychiatry 51:487–494

Jacobson GP, Tew JM (1987) Intraoperative evoked potential monitoring. J Clin Neurophysiol 4:145–176

James PB (1988) Late changes in the motor unit after acute poliomyelitis. Muscle Nerve 4:524–528

Janko M, Trontelj JV, Gersak K (1989) Fasciculation in motor neuron disease: discharge rate reflects extent and recency of collateral sprouting. J Neurol Neurosurg Psychiatry 52:1375–1381

Jellinek EH, Tulloch WS (1976) Herpes zoster with dysfunction of bladder and anus. Lancet 2:1219–1222

Jones SJ (1977) Short latency potentials recorded from the neck and scalp following median nerve stimulation in man. Electroencephalogr Clin Neurophysiol 43:853–863

Kakigi R, Shibasaki H, Kuroda Y, et al. (1988) Multimodality evoked potentials in HTLV-1 associated myelopathy. J Neurol Neurosurg Psychiatry 51:1094–1096

Kaplan PW, Hosford DA, Werner MH, et al. (1988) Somatosensory evoked potentials in a patient with a cervical glioma and syrinx. Electroencephalogr Clin Neurophysiol 70:563–565

Katifi HA, Sedgwick EM (1986) Somatosensory evoked potentials from posterior tibial nerve and lumbosacral dermatomes. Electroencephalogr Clin Neurophysiol 35:249–259

Kimura J (1983) F wave determination in nerve conduction studies. In: Desmedt JE (ed) Motor control mechanisms in health and disease. Raven, New York, pp 961–975

Kimura J (1985) Abuse and misuse of evoked potentials as a diagnostic test. Arch Neurol 42:78–80

Kimura J (1989) Electrodiagnosis: in diseases of nerve and muscle, 2nd edn. Davis, Philadelphia

Kitagawa H, Itoh T, Takano H, et al. (1989) Motor evoked potential monitoring during upper cervical spine surgery. Spine 14:1078–1083

Lesser RP, Lueders H, Dinner DS, et al. (1985) Technical aspects of surgical monitoring using evoked potentials. In: Struppler A, Weindl A (eds) Electromyography and evoked potentials. Springer-Verlag, Berlin, pp 177–180

Lesser RP, Randzens P, Lueders H, et al. (1986) Postoperative neurological deficits may occur despite unchanged intraoperative somatosensory evoked potentials. Ann Neurol 19:22–25

Levy WJ (1984) Clinical experience with motor and cerebellar evoked potential monitoring. Neurosurgery 20:169–182

Masur H, Elgar CE, Render K, et al. (1989) Functional deficits of central sensory and motor pathways in patients with cervical spinal stenosis: a study of SEPs and EMG responses to non-invasive brain stimulation. Electroencephalogr Clin Neurophysiol 74:450–457

Matthews WB, Beauchamp M, Small DG (1974) Cervical somatosensory evoked responses in man. Nature 252:230–232

Matthews WB, Wattam-Bell JRB, Pountney E (1982) Evoked potentials in the diagnosis of multiple sclerosis; a follow up study. J Neurol Neurosurg Psychiatry 45:303–307

Matthews WB, Acheson ED, Batchelor JR, Weller RO (1985) McAlpine's multiple sclerosis. Churchill Livingstone, Edinburgh

Mayer RF (1965) Peripheral nerve function in vitamin B12 deficiency. Arch Neurol 13:355–362

McLeod JG (1971) An electrophysiological and pathological study of peripheral nerves in Friedreich's ataxia. J Neurol Sci 12:333–349

Merton PA, Morton HB (1980a) Stimulation of the cerebral cortex in the intact human subject. Nature 285:227

Merton PA, Morton HB (1980b) Electrical stimulation of human motor and visual cortex through the scalp. J Physiol 305:9–10

Mills KR, Murray NMF (1986) Electrical stimulation over the human vertebral column: which neuronal elements are excited? Electroencephalogr Clin Neurophysiol 63:582–589

Nurmikko T, Bowsher D (1990) Somatosensory findings in post-herpetic neuralgia. J Neurol Neurosurg Psychiatry 53:135–141

Oppenheimer DR (1978) The cervical cord in multiple sclerosis. Neuropathol Appl Neurobiol 4:151–162

Panayiotopoulos CP (1979) F chronodispersion: a new electrophysiologic method. Muscle Nerve 2:68–72

Pedersen L, Trojaborg W (1981) Visual, auditory and somatosensory pathway involvement in hereditary cerebellar ataxia, Friedreich's ataxia and familial spastic paraplegia. Electroencephalogr Clin Neurophysiol 52:283–297

Peiogolu-Harmoussi S, Fawcett PRW, Howel D, et al. (1989) F response frequency in motor neuron disease and cervical spondylosis. J Neurol Neurosurg Psychiatry 50:593–599

Petito CK, Cho E-S, Lemann W, et al. (1988) Neuropathology of acquired immunodeficiency syndrome (AIDS): an autopsy review. J Neuropathol Exp Neurol 45:636–646

Roth G (1984) Fasciculations and their F response. J Neurol Sci 63:299–306

Rothwell JC, Thompson PD, Day BL, et al. (1987) Motor cortex stimulation in intact man. 1. General characteristics of EMG responses in different muscles. Brain 110:1173–1190

Schriefer TN, Hess CW, Mills KR, et al. (1989) Central motor conduction studies in motor neuron disease using magnetic brain stimulation. Electroencephalogr Clin Neurophysiol 74:431–437

Schwartz MS, Swash M (1982) Pattern of involvement in the cervical segments in the early stage of motor neuron disease – a single fibre EMG study. Acta Neurol Scand 65:424–431

Schwartz MS, Stalberg E, Swash M (1980) Pattern of segmental motor involvement in syringomyelia: a single fibre EMG study. J Neurol Neurosurg Psychiatry 43:150–155

Sclabassi RJ, Namerow NS, Enns NF (1974) Somatosensory response to stimulus trains in patients with multiple sclerosis. Electroencephalogr Clin Neurophysiol 37:23–33

Sedgwick EM, Katifi HA (1987) How to record and interpret dermatomal somatosensory evoked potentials (DSEP). J Electrophysiol Technol 13:51–60

Smith SJM, Claus D, Hess CW, et al. (1989) F responses and central motor conduction in multiple sclerosis. Electroencephalogr Clin Neurophysiol 74:438–443

Smith T, Trojaborg W (1988) Somatosensory evoked potentials and spinal decompression sickness. Lancet 1:364–365

Snooks SJ, Swash M (1985) Motor conduction velocity in the human spinal cord: slowed conduction in multiple sclerosis and radiation myelopathy. J Neurol Neurosurg Psychiatry 48:1135–1139

Stalberg E (1982) Macroelectromyography in reinnervation. Muscle Nerve 5:S135–S138

Stalberg E, Thiele B (1975) Motor unit fibre density in the extensor digitorum communis muscle. J Neurol Neurosurg Psychiatry 38:874–880

Stalberg E, Schwartz MS, Trontelj JV (1975) Single fibre electromyography in various processes affecting the anterior horn cell. J Neurol Sci 24:403–415

Stark RJ, Kennard C, Swash M (1981) Hand wasting in spondylitic high cord compression. Ann Neurol 9:58–62

Stöhr M, Büttner UW, Riffel B, et al. (1982) Spinal somatosensory evoked potentials in cervical cord lesions. Electroencephalogr Clin Neurophysiol 54:251–265

Swash M, Schwartz MS (1982) A longitudinal study of changes in motor units in motor neuron disease. J Neurol Sci 56:185–197

Swash M, Schwartz MS (1988) Neuromuscular diseases, 2nd edn. Springer-Verlag, London

Swash M, Schotz CL, Vowles G, et al. (1988) Selective and asymmetric vulnerability of corticospinal and cerebellar tracts in motor neuron disease. J Neurol Neurosurg Psychiatry 51:785–789

Tang L-M, Schwartz MS, Swash M (1988) Postural effects on F wave in lumbosacral root compression and canal stenosis. Brain 111:13–19

Thompson PC, Dick JPR, Asselman P, et al. (1987) Examination of motor function in lesions of the spinal cord by stimulation of the motor cortex. Ann Neurol 21:389–396

Tomado H, Shibasaki H, Hirata J, et al. (1988) Central versus peripheral nerve conduction before and after treatment of subacute combined degeneration. Arch Neurol 45:526–529

Ugawa Y, Kohara N, Shimpo T, et al. (1988) Central motor and sensory conduction in adrenoleucomyeloneuropathy, cerebrotendinous xanthomatosis, HTLV-1 associated myelopathy and tabes dorsalis. J Neurol Neurosurg Psychiatry 51:1069–1074

Uhthoff W (1889) Untersuchungen über die bei der multiplen Herdsklerose vorkommenden Augenstörungen. Arch Psychiatr Nervenkr 21:55–116, 303–410

Vanasse M, Garcia Larrea L, Neuschwander P, et al. (1988) Evoked potential studies in Friedreich's ataxia and progressive early-onset cerebellar ataxia. Can J Neurol Sci 15:292–298

Weichers DO, Hubbell ST (1981) Late changes in the motor unit after acute poliomyelitis. Muscle Nerve 4:524–528

Weir A, Hansen S, Ballantyne JP (1979) Single fibre electromyographic jitter in multiple sclerosis. J Neurol Neurosurg Psychiatry 42:1146–1150

Williams C, Kozlowski MA, Hinton DR, et al. (1990) Degeneration of spinocerebellar neurons in amyotrophic lateral sclerosis. Ann Neurol 27:215–225

Zegers de Beyl D, Delecluse F, Verbanck P, et al. (1988) Somatosensory conduction in vitamin B12 deficiency. Electroencephalogr Clin Neurophysiol 69:313–318

Chapter 10

Radiculopathy due to Diseases other than Disc Disease

A.A. Eisen

By definition a radiculopathy involves the dorsal and/or ventral roots. One or more segmental levels may be affected depending upon the nature of the disease. Some diseases, for example, disc diseases, may involve several roots at the same time or different roots sequentially.

Resulting motor deficit is restricted to those muscles sharing a common innervation through a particular root (a myotome). However, because most muscles derive their innervation through two or more roots, the motor deficit that arises as a result of disease involving a single root is often incomplete and may be extremely mild.

The sensory deficit associated with disease of the dorsal root is restricted to an area of skin innervated through that root (a dermatome). The territory of most dermatomes overlaps so that in a single root lesion the involved area of sensory deficit is usually incomplete. The extent to which different sensory modalities are affected in root lesions depends largely upon the underlying cause. Compressed lesions mainly affect the largest diameter nerve fibres; the Ia and type II cutaneous afferents. This results in loss of the segmental stretch reflex, and altered vibration and touch in the relevant dermatome(s).

The efferent and afferent arcs subserving the monosynaptic stretch reflex leave and enter the spinal cord through the ventral and dorsal roots respectively. This reflex is usually decreased and may be lost early in a root lesion.

Investigation of radiculopathies should include electromyography, CT scanning and/or MRI. Myelography should only be considered after these non-invasive procedures have failed to confirm the diagnosis. Although there are many causes of radiculopathy (Table 10.1), compressive (entrapment) radiculopathy due to disc degeneration and/or spondylosis is the commonest. This is described elsewhere and in this chapter other causes of radiculopathy and diseases with which they are easily confused will be discussed.

Diabetic Radiculopathies

Radicular-plexopathies (polyradiculopathy) frequently complicate diabetes. Elderly men with type II diabetes are particularly prone to this neuropathy which most frequently involves the myotomes of the anterior thigh (L2, L3,

Table 10.1.   Some causes of radiculopathy

Diabetes
   Diabetic amyotrophy
   Thoracoabdominal radiculopathy
Sensory neuronopathies (ganglionopathies)
   Subacute
     Lymphoma
     Leukaemia
     Carcinoma
   Acute
     Antibiotics (penicillin)
     Idiopathic
Carcinomatous radiculopathy ("seeding")
Primary tumours of nerve roots
   Schwannoma
   Neurofibromatosis
Infectious/granulomatous radiculopathy
   Lyme disease
   Brucellosis
   Histiocytosis X
   AIDS
Spinal epidural abscess – tuberculosis
Zoster radiculitis
Spinal stenosis
Arachnoiditis
Non-degenerative bony root compression
   Rheumatoid arthritis
   Paget's disease
   Ankylosing spondylitis
   Bony malignancy
   Achondroplasia
Angiomatous malformation of root
Cervical-brachial neuritis
Thoracic outlet syndromes
   Neurogenic thoracic outlet
   Droopy shoulder syndrome

L4) (Wilbourn 1987). Although usually unilateral at onset, many cases go on to involve the contralateral side, not necessarily in a symmetrical fashion. Pain which is typically acute in onset is followed by muscle wasting and weakness, depression or loss of reflexes and sensory loss. Clinical and electrophysiological localization indicate that there may be involvement of root, plexus or nerve or more usually combinations of these. Proximal diabetic radicular-plexopathies often occur on a background of the much commoner diabetic symmetrical polyneuropathy (Asbury 1977; Bastron and Thomas 1981; Brown and Asbury 1984).

Lower lumbar, sacral and cervical roots are affected rarely compared to the upper lumbar myotomes and severe involvement of, for example, the C5, C6 roots should prompt one to seek an alternative cause for the radiculopathy. Diabetic amyotrophy, described originally by Garland (1955), can be reasonably regarded as a specific variant of diabetic polyradiculopathy.

Diabetes can also involve the thoracic roots (thoracic polyradiculopathy, thoracoabdominal radiculopathy). The usual presenting symptoms are pain and dysaesthesia involving the chest wall or abdomen (Sun and Streib 1981; Streib et al. 1986; Sellman and Mayer 1988; Stewart 1989). When pain predominates and is restricted to the abdomen, especially if limited to one quadrant, the disease may be misinterpreted as "an acute abdomen". In some cases abdominal swelling due to abdominal muscle weakness ensues which may further confound the situation. Electromyography shows active denervation (fibrillation and positive sharp waves) in the paraspinal muscles which are innervated by the diseased roots. Persistent pain, which is often debilitating, frequently responds to anti-inflammatory therapy in combination with phenytoin, carbamazepine or amitriptyline.

Ultimately drugs will be available that will prevent the metabolic derangements causing the complications of diabetes (see below). Meanwhile control of hyperglycaemia, hypertension and obesity is essential. Recognizing the potentially life-endangering threat posed by hypoglycaemia, intensive insulin therapy has been repeatedly shown to be effective in prevention of diabetic complications. Insulin therapy is required for all type I diabetics and may be appropriate therapy for all type II patients who do not become rapidly normoglycaemic with diet and oral sulphonylurea (Flint and Clements 1988).

The chronic complications of diabetes result from the interaction of hyperglycaemia and other metabolic consequences of insulin deficiency as well as poorly understood but independent genetic and environmental factors. Rise in tissue sorbitol secondary to concentration-dependent activation of polyol pathway activity by glucose and an accompanying fall in tissue myo-inositol and Na-K-ATPase activity have been linked to a self-reinforcing cyclic metabolic defect that accounts for rapidly reversible slowing of conduction in peripheral nerve (Greene 1988; Greene et al. 1988). Treatment aimed at neutralizing this series of events is the obvious approach for the future. Pancreatic transplant has been shown to prevent development of neuropathy in inbred diabetic rats (Orloff et al. 1988; Sima et al. 1988) and to ameliorate complicating neuropathy in humans (Sutherland et al. 1988; Van der Vliet et al. 1988).

Sensory Neuronopathies (Ganglionopathies)

Sensory neuronopathy is distinguishable from sensory neuropathy by the global, rather than distal, distribution of sensory loss, total areflexia and the absence of recordable sensory nerve action potentials in the face of normal muscle strength and compound motor action potentials, normal motor conduction velocities and needle electromyography (Asbury 1987; Donofrio et al. 1989). These electrophysiological features point to the dorsal root ganglion cell as the site of primary pathology (Fagius et al. 1983). The disease is usually subacute most often being associated with lymphoma, chronic lymphatic leukaemia and carcinoma (in particular oat cell carcinoma); it affects women more frequently than men and may precede the underlying malignancy by several months. Paraesthesia, dysaesthesia, aching in the limbs and ataxia of gait due to impairment of vibration and position sense are the cardinal clinical features. Cutaneous sensation may be relatively preserved.

Rarely an acute form of the disease occurs (Dawson et al. 1988; Knazan et al. 1990). It has most frequently but not invariably been associated with systemic antibiotic therapy especially penicillin. Occasionally, acute sensory neuronopathy has been reported in the absence of associated factors (Knazan et al. 1990). Nosologically it may form part of a broader spectrum of radiculo-neuropathies including acute pandysautonomia with severe sensory deficit (which involves both dorsal root ganglia and peripheral nerve) and possibly Guillain-Barré syndrome with sensory predominance (Hodson et al. 1984).

Carcinomatous Radiculopathy

A variety of primary tumours may be associated with secondary seeding around the spinal roots. Most common are secondary deposits from primary tumours of the breast, lung, prostate, kidney and lymphomas. When cancer is complicated by seeding of cells within the spinal dural sac pain is predominant occurring in almost every case (Gilbert et al. 1978). The pain is of two types: local and radicular. Most patients complain of local pain which usually is experienced near the site of the lesion as identified myelographically. Radicular pain is localized within one or two vertebral segments of the lesion and is most frequent in the cervical or lumbosacral regions and less common in the thoracic segments. The pain is often bilateral and felt as a girdle radiating from the back to the front of the chest or abdomen. Unlike that associated with herniated intervertebral discs, pain due to carcinomatous seeding is typically made worse by lying down and frequently awakens the patient from sleep.

Carcinomatous radiculopathy of this type is not necessarily associated with signs of spinal cord compression; about 50% of patients presenting with back pain associated with a known cancer have a radiculopathy (Rodichok et al. 1986; Ruff and Lanska 1989).

Primary Tumours of the Spinal Roots

In comparison to secondary tumour invasion of roots, primary spinal root neoplasm is uncommon. The most common benign nerve tumour that affects the spinal roots is a schwannoma (a nerve sheath tumour). They are slowly growing, usually presenting with radicular pain. Although usually solitary they may be multiple in association with neurofibromatosis (von Recklinghausen's disease) where they also may be malignant. Any spinal segment can be involved by schwannomas but they are most frequent in the thoracic segments. If large they can cause secondary cord compression. Neurofibromas are typically as-sociated with von Recklinghausen's disease and can occur on virtually any nerve including the ventral and dorsal spinal roots. Lipomas are other, but rarer, benign tumours recognized as a cause of radiculopathy. Most are within the lumbosacral spinal canal and cause symptoms which vary from discrete intermittent uni- or bilateral sciatica to severe flaccid paraplegia with sensory and bladder dysfunction (Lassman and James 1967).

Myeloradiculopathies: Infectious and Granulomatous Radiculopathy

There are a variety of inflammatory conditions which result in radiculitis, myelitis and frequently a combination of the two: myeloradiculitis. Many are referred to in Chapter 14. In this section emphasis will be placed on the extent to which these disorders involve the spinal roots.

Lyme Disease

This occurs worldwide as a multisystem disorder caused by a recently recognized tick-transmitted spirochete, *Borrelia burgdorferi*. Transmission is from a bite, usually during summer months, by *Ixodes dammini* or related ixodid ticks (Benhamou et al. 1988; Editorial, Lancet 1989). Typically it induces fever, chills, malaise, headache, a characteristic rash and polyarthritis (stage 1). The acute form is usually benign and responds favourably to therapy with tetracycline. Weeks to months later neurological involvement occurs in about 15% of patients (stage 2). This may happen in the absence of the familiar systemic manifestations or the skin rash typical of stage 1.

The triad of lymphocytic meningitis, cranial nerve involvement and radiculopathy (Bannwarth's syndrome) are the usual neurological features (Pachner and Steere 1985; Midgard and Hofstad 1987; Pachner et al. 1989; Wilder-Smith and Roelke 1989). Facial palsy, often bilateral, thoracic sensory radiculitis, motor radiculitis in the extremities, brachial plexitis, mononeuritis and mononeuritis multiplex are the commonest peripheral nerve manifestations. Rarely, painful and even persistent radiculopathy may be the sole presenting feature.

CSF examination reveals pleocytosis, raised spinal protein levels and oligoclonal bands. The diagnosis is confirmed by demonstrating antibodies to *B. burgdorferi* in the CSF and serum. Neurological manifestations are usually self-limiting resolving in several months but respond to IV penicillin G, 20 million U/day in divided doses over 10 days. In patients allergic to penicillin, tetracycline should be tried. Arthritis and acrodermatitis occurring months or years after the initial infection typify stage 3 of the disease. Therapy with third-generation cephalosporins should be considered to treat the late stages of the disease (Czachor and Gleckman 1989). These drugs can, however, cause side effects including bleeding (with use of Moxalactam or Cefoperazone) and a reaction akin to that induced by disulfiram (Antabuse) if taken in association with alcohol. Prolonged therapy is presently expensive.

Brucellosis

The neurological complications of brucellosis are protean and pathogenic mechanisms diverse (Bahemuka et al. 1988; Al Deeb et al. 1989). Neurological manifestations may be the presenting feature and include transient ischaemic attacks and stroke, encephalopathy, motor neurone disease, a cauda equina syndrome and radiculopathy. The disease can be difficult to diagnose and is usually confused with tuberculosis. Serology and culture are superior to radiography and scanning in the diagnosis of brucellosis (Lifeso et al. 1985). There is often a good response to antibiotic therapy but it is important that therapy be continued for a reasonable duration and best monitored with repeated agglutination titres.

Histiocytosis X

This group of diseases encompasses unifocal eosinophilic granuloma, Hans-Schuller-Christian disease (multifocal eosinophilic granuloma) and Letterer-Siwe disease. "X" refers to the frequent but not invariable presence of xanthomata. Common to all three of the histiocytoses is the existence of granulomatous infiltration of histiocytes. There have been several reports of single eosinophilic granulomas causing a compressive radiculopathy (Eil and Adornato 1977; Padovani et al. 1988). Radiotherapy has been found useful in therapy either alone or in addition to surgery.

AIDS

Inflammatory polyradiculopathy infrequently complicates AIDS in the absence of other neurological involvement (Eidelberg et al. 1986; Behar et al. 1987). There is usually progressive, multiple root disease with CSF pleocytosis and elevated protein. The onset is usually insidious and most frequently involves the lumbar and sacral roots leading to a progressive paraparesis and areflexia. A cauda equina syndrome may occur. There may be eventual spread to involve the thoracic and cervical roots. Autopsy studies reveal extensive necrosis, inflammatory infiltrates and focal vasculitis of the involved spinal roots.

Spinal Epidural Abscess

Spinal epidural abscesses are infections in the space between the dura mater and the surrounding vertebral bodies. Purulent liquid or granulomatous tissue, located in the posterior portion of the epidural space of the thoracic or lumbar spine, spans several vertebral levels. The prominent clinical features are fever, spine pain with a radicular distribution and, if untreated, subsequent paraparesis from cord compression. Mild blunt spinal trauma often provides a devitalized site susceptible to transient bacteraemia with subsequent abscess formation. In such cases the infecting organism is frequently *S. aureus* (Kaufman et al. 1980). Epidural abscess and disc space infection of this type had, until recently, declined markedly in frequency (Verner and Musher 1985; Danner and Hartman 1987). However, with the abundance of drug abuse there has been a resurgence of these conditions especially amongst intravenous drug users and patients with human immunodeficiency virus (HIV) syndrome (Koppel et al. 1988). In many patients so affected, the course is subacute developing over several months with radicular pain commonly occurring. A preceding or associated fever is frequently absent or temperature may be only minimally elevated. The lower thoracic or lumbosacral spines are most commonly involved. Diagnostic evaluation should include spine radiographs, myelography with or without CT, nuclear bone scanning and radioactive gallium scanning. Staphylococcal infection is the commonest infective agent causing abscess amongst drug users.

Spinal tuberculous abscesses usually occur as a single small focus of infection; there is seldom evidence of active TB in another site and chest X-rays may be normal. Compared to bacterial infection, patients are younger (unless the abscess is associated with drug abuse) and back pain is usually much more chronic.

Zoster Radiculitis

Herpes zoster (shingles) represents latent reactivation of the varicella virus which has remained dormant in trigeminal or dorsal root ganglia following childhood chickenpox. Herpes zoster occurs in about 1% of the population. It is commoner in older subjects and occurs in about 25% of patients with cancer, especially lymphoma, and in immunocompromised patients including those with AIDS (Tenser 1984).

Radicular symptoms (pain, sensory deficit, weakness, depression or loss of appropriate reflexes) usually accompany the presence of vesicles in the relevant dermatome (Burkman et al. 1988). However, they may be absent or scanty and go unnoticed by the patient (zoster sine herpete) (Lewis 1958; Mayo and Booss 1989). Mid thoracic and trigeminal involvement is common, but when lumbosacral roots are involved, especially if there is associated motor deficit, the diagnosis may be easily confused with commoner causes of radiculopathy.

Spinal Stenosis

Mechanical compression of spinal roots from protruding discs or narrowed intervertebral foramina are the commonest causes of radiculopathy. These are largely dealt with elsewhere in this text. Mention here will only be made of spinal stenosis which typically affects elderly men (about 65 years old) more frequently than women. Intermittent *neurogenic* claudication with pain in the hips, thighs or legs brought on by walking are characteristic features (Lipson 1987; Torg and Pavlov 1987; Winter and Jani 1989). However, pain may also be initiated by lying supine and awaken the patient from sleep. Pain or numbness in the feet may also occur and when persistent can mimic and cause confusion with peripheral neuropathy. Most cases of spinal stenosis affect the lumbar spine and roots (L3/4 and L5/S1) at the rostral end of the cauda equina. Often the neurological examination is normal but objective deficit can be precipitated by mild or moderate exertion such as walking a few stairs. Occasionally the cervical cord may be involved. When this happens, transient reversible quadriplegia due to cervical cord neurapraxia occurs. In congenital spinal stenosis the whole spinal canal may be narrowed and cervical cord and cauda equina root compression become evident at a much younger age.

Arachnoiditis

Although this can occur anywhere in the meninges, the lumbosacral region is most commonly affected. The arachnoid becomes thickened and scarred, becoming adherent to the pia and dura. There is secondary obliteration of the meningeal vasculature. Single or multiple spinal roots become entrapped in the adhesions. The underlying mechanism(s) causing arachnoiditis is poorly understood but when experimentally induced in animals it is associated with decreased beta-endorphin in the CSF (Lipman and Haughton 1988).

The causes of arachnoiditis are varied and may follow trauma (including disc herniation) or spinal surgery, intrathecal injections including radiological contrast media or epidural anaesthesia (Sghirlanzoni et al. 1989). The latent period between the original insult and development of symptoms varies from a few months to several years. Spinal meningeal infections, particularly tuberculosis, syphilis and cryptococcosis or rarely cysticercosis, may be also complicated by arachnoiditis as can subarachnoid haemorrhage (Tjandra et al. 1989). Frequently, however, arachnoiditis seems to develop de novo, without apparent cause.

The clinical features of arachnoiditis are those of single or multiple root compression. Later a cauda equina syndrome develops and if the brunt of the disease is rostral to L2/L3 the cord may eventually be compressed. Chronic back pain with radiation down both legs is a prominent feature which early on in the disease may be the only symptom and unaccompanied by objective neurological deficit. Arachnoiditis is usually easily visible on enhanced CT scan. Whereas MRI is superior to CT in visualizing cord enlargement, compression or atrophy, it is not as sensitive as CT for documenting arachnoiditis (Karnaze et al. 1988).

Non-degenerative Bony Compression of Roots

Several conditions other than disc degeneration or degenerative spondylosis may cause radiculopathy from bony encroachment upon the spinal roots. The commonest of these include rheumatoid arthritis, Paget's disease, bony malignancy and achondroplasia. Secondary invasion of bone from primary tumours of the breast, lung, prostate, kidney and bowel are also common. Usually local pain with subsequent radicular pain indicates that there has been vertebral collapse entrapping the root. This may then go on to compression of the cord.

In rheumatoid arthritis and other arthropathies vertebral deformities may result in isolated nerve root compression, subluxation with secondary cord compression and susceptibility to trauma. Lesser trauma than usual can result in fractures of an arthritic spine and extradural haematoma. Ankylosing spondylitis shares similar potential complications. A cauda equina syndrome, commencing as single- or multi-level radiculopathy, at times unilaterally, can occur several years after the onset of the spondylitis. This complication is more common in ankylosing spondylitis than in the other arthropathies (Kramer and Krouth 1978). An unusual cause of mechanical root compression is a synovial cyst associated with the apophyseal joint (Hammer 1988).

Paget's disease is frequently complicated by neurological disturbances (Chen et al. 1979). This chronic progressive disease of bone is characterized by an abnormally rapid rate of bone resorption and unregulated reparative bone formation causing gross deformities of the skeleton. Neurological complications are often serious and given their potential reversibility by therapeutic agents such as calcitonin, mithramycin and etidronate require careful and early recognition. The most common picture associated with spinal root involvement due to Paget's disease is low back pain with radicular spread, leg weakness and sensory changes. In contrast, spinal cord compression is most frequent in the thoracic region where the highest ratio of cord to spinal canal cross-sectional area exists.

Neurological disorders in achondroplasia are produced by structural anomalies of the cranium (resulting in hydrocephalus) and spinal canal (producing spinal and radicular compression). The spinal canal in this disease has a decreased cross-sectional area and the intervertebral foramina are narrowed (Blondeau et al. 1984; Lonstein 1988). These changes reduce the area for the dural sac and exiting spinal nerves. Cervical-occipital compression is more frequent in childhood and may occur in the first months of life (Hecht et al. 1984). Decompressive surgery is successful in preventing these complications (Shikata et al. 1988). In later years disc degeneration with disc space narrowing and osteophyte formation further complicate an already compromised spinal canal and intervertebral foramina.

Angiomatous Radiculopathy

Angiomatous malformations of the spinal cord usually result in cord compression or ischaemia resulting in long tract signs or sometimes a mixture of upper and lower motor neurone dysfunction (see Chapter 18). Rarely, angiomas may primarily involve the cauda equina or occasionally only a single spinal root (Browne et al. 1976; Gennuso et al. 1989). Extramedullary-intradural haemangioblastomas are often attached to posterior nerve roots and radicular pain, posterior column sensory loss or both are frequent presenting symptoms. Equally unusual is lumbosacral plexopathy or painful radiculopathy secondary to abdominal aneurysm (Lainez et al. 1989)

Brachial Neuritis

Paralytic brachial neuritis (also referred to as neuralgic amyotrophy and the Parsonage-Turner syndrome) can closely mimic cervical radiculopathy and brief commentary is required given the relevance of this disease in the differential diagnosis of cervical root lesions (Parsonage and Turner 1948; Turner and Parsonage 1957).

Characteristically, the syndrome is of acute onset, often with severe pain, accompanied, or more usually followed in several days, by the onset of weakness and subsequent muscle wasting. Mild cases develop pain and weakness but do not go on to develop muscle wasting. The distribution of the pain and weakness is variable, characteristically being poorly localized in terms of peripheral anatomy, involving rather combinations of different peripheral nerves and various components of the brachial plexus. Careful clinical analysis suggests that the lesion in many cases of paralytic brachial neuritis is localized to branching points of the brachial plexus or its major peripheral nerves (England and Sumner 1987).

The aetiopathogenesis of this disease is not known, however, about 50% of cases are associated with antecedent events, such as immunization, viral infections, surgery, trauma, pregnancy, drug abuse and collagen vascular diseases. There is a rare familial form (Dunn et al. 1978), some cases of which have proven to have tomacular neuropathy (Madrid and Bradley 1975) and occasionally the condition is recurrent (Bradley et al. 1975). The majority of patients make a satisfactory, but usually slow, recovery taking one to three years. About 10% of patients do not regain useful function of the involved muscles.

Pathological observations in brachial neuritis are rare (Tsairis et al. 1972). A recent report of two patients with recurrent symptoms who, because of developing a tender supraclavicular mass underwent surgery, showed macroscopic fusiform segmental swelling of the trunks of the brachial plexus. Microscopically the lesions were characterized by oedema, onion bulb formation and marked focal chronic inflammatory infiltrates with lymphoid follicle formation, limited to the endoneurial compartment (Cusimano et al. 1988).

Thoracic Outlet Syndromes

The concept of thoracic outlet has evolved over the past century. Controversy surrounds virtually every aspect of it (Cuetter and Bartoszek 1989). However, in the context of the present chapter the critical issue lies in the differential diagnosis of root lesions, especially involvement of C8, T1 cervical roots. Pragmatically it can be argued that most, if not all, thoracic outlet syndromes are of two types. The very rare *true neurogenic thoracic outlet syndrome* and the very common *droopy shoulder syndrome*.

Neurogenic thoracic outlet syndrome has been well delineated (Gilliatt 1976; Gilliatt et al. 1978). It is rare and the author has seen fewer than 20 cases in 25 years of neurological and electromyographic practice. Typically it affects young women and presents with painless, partial, thenar wasting. But in contradistinction to carpal tunnel syndrome, sensory complaints, when they occur, involve the medial aspect of the forearm and ulnar side of the hand. The symptoms are directly due to pressure or stretching of the lower trunk or C8, T1 roots from a fibrous band attached to a supernumerary rib or elongated C7 transverse process. When extra ribs are present, they often occur bilaterally, but usually it is the less prominent rib (with the longer fibrous band) that is the one responsible for symptoms. X-ray or CT scan does not invariably reveal an extra rib or elongated C7 transverse process and therefore normal radiological studies do not rule out neurogenic thoracic outlet syndrome.

Electrophysiological studies are helpful in the diagnosis and localization of the lesion (Wilbourn 1982, 1988). A constellation of characteristic abnormalities have evolved. They are:

1. A much reduced median motor compound action potential in the face of a normal median sensory compound action potential.
2. A reduced or absent ulnar sensory compound action potential in the face of a normal or only modestly reduced ulnar motor compound action potential.

3. A prolonged or absent ulnar F wave.
4. A prolonged and/or small ulnar somatosensory evoked potential.
5. Needle EMG evidence for chronic partial denervation in the C8 and T1 supplied muscles.

In contrast to the above, the droopy shoulder syndrome, a term coined by Swift and Nichols (1984), is common and accounts for many if not most other cases of thoracic outlet syndrome. This syndrome is virtually limited to women. The following are the criteria for droopy shoulder syndrome:

1. Pain or paraesthesia occurring in the shoulder, arm, forearm or hand.
2. Long, graceful and swan-like neck; low set shoulders, and horizontal or downsloping clavicles.
3. Exacerbation of symptoms on palpation of brachial plexus or passive downward traction of the arms.
4. Immediate relief of symptoms by passive shoulder elevation.
5. Absence of vascular phenomena, muscle atrophy, sensory loss or reflex changes.
6. Normal electrophysiological studies.
7. The second thoracic or lower vertebrae are visible above the shoulders on lateral cervical spine X-rays.

Electrophysiological Investigation of Radiculopathies

CT scanning and MRI give excellent visualization of the nerve root and spinal cord and it is relevant to ask what, if any, is the role of electrophysiology in an era of these advanced radiological techniques. The presence of a radiological and clinical defect do not always go hand in hand. In older subjects silent radiological defects commonly occur in the absence of clinically obvious disease. In contrast, many of the inflammatory radiculopathies are not accompanied by radiological abnormalities. Radiological abnormalities give little or no information regarding severity and potential for prognosis and when several segmental levels are involved it is often not possible to determine on radiological grounds which or how many levels have clinical relevance.

Several different electrophysiological techniques are available for the assessment of root lesions (Tonzola et al. 1981; Eisen 1987; Wilbourn and Aminoff 1988). Each will be discussed briefly.

Motor and Sensory Conductions

Usually, these are normal in root lesions. If axonal destruction or loss has been marked there may be moderate slowing of motor conduction velocity in relevant nerves. More importantly, axonal loss is accompanied by reduced amplitude of the compound muscle action potential and side-to-side comparison of homologous muscles is useful in unilateral lesions. A reduction of greater than

50% indicates that there has been a considerable loss of axons and consequently, if spontaneous recovery is to be anticipated, it is likely to be delayed and incomplete. In the majority of root lesions, those due to mechanical causes, the dorsal root ganglion lies distal to the site of compression or entrapment. As a result the sensory nerve action potential remains normal. A reduced, or absent sensory nerve action potential indicates that either the lesion is distal to the dorsal root or that one is dealing with a true ganglionopathy in which there has been ganglion cell loss.

Needle Electromyography

This is by far the most useful of the various electrophysiological tests available for assessing root lesions. It is rare for other tests to be abnormal in the face of a normal needle EMG. The presence of fibrillation or positive sharp waves is proof positive that there is ongoing, or previous, axonal damage with resulting muscle denervation. This then becomes an important issue in prognosis (not available through imaging). Unfortunately fibrillation takes time to develop. It develops first in the paraspinal muscles which are innervated directly from the spinal root through the medial branch of its posterior primary ramus. In these muscles it can take up to a week to 10 days before fibrillation becomes evident. In distal limb muscles development of fibrillization can take as long as 6 weeks. Paraspinal needle EMG is not only a useful prognostic feature but is also valuable in localization. In the lumbosacral region there is reasonable specificity as to segmental level especially in the deeper muscle layers (multifidi). In the cervical region there is considerably more overlap and segmental specificity is limited. For this reason it is common for quite severe cervical root lesions to occur without the developing fibrillation.

Proximal Conduction Studies

Various methods have been employed specifically to evaluate conduction slowing and/or block through the root. In single root lesions conduction block is reflected clinically by depression or loss of the relevant deep tendon reflex but because of shared innervation muscle weakness, if present, is modest and incomplete. Two methods in particular have proved of limited value in the assessment of radiculopathies. They are the *F response* and *somatosensory evoked potentials*. It is beyond the scope of this chapter to detail these techniques and controversies surrounding their use for which the reader is referred to more comprehensive texts. Essentially the F response is an antidromically induced excitation of the anterior horn cell resulting from supramaximal stimulation of a peripheral motor nerve. In root lesions its latency is sometimes prolonged or it may become unrecordable. The somatosensory evoked potential (SEP), is the measurable cortical response to a sensory, predominantly Ia afferent, stimulus. Because its impulse traffic traverses the root it can be used to assess conduction through the dorsal root fibres. Both techniques suffer from the fact that they attempt to measure slowed conduction or block through a very short segment of nerve, the root, diluted in a long length of normally conducting distal stretch of nerve. One other technique, the H reflex, shares the same limitations and additionally can only be easily applied to lesions of the S1 or the L5 roots.

Electrophysiological Confirmation of Root Avulsion

Root avulsion is important to diagnose since it precludes any attempt at neurosurgical reconstruction. Radiological confirmation using myelography usually delineates the extent of root injury. However, pseudomeningoceles with intact roots and root avulsion without characteristic radiological changes both occur. Electrophysiologically, root avulsion is associated with paraspinal and limb muscle denervation in the relevant myotome(s). A normal sensory nerve action potential in the presence of an anaesthetic and paretic limb reflects that the dorsal root has been separated from its central connections. For the same reason the histamine response (skin flare induced by intradermal histamine) remains intact. Absence of a SEP and inability to record a muscle action potential using cortical (magnetic) stimulation are further proof that the dorsal and ventral roots have been severed.

References

Al Deeb SM, Yaqub BA, Sharif HS, et al. (1989) Neurobrucellosis: clinical characteristics, diagnosis, and outcome. Neurology 39:498–501

Asbury AK (1977) Proximal diabetic neuropathy. Ann Neurol 2:179–180

Asbury AK (1987) Sensory neuropathy. Semi Neurol 7:58–66

Bahemuka M, Shemena AR, Panayiotopoulos CP, et al. (1988) Neurological syndromes of brucellosis. J Neurol Neurosurg Psychiatry 51:1017–1021

Bastron JA, Thomas JE (1981) Diabetic polyradiculopathy. Mayo Clin Proc 56:725–732

Behar R, Wiley C, McCutchan JA (1987) Cytomegalovirus polyradiculoneuropathy in acquired immune deficiency syndrome. Neurology 37:557–561

Benhamou Cl, Gauvain JB, Calamy G, Lemaire JF (1988) Lyme disease: clinical, biological and developmental aspects. 29 cases in the Orleans region. Rev Rhum Mal Osteoartic 55:647–653

Blondeau M, Brunet D, Blanche JM, et al. (1984) Compression of the cervical spinal cord in achondroplasia. Sem Hop Paris 60:771–775

Bradley WG, Madrid R, Thrush DC (1975) Recurrent brachial plexus neuropathy. Brain 98:381–398

Brown MJ, Asbury AK (1984) Diabetic neuropathy. Ann Neurol 15:2–12

Browne TR, Adams RD, Roberson GH (1976) Hemangioblastoma of the spinal cord. Review and report of five cases. Arch Neurol 33:435–441

Burkman KA, Gaines Jr RW, Kashani SR, Smith RD (1988) Herpes zoster: a consideration in the differential diagnosis of radiculopathy. Arch Phys Med Rehabil 69:132–134

Chen J, Rhee RSC, Wallach S, et al. (1979) Neurologic disturbances in Paget disease of bone: response to calcitonin. Neurology 29:448–457

Cuetter AC, Bartoszek DM (1989) The thoracic outlet syndrome: controversies, overdiagnosis, overtreatment and recommendations for management. Muscle Nerve 12:410–419

Cusimano MD, Bilbao JM, Cohen SM (1988) Hypertrophic brachial plexus neuritis: a pathological study of two cases. Ann Neurol 24:615–622

Czachor JS, Gleckman RA (1989) Third-generation cephalosporins. A plea to save them for specific infections. Postgrad Med 85:169–172, 175–176

Danner RL, Hartman BJ (1987) Update of spinal epidural abscess: thirty-five cases and review of the literature. Rev Infect Dis 9:265–274

Dawson DM, Samuels MA, Morris J (1988) Sensory form of acute polyneuritis. Neurology 38:1728–1731

Donofrio PD, Alessi AG, Albers JW, Knapp RH, Blaivas M (1989) Electrodiagnostic evolution of carcinomatous sensory neuronopathy. Muscle Nerve 12:508–513

Dunn HG, Daube JR, Gomez MR (1978) Heredofamilial brachial plexus neuropathy (hereditary neuralgic amyotrophy with brachial predilection) in childhood. Dev Med Child Neurol 20:28–46

Editorial (1989) Lancet 2:198–199

Eidelberg D, Sotrel A, Vogel H, Walker P, Kleefield J, Crumpacker CS (1986) Progressive polyradiculopathy in acquired immune deficiency syndrome. Neurology 36:912–916

Eil C, Adornato BT (1977) Radicular compression in multifocal eosinophilic granuloma. Successful treatment with radiotherapy. Arch Neurol 34:786–787

Eisen A (1987) Radiculopathies and plexopathies. In: Brown WF, Bolton CF (eds) Clinical electromyography. Butterworths, Boston, Toronto, pp 51–73

England JD, Sumner AJ (1987) Neuralgic amyotrophy: an increasingly diverse entity. Muscle Nerve 10:60–68

Fagius J, Westerberg CE, Olsson Y (1983) Acute pandysautonomia and severe sensory deficit with poor recovery. A clinical, neurophysiological and pathological case study. J Neurol Neurosurg Psychiatry 46:725–733

Flint MA, Clements RS (1988) Prevention of the complications of diabetes. Prim Care 15:277–284

Garland H (1955) Diabetic amyotrophy. Br Med J 2:1287–1290

Gennuso R, Zappulla RA, Strenger SW (1989) A localized lumbar spinal root arteriovenous malformation presenting with radicular signs and symtoms. Spine 14:543–546

Gilbert RW, Kim JH, Posner JB (1978) Epidural spinal cord compression from metastatic tumor: diagnosis and treatment. Ann Neurol 3:40–51

Gilliatt RW (1976) Thoracic outlet compression syndrome. Br Med J 1:1274–1275

Gilliatt RW, Willison RG, Dietz V, Williams IR (1978) Peripheral nerve conduction in patients with cervical rib and band. Ann Neurol 4:124–129

Greene D (1988) The pathogenesis and prevention of diabetic neuropathy and nephropathy. Metabolism 37:25–29

Greene DA, Lattimer SA, Sima AA (1988) Pathogenesis and prevention of diabetic neuropathy. Diabetes Metab Rev 4:201–221

Hammer AJ (1988) Synovial cyst: an unusual cause of nerve root compression. A case report. S Afr Med J 73:44–45

Hecht JT, Butler IJ, Scott CI (1984) Long-term neurological sequelae in achondroplasia. Eur J Pediatr 143:58–60

Hodson AK, Hurwitz BJ, Albrecht R (1984) Dysautonomia in Guillain-Barré syndrome with dorsal root ganglioneuropathy, Wallerian degeneration, and fatal myocarditis. Ann Neurol 15:88–95

Karnaze MG, Gado MH, Sartor KJ, Hodges FJ (1988) Comparison of MR and CT myelography in imaging the cervical and thoracic spine. Am J Roentgenol 150:397–403

Kaufman DM, Kaplan JG, Litman N (1980) Infectious agents in spinal epidural abscesses. Neurology 30:844–850

Knazan M, Bohlega S, Berry K, Eisen A (1990) Acute sensory neuronopathy with preserved SEPs and long-latency reflexes. Muscle Nerve 13:381–384

Koppel BS, Tuchman AJ, Mangiardi JR, Daras M, Weitzner I (1988) Epidural spinal infection in intravenous drug abusers. Arch Neurol 45:1331–1337

Kramer LD, Krouth GJ (1978) Computerized tomography. An adjunct to early diagnosis in the cauda equina syndrome of ankylosing spondylitis. Arch Neurol 35:116–118

Lainez JM, Yaya R, Lluch V, et al. (1989) Lumbosacral plexopathy caused by aneurysms of the abdominal aorta. Med Clin (Barc) 92:462–464

Lassman LP, James CCM (1967) Lumbosacral lipomas: critical survey of 26 cases submitted to laminectomy. J Neurol Neurosurg Psychiatry 30:174–181

Lewis GW (1958) Zoster sine herpete. Br Med J 2:418–421

Lifeso RM, Harder E, McCorkell SJ (1985) Spinal brucellosis. J Bone Joint Surg (Br) 67:345–351

Lipman BT, Haughton VM (1988) Diminished cerebrospinal fluid beta-endorphin concentration in monkeys with arachnoiditis. Invest Radiol 23:190–192

Lipson SJ (1987) Spinal stenosis. Rheum Dis Clin North Am 14:613–618

Lonstein JE (1988) Treatment of kyphosis and lumbar stenosis in achondroplasia. Basic Life Sci 48:283–292

Madrid R, Bradley WG (1975) The pathology of tomaculous neuropathy: studies on the formation of the abnormal myelin sheath. J Neurol Sci 25:415–448

Mayo DR, Booss J (1989) Varicella zoster-associated neurological disease without skin lesions. Arch Neurol 46:313–315

Midgard A, Hofstad H (1987) Unusual manifestations of nervous system *Borrelia burgdorferi* infection. Arch Neurol 44:781–783

Orloff MJ, Macedo A, Greenleaf GE (1988) Effect of pancreas transplantation on diabetic somatic neuropathy. Surgery 104:437–444

Pachner AR, Steere AC (1985) The triad of neurological manifestations of Lyme disease: meningitis, cranial neuritis and radiculoneuritis. Neurology 35:47–53

Pachner AR, Duray P, Steere AC (1989) Central nervous system manifestations of Lyme disease. Arch Neurol 46:790–795

Padovani R, Cavallo M, Tonelli MP, et al. (1988) Histiocytosis-X: a rare cause of radiculopathy. Neurosurgery 22:1077–1079

Parsonage MJ, Turner JWA (1948) Neurologic amyotrophy: the shoulder-girdle syndrome. Lancet 1:973–978

Rodichok LD, Ruckdeschel JC, Harper GR, et al. (1986) Early detection and treatment of spinal epidural metastases: the role of myelography. Ann Neurol 20:696–702

Ruff RL, Lanska DJ (1989) Epidural metastases in prospectively evaluated veterans with cancer and back pain. Cancer 63:2234–2241

Sellman MS, Mayer RF (1988) Thoracoabdominal radiculopathy. South Med J 81:199–201

Sghirlanzoni A, Marazzi R, Pareyson D, et al. (1989) Epidural anaesthesia and spinal arachnoiditis. Anaesthesia 44:317–321

Shikata J, Yamamuro T, Iida H, et al. (1988) Surgical treatment of achondroplastic dwarfs with paraplegia. Surg Neurol 29:125–130

Sima AA, Zhang WX, Tze WJ, et al. (1988) Diabetic neuropathy in STZ-induced diabetic rat and effect of allogenic islet cell transplantation. Morphometric analysis. Diabetes 37:1129–1136

Stewart JD (1989) Diabetic truncal neuropathy: topography of the sensory deficit. Ann Neurol 25:233–238

Streib EW, Sun SF, Paustian FF, Gallagher TF, Shipp JC, Ecklund RE (1986) Diabetic thoracic radiculopathy: electrodiagnostic study. Muscle Nerve 9:548–553

Sun SF, Streib EW (1981) Diabetic thoracoabdominal neuropathy: clinical and electromyographic features. Ann Neurol 9:75–79

Sutherland DE, Kendall DM, Moudry KC, et al. (1988) Pancreas transplantation in nonuremic, type I diabetic recipients. Surgery 104:453–464

Swift TR, Nichols FT (1984) The droopy shoulder syndrome. Neurology 34:212–215

Tenser RB (1984) Herpes simplex and herpes zoster: nervous system involvement. Neurol Clin 2:215–240

Tjandra JJ, Varma TR, Weeks RD (1989) Spinal arachnoiditis following subarachnoid haemorrhage. Aust NZ J Surg 59:84–87

Tonzola RJ, Ackel AA, Shahani BT, Young RR (1981) Usefulness of electrophysiological studies in the diagnosis of lumbosacral root disease. Ann Neurol 9:305–308

Torg JS, Pavlov H (1987) Cervical spinal stenosis with cord neurapraxia and transient quadriplegia. Clin Sports Med 6:115–133

Tsairis P, Dyck P, Mulder DW (1972) Natural history of brachial plexus neuropathy. Arch Neurol 27:109–117

Turner JWA, Parsonage MJ (1957) Neurologic amyotrophy (paralytic brachial neuritis). Lancet 2:209–212

Van der Vliet JA, Navarro X, Kennedy WR, et al. (1988) The effect of pancreas transplantation on diabetic polyneuropathy. Transplantation 45:368–370

Verner EF, Musher DM (1985) Spinal epidural abscess. Med Clin North Am 69:375–384

Wilbourn AJ (1982) True neurogenic thoracic outlet syndrome. American association of electromyography and electrodiagnosis, Rochester MN

Wilbourn AJ (1987) The diabetic neuropathies. In: Brown WF, Bolton CF (eds) Clinical electromyography. Butterworths, Boston, Toronto, pp 329–364

Wilbourn AJ (1988) Thoracic outlet syndrome surgery causing severe brachial plexopathy. Muscle Nerve 11:66–74.

Wilbourn AJ, Aminoff MJ (1988) The electrophysiologic examination in patients with radiculopathies. AAEE minimonograph 32. Muscle Nerve 11:1099–1114

Wilder-Smith E, Roelke U (1989) Meningopolyradiculitis (Bannwarth syndrome) as a primary manifestation of a centrocytic-centroblastic lymphoma. J Neurol 236:168–169

Winter M, Jani L (1989) The narrowed spinal canal. Dtsch Med Wochenschr 114:756–758

Chapter 11

Disc and Degenerative Disease: Stenosis, Spondylosis and Subluxation

C.H.G. Davis

More than a century ago, Godlee removed the first brain tumour (Davis and Bradford 1986); yet it was over 50 years later before the first extruded lumbar intervertebral disc was excised (Mixter and Barr 1934). Since the Second World War degenerative and disc disease affecting the contents of the spinal column, i.e. the spinal cord and cauda equina, has received increasing recognition and appears to be ever more common. As late as the 1930s, sciatica was thought to originate within the sciatic nerve and was treated with bizarre methods such as high pressure oxygen insufflation.

A static anatomical view of the vertebral column is relevant only to the narrow and relatively immobile thoracic canal. Degenerative disease occurs particularly in the lumbar region and within the more capacious and mobile cervical spine where the cervical nerve roots are able to move up to 3 cm within their dural sheaths during everyday life (Adams and Logue 1971). Although lacking the remarkable mobility of the upper cervical spine, the lumbar canal is also relatively mobile and capacious. Occasionally, narrowing of the cervical or lumbar canals may arise as a result of congenital or acquired disease, or from a combination of pathologies. In the cervical spine, degenerative changes may compress both the spinal cord and/or the exiting nerve roots. In the lumbar region, the spinal cord terminates at L2, (unless there is spinal dysraphism), and the single nerve roots, which run a long angulated course, are more at risk from degenerative disease than the main bulk of the cauda equina.

There is often considerable confusion over the nomenclature of degenerative disease. Spondylosis, disc disease and degenerative or osteoarthritic changes are interchangeable terms and are applied to radiological rather than to symptomatic features. "Radiculopathy" is commonly used to indicate neural compression of the cervical nerve roots and "sciatica" to indicate compression of the lower lumbar or first sacral nerve roots; yet it is highly probable that most pain in the upper and lower limbs associated with spinal degenerative disease does not arise from neural compression but from facet joints, the discs or soft tissues. "Stenosis" in its radiological sense is used to describe a narrowing of the axial plane of the spinal column by bone or soft tissue, or by subluxation.

Pathophysiology

The pathophysiology of spinal degenerative disease is reasonably understood and may indeed be considered to be part of the natural process of ageing. Clinical and radiological investigators tend to concentrate their attention on a particular problem as it arises and thus gain a static image which may not relate clearly to a patient's symptoms and signs. The function and efficiency of the spinal column depends on the mobility and integrated movements of the various soft tissues, joints and bones which also serve to protect the spinal cord and its emerging nerve roots. These tissues, particularly where the spine is most mobile, are also involved in the degenerative changes along with the intervertebral discs.

An intervertebral disc consists of three parts.

1. The annulus fibrosus with its tough fibrous tissue acts as a restraint between the vertebral bodies and contains the nucleus pulposus of the disc. The annulus can be penetrated by ruptured degenerate nuclear material posteriorly giving rise to central and lateral disc protrusions and extrusions.

2. The nucleus pulposus likewise contains a tough fibrous material and is compressible within the annulus fibrosus.

3. The hyaline cartilage end plates of the adjacent vertebral bodies are attached to the annulus peripherally.

When the nucleus of an intervertebral disc degenerates it assumes the quality of "crabmeat" tending to collapse on itself and so loses its ability to act as an hydrostatic shock absorber. As a disc space collapses and disc protrusions and extrusions occur, the annulus fibrosus has to take the additional strain which is transmitted to the hyaline cartilage end plates, and stimulates the formation of osteophytes (Findlay 1987). A vicious cycle is set up resulting in further collapse of the disc space. Facet joints at the same level are thrown out of alignment, and additional tension is placed upon the adjacent joints, disc spaces, ligaments and muscles. Pain may arise from distortion of soft tissues, facet joints and disc spaces (discogenic pain) and may be referred to distant sites, particularly if nerve roots are also compressed.

Cervical Spondylosis and Disc Disease

Although the cervical spine does not carry the weight of the lumbar spine it should not be forgotten that the cranium and its contents weigh something in the region of 6.5 kg and that the cervical spine is constantly moving through a greater range of movement than other parts of the vertebral column. The upper cervical spine (Cl–C3) is chiefly responsible for rotatory movements. At this level the spinal canal is at its widest, spondylotic disease is rare, and impingement on the spinal cord is unusual.

Anterior osteophyte formation rarely causes any problem except for the occasional case of dysphagia. However, lateral osteophyte and degenerative changes in the associated joints may predispose to neurological symptomatology where there is concomitant vascular disease as, for example, through compression of atherosclerotic or ectatic vertebral arteries.

Posterior disc protrusion with osteophyte formation will impinge either on the spinal cord causing a myelopathy or in the region of the exit root canal causing a radiculopathy; a combination of both is often demonstrable radiologically but not usually clinically (Brain et al. 1952; Adams and Logue 1971; Nurick 1972; Ogino et al. 1983; Yu et al. 1986a,b, 1987). Degenerative changes can result in fusion of vertebrae as a disc space collapses, and this in turn may place additional strain on the cervical spine. Subluxation is not uncommon, and may be either fixed or mobile.

It is well known that C4/5 and C5/6 levels are most commonly affected in degenerative disease and that C6/7 is less often involved. In the elderly, and particularly the very old, it has become increasingly recognized that the C3/4 level is frequently affected, possibly due to degeneration of the cervical spine resulting in spontaneous fusions at lower levels thereby leaving C3/4 as the only flexion-extension joint. Lateral disc protrusion is usually the only recognized change at C7/T1. Above C3 spondylitic changes may give rise to occipital neuralgia but surgery on the canal itself is rarely required.

Some people are born with a congenitally narrow cervical spine but symptoms rarely develop until the ligamentum flavum becomes thickened with advancing age. At this stage cervical canal stenosis may be diagnosed radiologically, and radiculopathy and myelopathy present clinically. It is not uncommon for canal stenosis to exist in both the cervical and lumbar regions, i.e. tandem stenosis.

Radiological features of degenerative cervical spine disease are present in more than 50% of the middle aged and elderly and indeed by the age of 80 there are very few members of the population who do not exhibit such radiological changes.

Predisposing Factors

It is generally accepted that wear and tear, and trauma, are common factors in the development of degenerative arthritis in association with joints. As far as the cervical spine is concerned, there is no question that severe trauma can result in degenerative changes occurring very rapidly, often in a period of months. Similarly, an anterior bone graft will produce vertebral fusion within 6 to 8 weeks. However, the majority of patients with symptomatic spondylosis have not suffered severe trauma, but careful questioning may reveal moderate trauma or repeated minor trauma. Manual workers such as miners often develop radiological signs of degenerative disease particularly as age advances. It is known that repeated moderate trauma may result in the speedy development of radiological spondylotic changes. The best example of this is to be found among National Hunt jockeys who suffer flexion injuries on several occasions through every riding season. Although none of these injuries on its own may require hospital admission, the cumulative effect of this trauma may become symptomatic within 5 to 10 years.

The time lag between trauma and the development of symptomatic disease may be several years. In the author's personal series of 200 patients requiring anterior cervical decompression, 7 were members of the Armed Services undertaking parachute jumps in the Second World War. None of these patients remembers suffering severe neck pain at any time. This extraordinarily high proportion of parachutists in an otherwise normal population would suggest that repeated moderate trauma may lead to degenerative changes 30 to 40 years later. There is also evidence that patients who experience what is generally thought to be minor trauma such as whiplash injuries may continue with symptomatic spondylotic symptoms after litigation has been settled. Patients with continual trauma such as those suffering from spasmodic torticollis and dystonia rapidly develop radiculopathy and myelopathy. It would thus seem that trauma is certainly the most common factor in the development of the degenerative process although the time interval may be extremely variable and it is impossible to predict which patients will be affected.

There are other predisposing factors. Patients with a congenitally narrow spinal canal such as achondroplastics (Spillane 1952) have a high incidence of cervical myelopathy. Patients with neurological disability affecting the lower limbs, e.g. following spinal cord injury or multiple sclerosis, tend to throw excessive strain on the cervical spine. Patients with congenital fusions (Klippel-Feil syndrome) and those who have had cervical spine surgery in childhood also tend to develop degenerative disease.

Cervical Radiculopathy

Natural History and Symptoms

It is important to recognize the natural history of cervical radiculopathy before embarking on unnecessary treatment and investigations. The majority of patients who suffer an acute neck pain do not have an acute disc protrusion. There are three types of presentation of cervical radiculopathy:

First – the acute cervical disc protrusion with radiculopathy (Findlay 1987). An acute disc protrusion may be extremely painful and is often associated with trauma. Although a history of trauma is usually obtained, the symptoms may not develop for hours or even days after the event. The patient complains of severe pain at the back of the neck immobilizing his neck and limbs and preventing sleep. Any movement is painful and the pain is made worse by coughing, sneezing and straining. There may also be a complaint of root pain in the appropriate dermatome radiating down the ipsilateral upper limb. Often there are paraesthesiae distally and weakness and sensory loss appropriate to the degree of nerve root compression.

Second – and much more common – is the subacute and relapsing or chronic variety of radiculopathy. As in the first category this may occur at any age. The symptoms are not as acute or severe as the acute lateral disc protrusion of the younger patient and are associated with a chronic relapsing course. The episodes tend to last days, and on occasions weeks, and then clear completely. There may be intervals of months or years between episodes and after several attacks the patient may complain of a constant neck pain which is relieved by rest.

Third – and more rare – is the silent radiculopathy occurring predominantly in the elderly. These patients may present with a sudden neurological deficit in an arm associated with little pain in the neck. Usually a history of previous neck problems is obtained, though these symptoms may not have caused medical consultation.

Signs

The patient with an acute cervical disc protrusion is usually in extreme pain, is unable to move his cervical spine, and holds his or her shoulder elevated on the ipsilateral side. Neck movements, coughing or straining result in radicular pain in a dermatomal distribution with spinothalamic sensory loss. The reflexes are absent or may be exaggerated at the affected level, depending on the exact anatomical site of the lateral disc protrusion in relation to the nerve root. A full neurological examination is mandatory and particular attention must be paid to the lower limbs to exclude a concomitant myelopathy.

The patient with a chronic relapsing radiculopathy is usually not in severe pain. The examination findings are similar to those for a patient with an acute cervical disc except that the neck movements are less severely affected. It is very common to find tender "fibrotic nodules" around the medial side of the scapula in the distribution of the appropriate dermatome. The older patient with a silent radiculopathy may have an obvious root neuropraxia accompanied by weakness, wasting or sensory loss.

Management, Differential Diagnosis and Investigation

Cervical radiculopathy is usually a benign disease. Hospitalization and surgery are rarely required. Symptoms often remit when treated with simple analgesics and rest, with or without a cervical collar. Investigation and management will depend on available facilities but must be complementary. There is no point in ordering an MR scan for a patient who has a mild neck problem.

Neurophysiological investigations are rarely necessary unless there is doubt as to the diagnosis – as may occur with a brachial plexus lesion or if multiple sclerosis, motor neurone disease, or other diffuse neurological conditions are suspected. Proximal nerve lesions at the nerve root may summate and be combined with more distal lesions, e.g. ulnar nerve compression at the medial epicondyle. Traumatic lesions to the neck may be combined with a brachial plexus lesion, and at other times it may be necessary to exclude the presence of a spinal tumour or infection involving the meninges.

In the presence of clinical evidence of radiculopathy or coexisting myelopathy, it is essential to perform detailed radiological investigations (Fig. 11.1). Plain X-rays (anteroposterior, lateral and oblique views) may confirm the level of involvement but do not alter management. Myelography, with or without CT scanning, or MRI is essential where there is weakness, wasting or objective sensory loss. Reflex changes on their own do not necessitate further investigation provided the patient is watched carefully.

A relative indication for further investigation is pain. The pain may be severe or less severe but episodic. If the patient's lifestyle is adversely affected

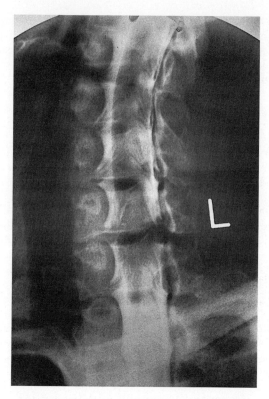

Fig. 11.1. Cervical radiculopathy. Myelogram oblique view; left lateral C6/7 disc protrusion.

and the symptoms are not improving or are worsening, either myelography or MR scanning is indicated.

Myelography still remains the best investigation for displaying nerve root compression in the cervical spine. With myelography it is possible to obtain flexion and extension views thus reproducing to a certain extent the physiological parameters for that patient. CT scanning (Yu et al. 1986a,b) without myelography is time consuming as it may be difficult to pinpoint which level to image and interpretation may be open to question. MR scanning (Modic et al. 1983), though ideal for imaging the spinal cord, requires axial views to image the nerve roots, and at present is of limited value in this respect. It is essential when the possibility of surgery arises that lateral plain X-rays in flexion and extension are obtained to show the degree of stability of the cervical spine.

Most patients respond to periods of analgesia and rest using a collar. Patients vary in their acceptance of collars. A substantial number will discard them after a few weeks; others become "addicts". There is some evidence that wearing a collar for very long periods results in a weakening of the cervical musculature. Isometric neck exercises are particularly useful in the management of painful radiculopathies as they encourage strengthening of the musculature without movement. Vigorous exercising and manipulation are to be avoided if a root lesion is suspected (Davis 1985). The length of time for which the patient should be observed prior to surgical referral will vary tremendously.

Surgery

The indications for surgery for cervical radiculopathy are progressive neurological signs and/or pain which has failed conservative treatment.

Where there is instability or subluxation, anterior discectomy by the anterior approach, using the natural plane between the carotid sheath and contents laterally, and pharynx and larynx medially, combined in most instances with fusion using autologous bone grafts (the Cloward procedure with the microscope), has found considerable favour (Cloward 1958; Lunsford et al. 1980; Grisoli et al. 1989). If there is instability without displacement, either the anterior approach or posterior approach (Henderson et al. 1983) i.e. foraminotomy with hemilaminectomy, will give similar results. Using the posterior approach, it is often not possible to remove disc material but an adequate nerve root decompression appears to achieve the same relief of symptoms.

Surgery for radiculopathy provides good relief in perhaps 75% of cases. The reason for lack of success in approximately a quarter of those operated upon may be that the nerve root has been irreparably damaged prior to operation. A more likely explanation arises from our lack of understanding of the mechanism of neck and upper limb pain. Where more than one intervertebral disc space is involved it may be necessary to perform a surgical procedure at several levels though care must be taken not to destabilize the spine. Fusion will throw additional strain over the coming years on the joints above and below perhaps resulting in later complications. Patients must be informed of the risks and the chances of success with any surgical procedure. In the older patient who has suffered a complete nerve root lesion of the silent variety, the outlook is ominous and it is debatable whether decompression has any place.

Cervical Spondylotic Myelopathy

Pathophysiology, Natural History and Symptoms

Cervical myelopathy tends to affect middle-aged and older patients, though younger patients can be affected by soft central disc protrusions. As with cervical radiculopathy, patients with a congenitally narrow canal with hypertrophy of the ligamentum flavum (stenosis), neurological disease affecting the central nervous system, or spinal cord injury, are prone to develop myelopathy (Brain et al. 1952; Nurick 1972; Kojima et al. 1989).

Cervical myelopathy due to disc protrusion and osteophyte formation, is not only the direct result of compression of the spinal cord but can also arise from vascular insufficiency, possibly due to compression of the anterior spinal artery. The presence of vascular changes may explain the occurrence of physical signs at a higher level than that demonstrated radiologically. Demyelination may also occur from compression, particularly in the older age group.

There are three clinical patterns of cervical spondylotic myelopathy. In the elderly especially, an acute episode may have a vascular basis. The patient awakes to find that he/she is unsteady in the lower limbs and has weakness with sensory loss in the hands. The patient may then remain on a plateau, perhaps with further acute episodes over months or years. The second form of myelopathy is an insidious progression over several months. The third and most common form is a mixture of episodic and progressive deterioration. However, some patients may appear to go into remission. All too often a careful history and examination will reveal that this is only an apparent remission. Where symptoms and signs continue for months or years, the results of decompressive laminectomy are disappointing. Thus, in the 1950s, neurologists were loath to send these patients for operation (Brain et al. 1952).

The symptoms of a cervical myelopathy are unsteadiness of gait usually affecting both lower limbs, difficulty with fine finger movement (e.g., doing up buttons, dropping objects), sensory loss in the hands, and uncomfortable peripheral dysaesthesiae. As the condition worsens there is a spastic quadriparesis with further sensory loss. Patients may occasionally present with a Brown-Séquard syndrome simulating a vascular accident. The initial complaints often appear to exceed recognizable neurological signs. Neck pain is not necessarily a feature of cervical myelopathy and is an unreliable prognostic indicator.

Signs

Neck movements are often normal. Neurological examination of the upper limbs will reveal weakness in the fingers with a lack of fine finger movement. When dressing, patients may fail to do up buttons whilst looking straight ahead. Wasting of the small muscles of the hand, if present, is more often due to disuse than to specific root involvement. Sensory loss to pinprick is often patchy and may suggest a peripheral neuropathy. Joint position sense is preserved except when the myelopathy affects the C3/4 level: the anatomy of this particular lesion is ill understood. Reflexes are increased below the highest level of cord compression but may be absent at the actual cervical level. In the lower limbs there is nearly always spasticity, with or without clonus, and the patient is unsteady. The unsteadiness is not just due to a spastic gait but appears to be out of proportion to any weakness or sensory loss that may be found. Careful neurological examination will give earlier diagnosis and consequently better results from treatment.

The differential diagnosis includes extradural and extramedullary spinal tumours, which are usually more dramatically painful; hereditary spastic paraparesis and spinocerebellar degeneration; subacute combined degeneration due to vitamin B12 deficiency; late onset demyelinating disease; and amyotrophic lateral sclerosis (motor neurone disease) with spasticity in the lower limbs and wasting of the upper limbs.

Investigation and Management

Surgery is the treatment of choice for cervical myelopathy. The results of surgery and the risks accompanying such procedures outweigh the dangers of leaving cervical myelopathy to progress. There is little place for conservative treatment unless the patient's general condition precludes anaesthesia. Myelography (Fig. 11.2A and B) with or without CT or MR scanning is

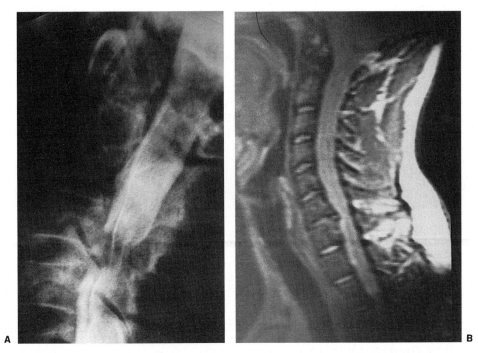

Fig. 11.2. Cervical myelopathy. **A** Myelogram lateral view; C3/4 disc protrusion. **B** MRI scan sagittal view; C6/7 disc protrusion.

mandatory (Modic et al. 1983; Yu et al. 1986a,b). Except where there is generalized cervical canal stenosis, compression usually arises at a single intra-vertebral space.

Surgery

If a single level of anterior compression can be identified, anterior de-compression is required. A posterior decompression could result in spinal cord infarction if there is considerable cord compression anteriorly from discs and bony excretions. If more than one level is involved or there is subluxation or instability, the anterior approach should also be employed using micro-discectomy or the Cloward procedure (1958). If there is cervical canal stenosis with ligamentous hypertrophy then the posterior approach – usually with cervical decompression from C3 to C7 inclusive – is required. A wide and lengthy decompressive laminectomy should be avoided in the younger age group as this can lead to deformity later in life. Where there is a combination of anterior and posterior compression then choices have to be made according to the exact anatomical problems relating to each individual patient (Symon and Lavender 1967; Jeffreys 1986). It is wise to remind the patient that not only does surgery near the spinal cord carry a morbidity and mortality but also late complications can occur from fusion.

Anterior spinal cord decompression for myelopathy should result in at least 80% of patients being stabilized as far as their neurological condition is concerned, though it must be admitted that surgeons tend to be overenthusiastic about their results. Not all the 80% will exhibit a marked neurological improvement. Cervical decompressive laminectomy for stenosis also gives reasonably favourable results. However, both the anterior and posterior approach carry a small risk of further neurological deterioration in 5% of cases and it is essential that only surgeons with experience operate in this field. The practice of a posterior approach with dural opening and division of the dentate ligaments has largely fallen into disuse as it has not been shown to carry superior results.

Thoracic Spine

The thoracic spine does not move and is rarely affected by degenerative disease causing compression of neural structures. Despite the high incidence of osteoporosis with vertebral body collapse, which can be considered an element in the degenerative process in women, an association with spinal cord compression is virtually unknown. The thoracic canal may be narrowed in achondroplasia (Spillane 1952), and ossification of the ligamentum flavum occurs in association with parathyroid disease (Kojima et al. 1989). These are rarities, but thoracic disc protrusion can occur and the condition is extremely difficult to diagnose without radiological confirmation.

Thoracic Disc Protrusion

This usually involves the lower thoracic spine and may present at any age. More often than not there is no preceding history of trauma or pain, thus the diagnosis is often extremely difficult. The patient usually presents with an insidious paraparesis of upper motor neurone type with pyramidal features. As compression progresses, sensory signs occur.

Disc calcification is seen with plain X-rays in at least 50% of cases. MR imaging is the investigation of choice where available; otherwise myelography should be combined with CT scanning (Figs. 11.3 and 11.4). It is important that axial views are taken to show in which direction the disc is protruded, i.e. laterally or centrolaterally. The thoracic disc protrusion usually consists of a firm extruded fragment which may penetrate the dura and indeed the spinal cord itself.

Surgery is required for thoracic disc protrusion (Findlay 1987). Conservative treatment will not prevent the development of a progressive irreversible disability. There is considerable controversy over the approach to thoracic disc protrusions and no surgeon can claim excellent results. It has always been considered surprising that such a small lesion can cause such disability. It is believed that part of the disability is due to direct compression of the anterior spinal artery. Other anterolaterally placed masses such as intradural tumours, e.g. meningiomas, usually reach a much larger size before causing an equivalent neurological deficit.

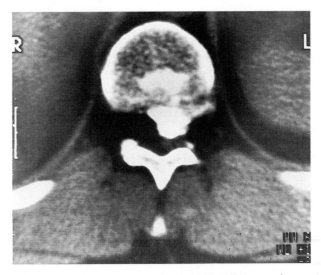

Fig. 11.3. Thoracic myelopathy. CT scan axial view; calcified disc protrusion.

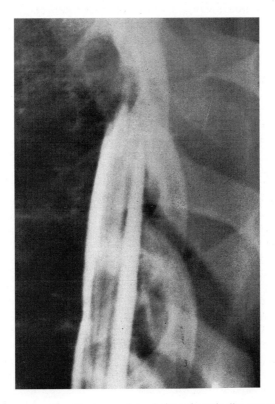

Fig. 11.4. Thoracic myelopathy. Myelogram lateral view; thoracic disc protrusion.

Laminectomy alone is liable to worsen the patient's condition. For centrolaterally placed discs a variety of approaches may be used: anterior thoracic, anterolateral (costotransversectomy), posterolateral with pediculectomy, or hemilaminectomy and intradural lateral excision. If the disc protrusion is central and known to be within the spinal cord substance then either the anterior transthoracic or anterolateral approach may be used.˙It may be impossible to remove disc material from within the spinal cord itself.

Lumbar Spondylosis and Disc Disease

Pathophysiology and Natural History

The pathophysiology of lumbar degenerative disease is similar to that of the cervical spine. Although the L4/5 and L5/S1 levels are the most mobile and are most frequently affected, the upper lumbar spine may be also involved, particularly in lumbar canal stenosis (Verbiest 1954). The lumbar spine has to bear the weight of the upper parts of the body and in consequence the bones, joints, ligaments and soft tissues are larger and stronger. The degenerative process probably starts in many cases at an early age, e.g. during adolescence, with degeneration of the nucleus pulposus of the intervertebral disc followed by disc protrusion and/or extrusion. From the clinical point of view the most important direction of protrusion is posteriorly in a central or lateral direction, initially stretching the annulus fibrosus and eventually tearing it (Maurice-Williams 1981; Findlay 1987). Anterior disc protrusion is of no consequence but extra posterolateral disc protrusion is now recognized as an uncommon cause of nerve root compression outside the spinal canal. As the process progresses, osteophyte formation begins in much the same manner as in the cervical spine. The facet joints become malaligned and overgrown, and there is thickening of the ligamentum flavum. In patients with a congenitally narrow canal (Critchley 1982; Ganz 1990), this process may occur throughout the lumbar spine and the canal loses its rounded appearance and assumes a "trefoil" axial shape. To a degree this is part of the natural process of ageing. Fortunately the lumbar spinal canal below L2 contains only the nerve roots of the cauda equina. Neural compression is thus mainly limited to the intervertebral exit root foraminae. Disc protrusion can affect either sex and may be related to obvious trauma. Lumbar canal stenosis is predominantly a disease affecting male manual workers around the age of retirement.

There are various predisposing factors to the development of lumbar degenerative disease. Patients with a congenitally narrow spinal canal, congenital spondylolisthesis or spinal dysraphism are at risk of developing lumbar canal stenosis. Pre-existing neurological conditions such as multiple sclerosis, shortening of one of the lower limbs, or kyphoscoliosis, are also more likely to result in lumbar degenerative disease (spondylosis) due to the asymmetrical forces exerted on the lower lumbar spine.

Low back pain and pain in one or both of the lower limbs is normally attributed to lumbar disc disease. However it must be emphasized that the lumbar disc is only one element of the lumbar spine liable to damage or disruption. The facet joints, ligaments and muscles may also show degenerative changes, with or without lumbar disc disease. Neural compression occurs in a minority of patients. Positive neurological signs are found only in a small percentage of those affected.

The differential diagnosis of lumbar disc disease must include infection (e.g. septic arthritis of the hip), tumours of the sacrum and pelvis, spinal intradural tumours (e.g. neuromas), sacroiliac disease, and extradural metastases of the lumbosacral bony spine.

Classification of Lumbar Degenerative Disease

For the purposes of classification, lumbar degenerative disease has been divided into seven varieties, although these may overlap:

1. Acute lumbar disc protrusion
2. Chronic lumbar disc protrusion and foraminal exit canal stenosis
3. Acute lumbar disc protrusion with neurological compression
4. Focal lumbar stenosis, lumbar spondylolisis, and spondylolisthesis
5. The failed back and pain syndromes
6. Lumbar canal stenosis
7. Extralateral (outside the spinal canal) lumbar disc protrusion

Acute Lumbar Disc Protrusion

The history of an acute lumbar disc protrusion is often of greater help in determining the diagnosis and management than the clinical examination (Maurice-Williams 1981). The onset begins with severe lumbar pain across the lower part of the lumbar spine. This is typically the case with a central disc protrusion at L4/5 level, but a more lateral protrusion is classically accompanied by sciatic pain radiating down one or both legs. If symptoms arise acutely, triggered by bending, twisting or lifting, the onset of pain is abrupt and the patient may be stuck in a particular position unable to straighten up.

Characteristically the pain of a lumbar disc protrusion is made worse by movement of the lumbar spine, by coughing and by sneezing. It is relieved by resting. Most patients get greatest relief when lying flat on their back, but others – particularly if an upper lumbar nerve root is involved – find it easier to lie in a lateral posture or prone with their hip flexed. The low back pain of an acute lumbar disc is mainly in the midline. Pain localized slightly to one side of the midline may suggest facet joint involvement or other pathology such as a tumour. At rest the pain is felt as a deep ache, but when the erector spinae muscles are thrown into spasm a sharp pain may radiate up the spine to the neck and the back may become acutely tender to touch. With time the patient may enter a chronic stage with a functional scoliosis and will limp when attempting to walk.

The "acute" lumbar disc is a disease of young and middle-aged adults. In the majority of cases of acute lumbar disc protrusion, a previous history of back strain is common. Indeed, the history may go back to injuries in the teens or during pregnancy. In the older age group the presentation is less likely to be acute but rather a combination of degenerative changes and chronic disc problems. The "sciatica" is a sharp pain, usually in the L5 or S1 distribution, radiating across the buttock passing down the outer border of the lower limb to the external malleolus and foot, often with gaps in the appropriate neurotome and associated with paraesthesia distally. The pain is made worse by movement of the lumbar spine and by flexion of the hip and dorsiflexion at the ankle, i.e. the straight leg raising test. The sciatic pain does not usually come on for some hours or sometimes days after the disc has prolapsed. In some cases, sciatica may be a more prominent feature than low back pain. The sudden disappearance of sciatica accompanied by a complaint of numbness or weakness, e.g. a footdrop, is frequently a sinister sign requiring urgent attention. A history of previous trauma, as opposed to backstrain, is present in 50% of patients and almost invariably associated with the patient's occupation. Nurses and others required to do heavy lifting should be specifically taught how to do so and should be encouraged to use any lifting aids available.

Signs, Investigations and Management

The patient with an acute lumbar disc protrusion may require opiate analgesia. Examination is often limited by the severity of the pain and hospital admission may be required for assessment. The test procedures used are in part mechanical looking for tension signs, and in part neurological.

Postural examination will reveal the presence of thoracolumbar scoliosis and spasm of the erector spinae muscles. Spinal movements may be assessed by marking the palpable spines and measuring the interspinous distances on flexion. Patients may compensate by moving or elevating a hip at the same time holding the lumbar spine immobile. In severe cases the patient may be bedridden. Straight leg raising is nearly always reduced on the appropriate side with lateral disc protrusions but may be normal with a central disc protrusion or extrusion. Dorsiflexion of the ankle, thereby stretching the sciatic nerve, will worsen sciatic pain; and higher disc protrusions at L3/4 can be recognized by the femoral stretch test. With experience it is possible to differentiate between a reduction in straight leg raising and spasm of the hamstrings (common with chronic disc protrusions) and arrive at a recordable clinical examination which can be compared with subsequent observations (Maurice-Williams 1981).

Neurological examination of the lower limbs is mandatory. A brief examination of the cranial nerves and upper limbs is required to exclude other neurological conditions. Localized muscle weakness and sensory loss in the appropriate dermatomes should be recorded. The reflexes in the lower limbs should be elicited and compared, if necessary asking the patient to kneel on a hard chair to obtain the ankle jerks. The lower sacral nerve roots must be examined with the patient turned on to his/her side. A rectal examination is also advisable to exclude the possibility of a tumour. Changes in neurological signs may indicate increased damage to the nerve root despite lessening of pain as the illness evolves.

The diagnosis of an acute lumbar disc protrusion where symptoms are severe and the signs demonstrable is usually not in doubt. However it must be

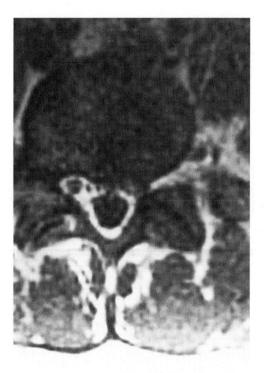

Fig. 11.5. Lumbar disc protrusion. MRI scan axial view; right lateral disc protrusion.

remembered that tumours within and without the spinal canal or of the pelvis and sacrum can present in a similar manner, though usually the history is more chronic.

In the United Kingdom it is generally accepted that a conservative course should be followed in the management of acute lumbar disc disease unless there is an indication to investigate early, e.g. the diagnosis is in doubt or there are hard neurological signs. However, this policy is questionable when considerations such as loss of employment and earnings are evaluated, and may do no more than mask delays in hospital referral. Early surgery may be helpful for sedentary workers but risk the livelihood of manual workers. In the majority of cases bed rest at home, analgesia and sometimes sedation, is usually enough to overcome an acute attack. If the pain is uncontrollable, hospital admission may be required. If there are positive neurological signs or the pain cannot be relieved, further investigation as a prelude to invasive treatment is required. Plain radiographs alone will not suffice. Myelography (Begg et al. 1946) with or without CT scanning or MRI may be performed according to the availability of these investigations and the certainty of diagnosis (Fig. 11.5).

If a small disc protrusion is found or the investigations prove to be negative, inpatient care with analgesia, epidural anaesthesia and facet joint anaesthetic blocks will be required. Manipulation may help occasionally. Referral to a pain clinic or a second opinion may be needed at this stage and the patient should be reassured that a positive approach to his complaint is being adopted and that he will not be forced into unnecessary treatment. Wrong decisions made at an early stage may prove difficult or impossible to rectify.

Invasive Treatment of Acute Lumbar Disc Protrusion

Before embarking on invasive treatment it is essential to take into account any psychological factors or pending litigation. The surgeon must get to know his patient well and explain thoroughly the positive and negative aspects of lumbar spine surgery and/or chemolysis. On occasion it may be useful to obtain a second opinion but this may often serve to cloud the patient's mind. A joint decision needs to be reached between patient and surgeon.

Chemonucleolysis is the least invasive procedure for soft protruded lumbar discs (McCulloch 1977). The procedure offers a 50% success rate for patients with low back pain, sciatica and a proven protrusion (but not for an extrusion as shown by CT scanning). However, it is not a completely safe procedure, neither is it painless. Under image intensification, chymopapain is injected into the ipsilateral side of the disc protrusion with the patient mildly sedated. The L5/S1 space is more difficult to inject than L4/5. Post-treatment analgesia is usually required for a few days before the patient is mobilized in a brace. Manual work must not be undertaken for 6 weeks post-treatment.

An alternative therapy is percutaneous lumbar discectomy using a rotating sucking side-cutting needle to evacuate the contents of a disc protrusion. Patients with a large disc protrusion or an extruded fragment are not suitable for such treatment. Both chemonucleolysis and percutaneous discectomy have gained in popularity in North America, whereas in the United Kingdom more conservative management is preferred. Open surgery aimed at early mobilization by means of microdiscectomy or fenestration procedures can be used for lateral disc protrusions. Patients should have at least 6 to 8 weeks off work and 12 weeks if heavy manual work is contemplated. It must be remembered that disc protrusions requiring surgery not only result in a focal lesion but also result in some derangement of the lumbar spine.

The results of surgery for large protrusions or extruded fragments are excellent with regard to pain relief, although the abolition of all low back pain cannot be guaranteed (O'Connell 1951). With a small disc protrusion, surgical results are less favourable. The risks of surgery, e.g. neuropraxia, infection, and nerve root scarring, should always be considered. Patients should be carefully selected for surgery and appropriate facilities for physiotherapy available. With centrolateral or central protrusions, bilateral microdiscectomies, bilateral fenestration operations, or a laminectomy of the L4/5 level may be indicated.

Chronic Lumbar Disc Protrusions and Foraminal Exit Canal Stenosis

Most patients with low back problems have more chronic symptoms punctuated by occasional relapses. There is often a background of low back pain, and each attack lasts days or weeks. Neurological signs may be absent and tension signs less obvious than expected from the patient's complaints. There is often a functional thoracolumbar scoliosis and unilateral facet joint pain causing the patient to limp. Pain from a facet joint may radiate into the ipsilateral leg as a dull ache but rarely extends below the knee. The pain is relieved by rest and lacks the characteristics of true sciatica. If the patient limps, a pelvic tilt will develop thereby throwing increased strain on to the contralateral leg which may also become painful. Hamstring spasm is common and may be mistaken for a true reduction in straight leg raising. A thorough neurological examination should be undertaken with each relapse to exclude the possibility of a slow-growing tumour in the spinal canal such as an ependymoma (Davis and Barnard 1985). As the patient's disease becomes more chronic the pain threshold drops and symptoms may summate warranting further radiological investigation. Many of the patients have a degree of exit root canal stenosis (Epstein et al. 1972; Crock 1981) due to bony overgrowth of the facet joints and osteophyte formation without soft disc protrusions.

It is essential that a psychological profile of the patient is understood. The role of a clinical psychologist in revealing sexual, marital, financial and other problems is not to be underestimated. The radiological investigations are the same as for an acute disc but the results of surgery are far less satisfactory.

Acute Disc Protrusion with Neurological Compression

A rare, but serious, manifestation of lumbar or lumbosacral disc protrusion is neurological compression. A central disc protrusion – most commonly at L4/5 – may cause acute compression of the cauda equina. Usually an extruded fragment affects all the roots of the cauda equina below the appropriate level giving rise to a lower motor neurone type of paraparesis with sphincter involvement. Symptoms may develop rapidly, and sometimes silently. A lateral disc protrusion causing compression of the L5 or S1 nerve root may produce an acute, and often painless, footdrop. If the clinical diagnosis is uncertain, neuropraxia may be differentiated from a lateral popliteal nerve palsy by nerve conduction studies.

Both acute cauda equina compression and acute footdrop need urgent admission and removal of the disc as an emergency measure (Jennett 1956) (Fig. 11.6). Unfortunately the results of surgery are not good if neurological signs have been present for more than 48 hours. Neural regeneration is poor with complete lesions, and in older patients there may be little point in offering surgery.

Focal Lumbar Stenosis, Lumbar Spondylolisis and Spondylolisthesis

Two types of vertebral subluxation are particularly associated with the lower end of the lumbar spine.

With the congenital variety there is an absence of the pars interarticularis, i.e. incomplete formation of part of the pedicle. Patients may present at a young age with bilateral sciatica or acute neurological compression. The absence of bone may not appear obvious on lateral radiographs, but at opera-

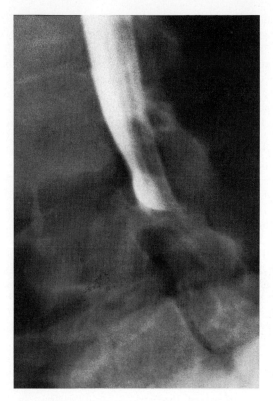

Fig. 11.6. Acute cauda equina compression. Lumbar myelogram lateral view; L4/5 disc protrusion migrating behind the body of L4.

tion one is often surprised by the presence of large bilateral defects, which unless replaced by a fibrous union may allow the lamina to hang loose.

In the acquired mature onset focal spondylolisis with focal stenosis the spine is usually stable. There is often a long history of low back pain with bilateral sciatica and neurogenic claudication. Symptoms develop in middle age with women more often affected than men. An element of stenosis usually exists at the affected level, which is commonly L4/5. The aetiology is probably of disc space narrowing at L5/S1 earlier in life followed by fusion; thus setting up a process of strain with excessive mobility of the proximal joint.

With both varieties intervertebral body subluxation can be seen radiographically and the degree of instability of the spine assessed by flexion/extension views (Fig. 11.7). Further investigation by myelography or MRI is mandatory prior to surgery which is the treatment of choice. A fusion operation is required for the younger patient with congenital spondylolisthesis, either by anterior interbody fusion or preferably by a posterior approach with instrumentation as well as an autologous bone graft. If more than half the anteroposterior surface of the vertebral body has slipped, the patient should be dealt with as an emergency. In the mature spondylolisis with focal stenosis, local decompression with undercutting facetectomy may be undertaken provided stability is assessed pre- and per-operatively. Both conditions respond well

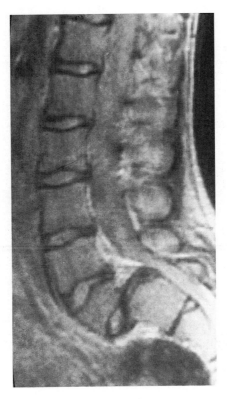

Fig. 11.7.   Spondylolisthesis. MRI sagittal view; congenital L4/5 spondylolisthesis.

to surgical treatment (Stauffer and Coventry 1972; Epstein et al. 1983; Markwalder and Reulen 1989).

The Failed Back and Pain Syndromes

With any longstanding chronic pain syndrome there are a minority of patients who fail to respond to treatment. This is particularly so with respect to the lumbar spine. Often the doctor is tempted to blame the patient's psyche and, indeed, there is no question that psychological evaluation can be most useful in assessing the patient's symptoms. Recurrent or continuing symptoms of low back pain and sciatica may be attributed to nerve root damage, reverberating circuits and changes in receptor sites within the spinal cord and brain; or to exaggeration of symptoms due to impending litigation, work avoidance, marital or sexual problems, etc. It is encumbent upon specialists who deal with lumbar degenerative disease to offer a service not only to their potentially successful patients, but also to their failures.

The degree to which one investigates patients with pain syndromes and those with poor surgical results will depend on personal preference. However, with the increasing availability of non-invasive investigations, e.g. MR scanning, it is not unreasonable to ascertain that the patient has not suffered a recurrent

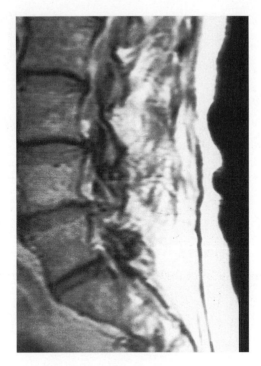

Fig. 11.8. Lumbar canal stenosis. MRI sagittal view; L3/4 and L4/5 canal stenosis.

disc protrusion at the previous surgical site, or even at another level. Once radiological investigation has excluded an obvious surgical target then evaluation by a clinical psychologist and pain specialist in a multidisciplinary approach may be most useful. Further conservative treatment such as epidural anaesthesia, acupuncture or antidepressants may be useful in the first instance and dorsal column stimulation and even deep brain stimulation helpful in a minority of carefully selected patients. Cordotomy and rhizotomy have no place in the treatment of benign pain as a recurrence of symptoms is inevitable within two years.

Lumbar Canal Stenosis

Lumbar canal stenosis is an underdiagnosed condition affecting the middle aged and elderly (Verbiest 1954; Blau and Logue 1961; Jones and Thompson 1968; Kavanagh et al. 1968; Critchley 1982). Such patients are considered to have a congenitally narrow lumbar canal. Achondroplastics are similarly affected (Spillane 1952). As the patient ages multiple disc protrusions with osteophytosis occur in conjunction with overgrown facet joints, and the ligamentum flavum becomes hypertrophied (Jones and Thompson 1968; Sortland et al. 1977). The lumbar spinal canal assumes a typical trefoil shape with a narrow anteroposterior diameter (Fig. 11.8).

The patient has two complaints. First, sciatic pain related to exercise (Verbiest 1954). Such pain is often bilateral and due to exit root canal stenosis.

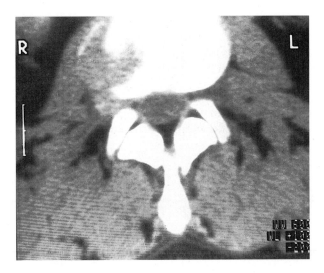

Fig. 11.9. Extralateral disc protrusion. CT scan axial view; right extralateral disc protrusion.

Second, typical neurogenic claudication where one or both the lower limbs become weak and floppy after walking a set distance (Blau and Logue 1961). These symptoms are relieved by sitting down and resting for 5 to 10 minutes and the patient is then able to walk a similar distance (Kavanagh et al. 1968). The vascular supply to the cauda equina is presumed to be affected and claudication may be eased by flexion opening up the exit root canals thereby relieving the compression caused by overgrowth of the ligamentum flavum (Ganz 1990). Occasionally as the disease progresses, the nerve roots become entrapped causing concomitant neurological signs. However, in general, the main feature of lumbar canal stenosis with claudication of the cauda equina is the absence of physical signs at rest, although an exercise test may reveal absent ankle reflexes. Straight leg raising is nearly always normal. Lumbar canal stenosis usually affects the L4/5 and L3/4 levels but later extends throughout the whole lumbar spine as the disease progresses.

Lumbar canal stenosis is treated by surgical decompression, usually with a laminectomy at the affected level and undercutting facetectomy (Verbiest 1977; Critchley 1982; Ganz 1990). The results of surgery are good with 80% of patients being relieved of their symptoms. However, if there is severe sciatica at rest with objective neurological signs, the results of decompression are not nearly as favourable. In patients with tandem stenosis, lumbar decompression may unmask upper motor neurone signs due to a disguised cervical myelopathy.

Extralateral Lumbar Disc Protrusion

It has recently become appreciated that extralateral lumbar disc protrusions may actually involve the nerve root one level above that expected (Frankhauser and de Tribolet 1987; Abdullah et al. 1988; Jane et al. 1990). Myelography is of no help in the diagnosis of this condition which is best seen on an axial CT scan (Fig. 11.9). When the diagnosis of an acute lumbar disc protrusion is expected but routine investigations are negative, axial CT scanning of adjacent intervertebral levels should be undertaken, if necessary at several levels. Surgical treatment may be confined to a lateral approach completely outside the lumbar canal (Jane et al. 1990).

Acknowledgements. I would like to thank Dr. C. Coutinho of the Neuro-Radiology Department, Royal Preston Hospital and Professor J. Edwards of the University of Liverpool for supplying the illustrative X-rays.

References

Abdullah AF, Wolber PGH, Warfield JR, Gunani IK (1988) Surgical management of extreme lateral lumbar disc herniations: review of 138 cases. Neurosurgery 22:648–653

Adams CBT, Logue V (1971) Studies in cervical spondylotic myelopathy. II The movement and contour of the spine in relation to the neural complications of cervical spondylosis. Brain 94:569–586

Begg AC, Falconer MA, McGeorge M (1946) Myelography in lumbar intervertebral disk lesions. A correlation with operative findings. Br J Surg 34:141–157

Blau JN, Logue V (1961) Intermittent claudication of the cauda equina. An unusual syndrome resulting from central protrusion of a lumbar intervetrebral disc. Lancet 1:1081–1086

Brain WR, Northfield D, Wilkinson M (1952) The neurological manifestations of cervical spondylosis. Brain 75:187–225

Cloward RB (1958) The anterior approach for removal of ruptured cervical disks. J Neurosurg 15:602–614

Critchley EMR (1982) Lumbar spinal stenosis. Br Med J 284:1588–1589

Crock HV (1981) Normal and pathological anatomy of the lumbar spinal nerve root canals. J Bone Joint Surg (Br) 63B:487–490

Davis C (1985) Osteopathic manipulation resulting in damage to spinal cord. Br Med J 291:1540–1541

Davis C, Barnard RO (1985) Malignant behaviour of myxopapillary ependymoma. J Neurosurg 62:925–929

Davis C, Bradford R (1986) A surgical history of Maida Vale Hospital. In: Walker MD, Thomas DGT (eds) Biology of brain tumour. Martinus Nijhoff, Netherlands, pp 245–249

Epstein JA, Epstein BS, Rosenthal AD, Carras R, Lavine LS (1972) Sciatica caused by nerve root entrapment in the lateral recess: the superior facet syndrome. J Neurosurg 36:584–589

Epstein NE, Epstein JA, Carras R, Lavine LS (1983) Degenerative spondylolisthesis with an intact neural arch: a review of 60 cases with an analysis of clinical findings and the development of surgical management. Neurosurgery 13:555–561

Findlay FG (1987) Spinal degenerative disease. In: Miller JD (ed) Northfield's surgery of the central nervous system. Blackwell Scientific, Oxford, pp 760–794

Frankhauser H, de Tribolet N (1987) Extreme lateral lumbar disc herniation. Br J Neurosurg 1:111–129

Ganz JC (1990) Lumbar spinal stenosis: postoperative results in terms of preoperative posture-related pain. J Neurosurg 72:71–74

Grisoli F, Graziani N, Fabrizi AP, Peragut JC, Vincentelli F, Diaz-Vasquez P (1989) Anterior discectomy without fusion for treatment of cervical lateral soft disc extrusion: a follow-up of 120 cases. Neurosurgery 24:853–859

Henderson CM, Hennessy RG, Shuey HM, Shackelford EG (1983) Posterior-lateral foraminectomy as an exclusive operative technique for cervical radiculopathy: a review of 846 consecutively operated cases. Neurosurgery 13:504–512

Jane JA, Haworth CS, Broaddus WC, Lee JH, Malik J (1990) A neurosurgical approach to far-lateral disc herniation. J Neurosurg 72:143–144

Jeffreys RV (1986) The surgical treatment of cervical myelopathy due to spondylosis and disc degeneration. J Neurol Neurosurg Psychiatry 49:353–361

Jennett WB (1956) A study of 25 cases of compression of the cauda equina by prolapsed intervertebral discs. J Neurol Neurosurg Psychiatry 19:109–116

Jones RAC, Thompson JLG (1968) The narrow spinal canal. A clinical and radiological review. J Bone Joint Surg (Br) 50B:595–605

Kavanagh GJ, Svien HJ, Holman CB, et al. (1968) "Pseudoclaudication" syndrome produced by compression of the cauda equina. JAMA 206:2477–2481

Kojima T, Waga S, Kubo Y, Kanamaru K, Shimosaka S, Shimizu T (1989) Anterior cervical vertebrectomy and interbody fusion for multi-level spondylosis and ossification of the posterior longitudinal ligament. Neurosurgery 24:864–872

Lunsford LD, Bissonette DJ, Jannetta PJ, Sheptak PE, Zorub DS (1980) Anterior surgery for cervical disc disease. Part I: treatment of lateral cervical disc herniation in 253 cases. J Neurosurg 53:1–11

Markwalder TM, Reulen HJ (1989) Translaminar screw fixation in lumbar spine pathology: technical note. Acta Neurochir 99:58–60

Maurice-Williams RS (1981) Spinal degenerative disease. Wright, Bristol

McCulloch JA (1977) Chemonucleolysis. J Bone Joint Surg (Br) 59B:45–52

Mixter WJ, Barr JS (1934) Rupture of the intervertebral disc with involvement of the spinal canal. N Engl J Med 211:210–215

Modic MT, Weinstein MA, Pavlicek W, Boumphrey F, Starnes D, Duchesneau PM (1983) Magnetic resonance imaging of the cervical spine: technical and clinical observations. Am J Roentgenol 141:1129–1136

Nurick S (1972) The pathogenesis of the spinal cord disorder associated with cervical spondylosis. Brain 95:87–100

O'Connell JEA (1951) Protrusions of the lumbar intervertebral discs: a clinical review based on five hundred cases treated by excision of the protrusion. J Bone Joint Surg (Br) 33B:8–30

Ogino H, Tada K, Okada K, Yonenobu K, et al. (1983) Canal diameter, anteroposterior compression ratio, and spondylotic myelopathy of the cervical spine. Spine 8:1–15

Sortland O, Magnaes B, Hauge T (1977) Functional myelography with metrizamide in the diagnosis of lumbar spinal stenosis. Acta Radiol (suppl) 355:42–54

Spillane JD (1952) Three cases of achondroplasia with neurological complications. J Neurol Neurosurg Psychiatry 15:246–252

Stauffer RN, Coventry MB (1972) Posterolateral lumbar-spine fusion: analysis of Mayo Clinic series. J Bone Joint Surg (Am) 54A:1195–1204

Symon L, Lavender P (1967) The surgical treatment of cervical spondylotic myelopathy. Neurology 17:117–127

Verbiest H (1954) A radicular syndrome for developmental narrowing of the lumbar vertebral canal. J Bone Joint Surg (Br) 36B:230–237

Verbiest H (1977) Results of surgical treatment of idiopathic developmental stenosis of the lumbar vertebral canal. A review of twenty-seven years' experience. J Bone Joint Surg (Br) 59B:181–188

Yu YL, du Boulay GH, Stevens JM, Kendall BE (1986a) Computer-assisted myelography in cervical spondylotic myelopathy and radiculopathy: clinical correlations and pathogenetic mechanisms. Brain 109:259–278

Yu YL, du Boulay GH, Stevens JM, Kendall BE (1986b) Computed tomography in cervical spondylotic myelopathy and radiculopathy: visualisation of structures, myelographic comparison, cord measurements and clinical utility. Neuroradiology 28:221–236

Yu YL, Woo E, Huang CY (1987) Cervical spondylotic myelopathy and radiculopathy. Acta Neurol Scand 75:367–373

Chapter 12

Craniocervical Anomalies and Non-traumatic Syringomyelia

R.A. Metcalfe

The majority of cases of syringomyelia are associated with abnormalities in the region of the foramen magnum but the reverse is not so and the true prevalence of structural anomalies in this region is unknown. It is difficult and somewhat artificial to analyse these disorders separately for many are found together in the same patient. There is also little genuine consensus of opinion about the cause of the anomalies or of related syringomyelia. In this review I have attempted to shed a little light by considering first the anomalies themselves and then proceeding to a more detailed discussion of syringomyelia.

Chiari Malformations

Chiari (1891, 1896) described a number of cases of childhood hydrocephalus with particular reference to changes which he observed in the cerebellum and lower brain stem. He divided his cases into four groups, only the first two being of contemporary relevance. Arnold (1894) presented a single case of Chiari's Type II deformity and his name has been frequently associated with the condition without evident justification. The chauvinistic reader might prefer the term Cleland-Chiari syndrome since the original description was by the Englishman John Cleland (1883). In the interests of simplicity only Chiari's name will be used in this article. Other authors have avoided eponyms in favour of descriptive titles – e.g. *primary cerebellar ectopia* (Spillane et al. 1957) and *hindbrain herniation* (Williams 1986). The problem with these terms is that they both imply that the primary defect relates to the hindbrain not the surrounding structures. This has not actually been established beyond doubt.

Baker (1963) showed that the condition was easily missed if myelography in the supine position was not performed and after this both recognition of the disorder and frequency of publications increased. This chapter will concentrate on recent publications but the reader interested in the older literature is referred to the papers by Gardner (1965), Conway (1967), Appleby et al. (1968) and Banerji and Millar (1974).

There are two components to the malformation:

1. A tongue of cerebellum posterior to the medulla and spinal cord extending through the foramen magnum.
2. Downward displacement of the medulla and sometimes the caudal portion of the fourth ventricle relative to the foramen magnum.

The mildest, Chiari Type I, refers to patients who have cerebellar tonsillar descent through the foramen magnum but no evidence of spina bifida or other dysraphism. In Type II, the herniation is more severe and is associated with spina bifida and pronounced medullary descent. The distinction is artificial but the more subtle Type I form is of interest in that it presents commonly in adult life (Mohr et al. 1977; Paul et al. 1983), is often unaccompanied by other disorders and indeed is sometimes encountered as an incidental finding at myelography and MRI. The prevalence of tonsillar herniation is unknown. The largest published series from the Cleveland Clinic (Levy et al. 1983) reports an average annual incidence of 3.5 new cases each year in a large neurosurgical department. This figure is likely to be an underestimate and increased availability of MRI will probably result in a higher proportion of cases, both symptomatic and incidental, being discovered.

Aetiology

There is considerable divergence of opinion about the aetiology. One theory proposes a primary distortion of neuronal tissue secondary to a failure of embryonic development of the hindbrain structures including cerebellum, medulla, fourth ventricle and also the occipital bone and cervical spine. This is the most widely held view (Salam and Adams 1978). Other suggestions include downward pressure from hydrocephalus and tethering of the spinal cord by a myelomeningocele. This latter suggestion elaborated by Roth (1986) requires that the normal craniocaudal skeletal development is prevented by tethering of the spinal cord at the level of the meningomyelocele and a compensatory reversal of growth direction results in the posterior fossa contents being assimilated into the spinal canal. It is an attractive concept which does not explain those Chiari malformations which are not associated with cord tethering. A careful neuropathological analysis of 25 children with severe Chiari II malformation including myelomeningocele and hydrocephalus demonstrated a wide range of associated malformations, including hypoplastic cranial nerve nuclei, cerebellar dysplasia, fusion of the thalami and agenesis of the corpus callosum (Gilbert et al. 1986). The authors reasonably suggest that the Chiari malformation is part of a spectrum of malformations caused by an unknown influence on the development of the central nervous system.

Recently a case has been advanced for a distortion of the bones forming the posterior fossa (occipital dysplasia) as the primary event with subsequent crowding of the posterior fossa structures leading to secondary neuronal distortion. Thus Marin-Padilla and Marin-Padilla (1981) treated pregnant hamsters with high dose Vitamin A on the eighth day of gestation and produced an underdeveloped basichondrocranium and cerebellar descent. Schady et al. (1987) made careful measurements of lateral skull radiographs of patients with the Chiari I malformation and found a high incidence of bony abnormalities in the posterior fossa. This positive result does not of course exclude the possibility that the bone changes are secondary to neural maldevelopment but a low incidence would have argued against the Marin-Padillas' assertion. Battersby and Williams (1982) advance the notion that distortion of the occipital bone during a traumatic birth may contribute to hindbrain herniation secondary to basilar impression.

Familial syringomyelia usually occurs on the basis of a craniocervical disorder (Schliep 1978). Coria et al. (1983) describe three generations of a family affected by occipital dysplasia and Chiari I malformation, postulating an autosomal dominant disorder with variable phenotypic expression, the bony abnormality being primary. It seems unlikely that a genetic factor is present in all cases but the hypothesis can now be tested with the advent of MRI.

Clinical Features

The more severe Type II Chiari malformations present as a rule in infancy with major deformities, spina bifida and hydrocephalus. Syringomyelia may present later in life and sometimes in patients who have forgotten or never been told about surgery on the spine early in life. Although Williams (1986) has emphasized the artificiality of the distinction between the two varieties, the clinical description given here refers primarily to the milder Type I herniation which presents in adult life.

Symptoms

Headache and neck pain are the commonest complaints followed by sensory disturbance in the arms, gait disorder and lower cranial nerve dysfunction (Paul et al. 1983; Levy et al. 1983). Nightingale and Williams (1987) draw attention to the clinical characteristics of "hindbrain hernia headache" – severe occipital headache provoked by measures which increase the pressure differential between head and neck. Rarely, syncope may also be the presenting feature of hindbrain herniation, perhaps related to impaction at the foramen magnum (Hampton et al. 1982). One case of central sleep apnoea in association with a Chiari malformation has been reported with clinical improvement after occipital decompression (Balk et al. 1985). Bullock et al. (1988) report two cases of central respiratory failure in the context of syringomyelia and a Chiari malformation.

Signs

The most common features on examination are: lower limb hyperreflexia, weakness and wasting in the arm and hand, nystagmus, dissociated sensory loss, lower cranial nerve palsy and a gait disorder due to varying combinations of cerebellar, posterior column and pyramidal tract disturbance.

Clinical Syndromes

All the recent papers on the adult Chiari malformation use slightly different classifications of the clinical manifestations but there are five main components which may present separately or in combination:

1. Syringomyelia – most probably related to obstruction of CSF flow from the fourth ventricle with subsequent development of fluid-filled cavities in the substance of the spinal cord.
2. Paraparesis – related to direct pressure on the spinal cord.
3. Cerebellar syndrome – usually a truncal ataxia due to disturbance of midline cerebellar function and spinocerebellar pathways.
4. Raised intracranial pressure – headache often exacerbated by exertion and presumed to relate to plugging of the foramen magnum with intermittent intracranial hypertension. Papilloedema may result from more protracted plugging and a dissociation between intracranial and spinal pressures should give a clue to the site of the lesion.
5. Cranial nerve disorder – this could relate to either syringobulbia or cranial nerve distortion due to the cephalad course of the lower cranial nerves frequently seen in the Chiari malformation.

Oculomotor Features

The classical disorder, downbeating nystagmus, was described by Cogan (1968) but a wide range of other features have been documented including side-beat, periodic alternating, divergent, gaze-evoked and rebound nystagmus, impaired saccadic, pursuit and vergence eye movements and internuclear ophthalmoplegia (Leigh and Zee 1983). One case of see-saw nystagmus has also been reported (Zimmerman et al. 1986). In practice the presence of genuine downbeating nystagmus should lead to a thorough search for a foramen magnum lesion. Oscillopsia is a frequent complaint and both this and the abnormal eye signs tend slowly to improve after surgical decompression.

Misdiagnosis

Foramen magnum disorders presenting with vague headache and odd sensory complaints without clear physical signs are quite likely to be misdiagnosed. Neurosis, multiple sclerosis and motor neurone disease are common errors (Levy et al. 1983).

Investigation

Plain radiology

Plain radiology has no real place in the investigation of the patient suspected of having a foramen magnum syndrome but the results are interesting and of some relevance to the aetiology.

The frequency of detection of bony abnormalities related to Chiari malformations depends on how hard one looks. Platybasia, basilar impression, concavity of the clivus and enlargement of the foramen magnum have all been reported, the largest series describing skull abnormalities in 36% of cases (Levy et al. 1983). Careful measurement of lateral skull radiographs increases this proportion to two-thirds (Schady et al. 1987). Cervical spine views may show assimilation of the atlas, a widened canal, altered cervical curvature (increased, decreased or reversed) or spina bifida. These changes are seen in 35% of cases (Levy et al. 1983).

Imaging

The hazardous and invasive investigations of oily contrast medium myelography, pneumoencephalography and vertebral angiography have now been superceded by two main investigations, water-soluble supine myelography with or without CT and MRI (Bosley et al. 1985). There is already an extensive literature on MRI in this region all of which confirms that MRI is now the investigation of choice (McManus and Bartlett 1986), although imaging abnormalities do not necessarily correlate with clinical features (Wolpert et al. 1988). A study of the position of cerebellar tonsils in the normal population compared with the Chiari malformation (Aboulezz et al. 1985) suggests that extension of the tonsils up to 3 mm below the foramen magnum is normal but clearly pathological beyond 5 mm. Barkovitch et al. (1986) produced similar findings. MRI's superiority is likely to be enhanced with further technical developments and the use of gadolinium as a contrast agent. Regrettably in the United Kingdom, the lack of easy access to MRI will ensure that many Chiari malformations will be detected by myelography for some time to come. Fig. 12.1 shows a water-soluble contrast supine myelogram and Fig. 12.2 the results of MRI in a similar patient.

Management

There are no controlled data available on this topic and even the natural history is difficult to establish in an area where there is such a wide range of severity and type of presentation. The management of *symptomatic* adult Chiari malformations without syrinx tends to be similar to that of syringomyelia – i.e. surgical in the presumption that the condition is likely to worsen with the passage of time and that operation stands a reasonable chance of stabilizing the condition and in some cases results in sustained improvement. Fig. 12.3 shows a view of a Chiari I malformation at operation.

Paul et al. (1983) reported the results of suboccipital decompression and C1–C3 laminectomy in 71 patients presenting in adult life; 65% had a central cord syndrome, 22% evidence of foramen magnum compression and 11% a pure cerebellar syndrome. At operation 41% had evidence of arachnoiditis in addition to tonsillar herniation, 30% had a constricting dural band at the foramen magnum or C1 and a variety of bony abnormalities were described, not all of which were evident on radiology. Respiratory depression was the most frequent operative complication (14%) and one patient died from this. About three-quarters of the whole group showed initial improvement but 20% subsequently relapsed, usually within 2–3 years of operation. Patients with a purely cerebellar presentation did not relapse.

Levy et al. (1983) reported a series of 127 patients who had had a similar procedure with or without an attempt to plug the central canal of the spinal

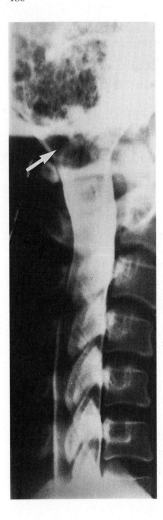

Fig. 12.1. Lateral view of myelogram demonstrating cerebellar tonsillar herniation below foramen magnum (arrow). (Radiograph by courtesy of Professor I. Isherwood.)

cord with muscle. Of these patients, 21 had no evidence of tonsillar descent at operation and in this group arachnoiditis was a universal finding often associated with a kinked brain stem or occlusion of the foramen of Magendie. In general the results were similar to those described by Paul with about half showing long-term benefit, a quarter unchanged and the remainder deteriorating. The attempt to block the central canal produced neither obvious benefit nor complication. The results of Saez et al. (1976) are in broad agreement with both these publications.

Dandy-Walker Syndrome

Although not strictly a craniocervical anomaly, it seems appropriate to mention this unusual disorder here since it may form part of the spectrum of hindbrain

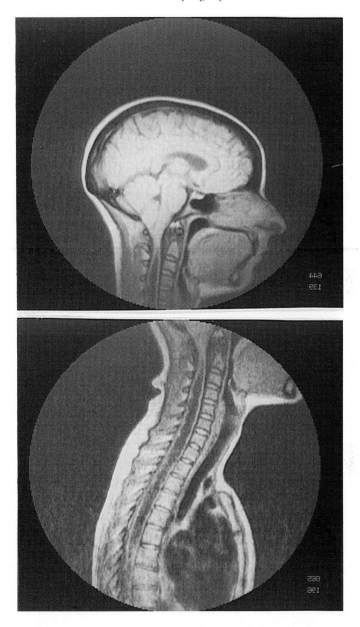

Fig. 12.2. Upper figure: MRI demonstrating Chiari I malformation with associated syringomyelia. Lower figure: MRI of the same patient demonstrating the extensive syrinx formation. (Radiograph by courtesy of Professor I. Isherwood.)

developmental disorders which include the Chiari malformation. Brown (1977) defines six major features: hydrocephalus; defective development of the cerebellar vermis; cyst-like enlargement of the fourth ventricle; enlargement of the posterior fossa; elevated location of the transverse sinuses and the

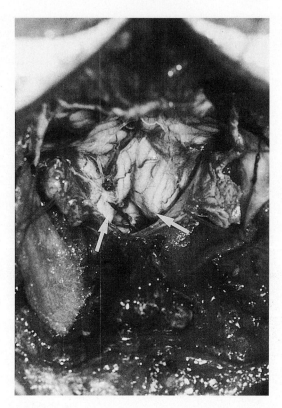

Fig. 12.3.   Operative view of a Chiari I malformation. The dura has been opened and the tips of the cerebellar tonsils are arrowed. (Illustration by courtesy of Mr. R. A. Johnston.)

tentorium; and usually lack of patency of the foraminae of Luschka and Magendie.

The syndrome was properly delineated in separate publications by Dandy and Blackfan (1914) and Taggert and Walker (1942). Gardner postulated a relationship between the Chiari malformations and the Dandy-Walker syndrome, suggesting that they both represented "failure of the outlets of the fourth ventricle to develop normally in the rhombic roof of the embryo" (Gardner et al. 1972; Gardner 1973). In his view if CSF, unable to exit from the fourth ventricle was retained in the lateral ventricles, then a small posterior fossa resulted with herniation through the foramen magnum. Retention in and hence expansion of the fourth ventricle would cause an enlarged posterior fossa with the Dandy-Walker cyst. This may explain some cases where there is evident hydrocephalus but cannot easily explain the small or distorted posterior fossa seen in the Chiari malformations without hydrocephalus. Barkovich et al. (1989) have studied 31 patients with posterior fossa CSF collections using MRI and conclude that the Dandy-Walker syndrome is part of a spectrum of posterior fossa developmental anomalies which include mega-cisterna magna.

Clinically the syndrome usually presents at birth or in infancy with hydrocephalus (about 60%), in childhood or adolescence with raised intracranial

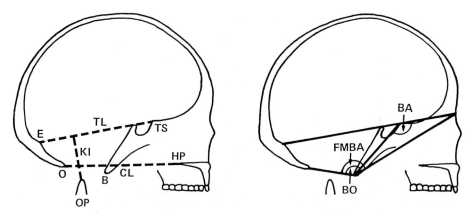

Fig. 12.4. Diagram to illustrate some of the relevant measurements indicating platybasia and basilar impression (the position of the odontoid peg has been shifted posteriorly to aid clarity). Key to abbreviations: B, Basion; E, Endinion; O, Opisthion, OP, Odontoid Peg, TL, Twining's line; TS, Tuberculum Sella; KI, Klaus Index; CL, Chamberlain's Line; HP, Hard Palate; BA, Basal Angle; BO, Boogaard's Angle; FMBA, Foramen Magnum Basilar Angle. (Reproduced by courtesy of Dr. W. Schady.)

pressure (35%) and the remainder in adult life. There seems to be a female excess in most series (Brown 1977). A variety of associated anomalies have been reported but syringomyelia occurs rarely. Management is by shunting to control intracranial pressure.

Bony Abnormalities at the Craniocervical Junction

A variety of different measurements have been applied to lateral skull radiographs in order to define disorders of the skull base (McRae 1953; Schmidt et al. 1978; Schady et al. 1987). Fig. 12.4 is taken from the paper by Schady et al. and demonstrates most of them. The reader is referred to the exhaustive account of Schmidt et al. (1978) for more details. *Platybasia* means flattening of the skull base with an increase in the basal angle (BA in the diagram), the angle between the planes of clivus and the floor of the anterior fossa. *Basilar invagination* or *impression* implies an upward bulging of the margins of the foramen magnum. In practice, the anterior margin of the foramen magnum is often displaced upwards to a greater degree than the posterior margin, thus increasing Boogaard's angle (BO), the angle between the plane of the clivus and the plane of the foramen magnum. The position of the odontoid peg relative to Chamberlain's line (CL) and Twining's line (TL) may also be used to indicate basilar impression. Hypoplasia of the occipital condyles is perhaps the mildest example of occipital dysplasia and marked asymmetries of development of the occipital bone are also recognized to occur (Schmidt et al. 1978).

The majority of cases of platybasia and basilar impression are congenital or possibly acquired during birth but a number of primary bone disorders can produce a secondary invagination during adult life. These include: Paget's disease, rickets, osteomalacia, hypothyroidism, osteogenesis imperfecta, fibrous dysplasia, gargoylism, achondroplasia and cleidocranial dysostosis. The proportion of cases of secondary basilar impression is probably between 4% and 8% of the total (Schmidt et al. 1978).

Occipitalization of the Atlas

Some degree of bony union between skull and atlas was recognized in 28 cases out of 66 discussed by McRae (1953). This was *not* commonly associated with platybasia and basilar impression but neurological symptoms and signs similar to those seen in the Chiari malformation were present in two-thirds. McRae reports the presence of the Chiari malformation and dural bands which may well contribute to symptomatology. A high, long or posteriorly angulated odontoid process was usually associated with symptoms.

Clinical Features

The proportion of cases of basilar impression presenting as a clinical problem varies in series depending largely on the derivation of patients. Series from departments attached to neuroscience units will naturally produce a higher frequency of patients with clinical problems. In the English literature, Moreton's (1943) figure of 20% symptomatic is representative of a general radiological series compared with McRae's (1953) suggestion of 62% in patients derived from a neurological institute. Peak onset appears to be in the fifth decade.

A number of authors have commented on the general appearance of many patients with basilar impression. These features are by no means invariable but the presence of a short neck should alert the clinician to the possible association. Neurological symptoms and signs cannot in general be distinguished from those outlined in the discussion of the Chiari malformation for the very good reason that the pathophysiology is essentially the same. However De Barros et al. (1968) felt that a pure pyramidal syndrome was more common in isolated basilar impression.

Association with Chiari Malformation and Syringomyelia

De Barros et al. (1968) reported a series of 66 patients with neurologically symptomatic basilar impression; 33 were subjected to surgical decompression and the Chiari malformation was found in 76% of these. Syringomyelia is also found in association with basilar impression but much less frequently; a figure of 15%–20% seems reasonable but clearly very much dependent upon the derivation of cases (Schmidt et al. 1978).

Management

There are no recent series on the management of bony craniocervical anomalies. The asymptomatic patient clearly presents no problem but a progressing and disabling neurological disorder usually requires surgical decompression. The outlook is clearly less good than for the Chiari malformation and will depend upon the degree of deformation of bone and neural tissue. The coexistence of the Chiari malformation may be protective by acting as a cushion between bone and medulla (De Barros et al. 1968) and in the same way the presence of a wide spinal canal may be helpful in reducing the likelihood of impaction in the Chiari malformation.

Birth Injury

The effects of perinatal trauma have been studied in basilar impression (Battersby and Williams 1982) and in syringomyelia (Williams 1977; Newman et al. 1981). The Chiari malformation has not been studied specifically but as the reader will be aware, there is a great deal of overlap and many of the cases cited in these three studies also had tonsillar herniation. Battersby and Williams derived a birth score based on such factors as prolonged labour, high birth weight, use of forceps and breech delivery and found a history of birth trauma to be four times more likely in patients with basilar impression than in control subjects. This study followed on from the earlier publication of Williams (1977) in syringomyelia. Overriding of the lateral and squamous portions of the occipital bones (occipital osteodiastasis) during birth is proposed as one of the mechanisms leading to foramen magnum distortion and syringomyelia.

   Newman et al. (1981) from data in their similar study suggest that traumatic birth is common in cases of syringomyelia and *either* Chiari malformation *or* basal arachnoiditis but no association was found with the Chiari malformation presenting in other ways. This finding requires confirmation but, if correct, suggests that birth trauma is a factor precipitating syringomyelia in individuals prone to this condition by virtue of the Chiari malformation.

Klippel-Feil Syndrome

This disorder, first described in 1912 by Klippel and Feil, consists of the clinical features of limited neck movements, a low hairline and a very short neck and radiology demonstrating fusion of vertebrae. Considerable variation in the degree of severity exists, a familial tendency has been recognized and the defect is generally thought to represent a defect of mesodermal segmentation, probably occurring before the eighth week of gestation. Many associated abnormalities have been described including hydrocephalus, syringomyelia and syringobulbia. Deafness is fairly common and a curious form of synkinesis or mirror movements of the arms has also been recognized (Wilkinson 1978).

Syringomyelia

The majority of cases of cord syrinx formation are related to obstruction to the outflow of CSF from the fourth ventricle and as such are associated with either craniocervical anomalies or arachnoiditis. As with the anomalies themselves the terminology is confused and confusing. Hydromyelia is used interchangeably with syringomyelia by some authors but by others to describe dilatation of the central canal without the formation of fluid-filled cavities outside the canal in the substance of the cord. Some prefer the combined term syringohydromyelia but the simple terms syringomyelia and syrinx will be used here to describe all fluid-filled cavities within the cord. The majority of syrinx, presenting usually with a. central cord syndrome, are secondary to obstruction of the foramen magnum ("communicating syringomyelia" in the terminology of Barnett et al. 1973). A small proportion are post-traumatic, relate to local arachnoiditis around the cord or are cystic central cord tumours ("non-communicating syringomyelia" according to Barnett et al. 1973). A variety of other disorders have been described in which syrinx formation has occurred. These include intradural extramedullary tumours, vertebral body fractures and disc protrusions. These relatively rare causes of syrinx formation are outside the scope of this article and will not be considered further here.

Aetiology

Like many neurological conditions whose origins are obscure, syringomyelia was first regarded as a degenerative disorder. This term prevented proper thought and active enquiry into its origins for many years. Gardner (1965, 1967) provided the first rational concept when he proposed his *hydrodynamic theory*. This asserted that the condition arose from an obstruction to the outflow of CSF from the fourth ventricle with a patent central canal (which normally closes early in embryonic life) providing an ingress for CSF at raised pressure into the substance of the cord. Arterial pulsations transmitted to the CSF were thought to be the source of the pressure differential. Foster and Hudgson (1973) reasonably nominate cord cavitation, ventricular outflow obstruction and a communication between cavity and fourth ventricle as *Gardner's triad*. They point out that whilst it may not be possible to demonstrate a communication between syrinx and ventricle at operation or post mortem, this does not mean that such a channel was never present.

In a development of this concept, Williams (1969, 1970, 1972) suggested that the major hydrodynamic event was a transfer of CSF from the spinal into the cranial subarachnoid space past the occluding cerebellar tonsils during Valsalva manouevres. The tonsils then re-impact in the foramen magnum leaving a pressure differential between cranial and spinal compartments. The presence of a patent canal leading from the fourth ventricle then encourages tracking of this CSF at raised pressure into the spinal cord. As Foster and Hudgson (1973) point out, this does not really explain every case of communicating syringomyelia especially those with adhesive arachnoiditis around the foramen magnum but the two concepts are not mutually exclusive and both mechanisms may operate.

There is a lack of pathological evidence of a connection between syrinx cavity and either a patent canal or the fourth ventricle itself. Protagonists of the hydrodynamic theory protest that a connection may have been present at some stage which was subsequently sealed off but this awkward fact remains a problem. Ball and Dayan (1972) avoided this difficulty by suggesting that fluid in the spinal subarachnoid space under increased pressure as a result of foramen magnum block, tracked into the substance of the spinal cord along the Virchow-Robin spaces and thus formed syrinx cavities independent of the central canal.

A number of authors have considered ischaemia of the cord to be important in the aetiology (see Foster and Hudgson (1973) for a discussion). Logue and Rice Edwards (1981) regard syringomyelia and the Chiari malformation as associated conditions without a causal link and point out that most of the improvement seen after operation is attributable to decompression of cerebellum and spinal cord rather than an improvement in syringomyelia. MRI of the syrinx before and after operation has however demonstrated reduction in syrinx size, at least initially (Grant et al. 1987a). Prevention of progression of syringomyelia would seem to be the important point here and a definite benefit is difficult to establish given the impossibility of performing a controlled study.

Clinical Features

The two large series of Barnett et al. (1973) and Logue and Rice Edwards (1981) are remarkably similar in the clinical features which they describe. Both describe patients from the era when investigations were not free of hazard and thus the clinical suspicion of syringomyelia had to be strong, i.e. usually a presentation conforming to the classical description. Mean duration of disease before diagnosis was 7.8 years in Logue's series. One must suspect that ready availability of MRI will alter our concepts of the clinical presentation and many more asymptomatic syrinx will be revealed.

Symptoms

Both series point out the extreme variability of both presentation and progression. Onset or deterioration of symptoms in relation to minor trauma, coughing or sneezing is commonplace. Stiffness of the legs, numb hands, pain in the neck and arms and headache are the common principal complaints. Others presented with symptoms of brain stem or lower cranial nerve involvement.

Signs

General appearance. A substantial minority of Barnett's patients had one or more of the following: large head, short neck, scoliosis, Morvan's acrodystrophy of the hands, a *main succulente* or a Charcot joint.

Neurological signs. About 75% of cases had classical syringomyelia with features of a central cord syndrome. The dissociated anaesthesia can be unilateral or bilateral, usually in a "cape", "*cuirasse*" or "suspended" distribution affecting the cervical and dorsal segments. Sensory loss which does not respect the conventional dermatomes may lead the unwary to conclude that a functional component is present. Spinothalamic sensory loss only affecting the leg caused by involvement of sensory long tracts rather than crossing fibres may be seen. Loss of all modalities of sensation in an arm due to root entry zone disease are also recognized to occur. Dissociated sensory loss involving the head and tending to spare the snout regions are a late feature. Somewhat surprisingly, in both series, joint position sense was found to be commonly impaired in both arms and legs. Barnett attributes this to cervical cord compression or upward extension of the syrinx whilst Logue found that proprioceptive loss in the hips is commoner than distal joint loss. This interesting observation is deserving of further study.

As for the sensory changes, lower motor neurone features in the upper limbs are a rule which is frequently broken with either preserved reflexes or frank upper motor neurone changes in the arms. Nine of Logue's 75 patients had complete preservation of upper limb reflexes. Normally the first dorsal segment of the spinal cord is involved early in the disease process producing intrinsic hand muscle wasting and a claw hand. Unless a lumbar syrinx is present, only upper motor neurone signs are found in the legs with a substantial number having no lower limb abnormality. Rarely, a patient may present with lower

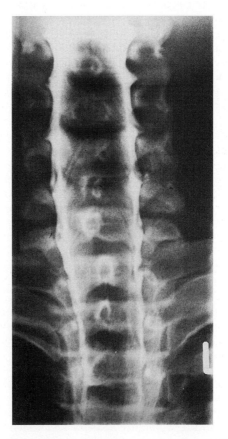

Fig. 12.5. Myelogram demonstrating enlarged cervical spinal cord containing a syrinx. (Radiograph by courtesy of Professor I. Isherwood.)

motor neurone features in the leg. Bladder, bowel and sexual dysfunction occur relatively late in most cases.

Roughly 25% of patients in these two series had symptoms attributable to brain stem involvement. What proportion if these features are truly due to syringobulbia rather than brain stem and lower cranial nerve distortion secondary to the Chiari malformation is another issue which should be resolvable in the future by MRI.

In general the oculomotor disorders seen in syringomyelia are due to a coexistent Chiari malformation and have already been described. The series of both Logue and Barnett mention nystagmus, commonly rotary or vertical in their patients. Clearly true syringopontis might produce a wide range of disorders of gaze but clear correlation of pathology with clinical signs is difficult to obtain. A unilateral Horner's syndrome is not uncommon and usually occurs in association with T1 lower motor neurone signs.

Differential Diagnosis

The patient presenting with a classical central cord syndrome, with or without features of the Chiari malformation, does not usually present much problem to the clinician. The real difficulty here lies with the radiologist who has to differentiate a communicating syrinx from intramedullary tumour, syrinx related to local arachnoiditis or that seen after spinal cord trauma.

Just as the Chiari malformation may present in subtle and insidious ways, so the diagnosis of syringomyelia can be difficult in the early stages. Pain is an early symptom and if unaccompanied by other complaints or definite signs, may be dismissed. Lower motor neurone signs in the arms with atypical sensory signs and a spastic paraparesis may be mistaken for cervical spondylosis in the elderly and multiple sclerosis in the young. Amyotrophy with complete absence of sensory changes can lead to the diagnosis of motor neurone disease being entertained.

Imaging

A full review of imaging of syringomyelia is beyond the scope of this article. The field is rapidly changing and the plethora of papers appearing in the radiologircal journals is testimony to this. Water-soluble contrast myelography in the supine position will usually demonstrate a Chiari malformation (Fig. 12.1) and sometimes a spinal cord of increased diameter (Fig. 12.5). CT of the spinal cord after myelography will often demonstrate the accumulation of contrast in the syrinx cavity, though there is debate about how it gets there. This is often best seen with delayed CT. There is however no doubt that MRI is the investigation of choice on grounds of image quality and the non-invasive nature of the procedure (Fig. 12.2). Patients suspected of syringomyelia should be referred to an appropriately equipped centre. Unfortunately a few patients are quite unable to tolerate the procedure because of the claustrophobia which is induced by the confined space within the scanner. The presence of aneurysm clips or cardiac pacemakers are also contraindications. MRI produces sagittal images which demonstrate the longitudinal extent of syrinx cavities and the degree of hindbrain or cerebellar herniation. A correlation of syrinx size with clinical features has not been demonstrated (Grant et al. 1987b). The presence of severe degrees of scoliosis may make it difficult to obtain these images. T1-weighted or proton density images provide the best anatomical demonstration of disordered anatomy (Sherman et al. 1986). The advent of gadolinium-DTPA as an intravenous contrast agent may contribute to the recognition of arachnoiditis and help in the differentiation of communicating syringomyelia from cavities related to intramedullary tumours.

Management

Gardner's approach to management followed naturally from his hydrodynamic theory of aetiology and consisted of an occipital decompression together with the insertion of a muscle plug into the central canal. Recently it has been recognized that the latter adds to the complications without improving results and in the majority of cases where a foramen magnum abnormality can be

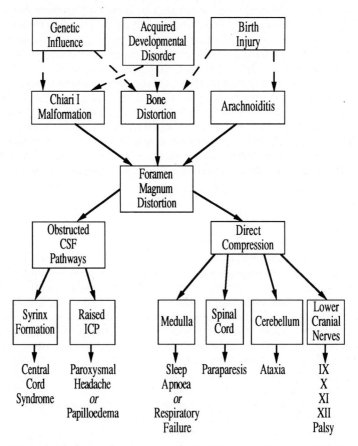

Fig. 12.6. A diagrammatic representation of some of the potential interreacting factors in the production of foramen syndromes.

recognized, simple occipital decompression is practised by many surgeons (Williams 1986). Syrinx drainage by myelotomy and insertion of a tube has been reported to be of benefit, either in combination with occipital decompression or as an isolated or secondary procedure. Drainage may be to the subarachnoid space (Tator et al. 1982) or the peritoneum (Barbaro 1984). Terminal ventriculostomy appears to have gone out of fashion.

Logue and Rice Edwards (1981) performed a decompression of the foramen magnum in the majority of their cases with removal of the lower two-thirds of the squamous portion of the occipital bone, the posterior margin of the foramen magnum and laminae of the upper cervical vertebrae so as to expose the cerebellar tonsils, leaving the dura open but avoiding disturbance of the arachnoid where possible. Syringostomy was performed in a minority. The authors acknowledge the difficulty of drawing conclusions from uncontrolled observations in a disorder with a long time course, variable outcome and natural fluctuations. Pain and paraparesis responded best and little change in sensation, lower motor neurone signs or brain stem features was recorded. Some patients reported sensory improvement but this was usually short-lived. Twenty-two of Logue's series improved after surgery with three relapses. Thirty-three were apparently stabilized and 19 deteriorated after surgery. One patient died. Logue suggests that surgery be avoided in patients who are severely disabled and in those in whom there is no evidence of deterioration.

Levy et al. (1983) provide a good review of the literature as well as reporting their own experience of the Chiari malformation. Comparison of series is very difficult because of varying case mixes but a rough guide suggests that, of patients with syringomyelia and associated Chiari malformation, presenting relatively early, about one-third will have lasting improvement, rather less than half will be stabilized and one-quarter will deteriorate despite surgery. When no foramen magnum lesion is present the much less satisfactory syrinx drainage procedures are the only real option and the possibility of the syrinx being an intramedullary tumour should be reconsidered. The presence of arachnoiditis will reduce the chances of success.

Conclusion

This brief chapter has attempted to identify a number of different clinical strands in a rather complex web of disorders. The central feature is a malformation at the foramen magnum producing a fascinating variety of effects which remain ill-understood and partly because of that lack of understanding, are difficult to manage. Fig. 12.6 is an attempt to illustrate some of the factors which may be important in the development of the clinical syndromes described. The relative importance of genetic, developmental and acquired factors is likely to remain unclear for some time and the challenge for treatment probably lies in the detection of people at risk for syrinx development and a better understanding of the pathophysiology involved, the hope being that early and appropriate intervention will help prevent the awful decline that was previously the lot of the patient with syringomyelia.

Acknowledgements. I am grateful to Professor Ian Isherwood of the Department of Diagnostic Radiology at Manchester University for the radiological illustrations. Mr. Robin Johnston kindly supplied the picture of the Chiari malformation at operation. Drs. Ian Bone and Donald Hadley reviewed the manuscript and provided much helpful comment. Any errors are my own.

References

Aboulezz AO, Sartor K, Geyer CA, Gado MH (1985) Position of cerebellar tonsils in the normal population and in patients with the Chiari malformation: a quantitative approach with MR imaging. J Comput Assist Tomogr 9(6):1033–1036

Appleby A, Foster JB, Hankinson J, Hudgson P (1968) The diagnosis and management of the Chiari anomalies in adult life. Brain 91:131–140

Arnold J (1894) Myelocyste, Transposition von Gewebskeimen und Sympodie. Beitr Path Anat 16:1

Baker HL (1963) Myelographic examination of the posterior fossa with a positive contrast medium. Radiology 81:791

Balk RA, Hiller FC, Lucas EA, Scrima L, Wilson FJ, Wooten V (1985) Sleep apnoea and the Arnold-Chiari malformation. Am Rev Respir Dis 132(4):929–930

Ball MJ, Dayan AD (1972) Pathogenesis of syringomyelia. Lancet 2:799

Banerji NK, Millar JHD (1974) Chiari malformation presenting in adult life – its relationship to syringomyelia. Brain 97:157–168

Barboro NM, Wilson CB, Gutin PH, Edwards MS (1984) Surgical treatment of syringomyelia. Favourable results with syringoperitoneal shunting. J Neurosurg 61:531–538

Barkovich AJ, Wippold FJ, Sherman JL, Citrin CM (1986) Significance of cerebellar tonsillar position on MR. AJNR 7:795–799

Barkovich AJ, Bent OK, Norman D, Edwards MS (1989) Revised classification of posterior fossa cysts and cystlike malformations based on the results of multiplanar MR imaging. AJNR 10:977–988

Barnett HJM, Foster JB, Hudgson P (1973) Syringomyelia. Saunders, London

Battersby RDE, Williams B (1982) Birth injury: a possible contributory factor in the aetiology of primary basilar impression. J Neurol Neurosurg Psychiatry 45:879–883

Bosley TM, Cohen DA, Schatz NJ, et al. (1985) Comparison of metrizamide computed tomography and magnetic resonance imaging in the evaluation of lesions at the cervicomedullary junction. Neurology 35:485–492

Brown JR (1977) The Dandy-Walker syndrome. In: Vinken PJ, Bruyn GW (eds) Handbook of clinical neurology vol 30. Elsevier/North-Holland, Amsterdam, pp 623–646

Bullock R, Todd NV, Easton J, Hadley D (1988) Isolated central respiratory failure due to syringomyelia and Arnold-Chiari malformation. Br Med J 297:1448–1449

Chiari H (1891) Über Veränderungen des Kleinhirns infolge Hydrocephalie des Grosshirns. Dtsch Med Wschr 17:1172–1175

Chiari H (1896) Über Veränderungen des Kleinhirns, des Pons und Medulla oblongata infolge von kongenitaler Hydrocephalie des Grosshirns. Denkschr Akad Wiss Wien 63:71

Cleland J (1883) Contribution to the study of spina bifida, encephalocoele and anencephalus. J Anat Physiol 17:257

Cogan DG (1968) Downbeating nystagmus. Arch Ophthalmol 80:757

Conway LW (1967) Hydrodynamic studies in syringomyelia. J Neurosurg 27:501–514

Coria F, Quintana F, Rebollo M, Combarros O, Berciano J (1983) Occipital dysplasia and Chiari type I deformity in a family. Clinical and radiological study of three generations. J Neurol Sci 62:147–158

Dandy WE, Blackfan KD (1914) Internal hydrocephalus: an experimental, clinical and pathological study. Amer J Dis Child 8:406–482

De Barros MC, Farias W, Ataide L, Lins S (1968) Basilar impression and Arnold Chiari malformation. J Neurol Neurosurg Psychiatry 31:596–605

Foster JB, Hudgson P (1973) The pathogenesis of communicating syringomyelia. In: Barnett HJM, Foster JB, Hudgson P (eds) Syringomyelia. Saunders, London, pp 104–123

Gardner WJ (1965) Hydrodynamic mechanisms of syringomyelia: its relationship to myelocele. J Neurol Neurosurg Psychiatry 28:247–256

Gardner WJ (1967) Myelocele: rupture of the neural tube? Clin Neurosurg 15:57

Gardner WJ (1973) The Dandy Walker malformation. The dysraphic states from syringomyelia to anencephaly. Excerpta Medica, Amsterdam, pp 127–143

Gardner WJ, Smith JL, Padget DH (1972) The relationship of Arnold-Chiari and Dandy-Walker malformations. J Neurosurg 36:481–486

Gilbert JN, Jones KL, Rorke LB, Chernoff GF, James HE (1986) Central nervous system anomalies associated with meningomyelocoele, hydrocephalus and the Arnold-Chiari malformation: reappraisal of theories regarding the pathogenesis of posterior neural tube closure defects. Neurosurgery 18(5):559–564

Grant R, Hadley DM, Lang D, et al. (1987a) MRI measurement of syrinx size before and after operation. J Neurol Neurosurg Psychiatry 50:1685–1687

Grant R, Hadley DM, Macpherson P, et al. (1987b) Syringomyelia: cyst measurement by magnetic resonance imaging and comparison with symptoms, signs and disability. J Neurol Neurosurg Psychiatry 50:1008–1014

Hampton F, Williams B, Loizou LA (1982) Syncope as a presenting feature of hindbrain herniation with syringomyelia. J Neurol Neurosurg Psychiatry 45:919–922

Leigh JR, Zee DS (1983) Diagnosis of central disorders of ocular motility. The neurology of eye movement. Davis, Philadelphia, pp 216–217

Levy WJ, Mason L, Hahn JF (1983) Chiari malformation presenting in adults: a surgical experience in 127 cases. Neurosurgery 12:377–390

Logue V, Rice Edwards M (1981) Syringomyelia and its surgical treatment – an analysis of 75 patients. J Neurol Neurosurg Psychiatry 44:273–284

Marin-Padilla M, Marin-Padilla TM (1981) Morphogenesis of experimentally induced Arnold-Chiari malformation. J Neurol Sci 50:29–55

McManus D, Bartlett P (1986) The role of nuclear magnetic resonance imaging in the diagnosis of the Arnold Chiari malformation. Radiography 52:275–80

McRae DL (1953) Bony abnormalities in the region of the foramen magnum: correlation of the anatomic and neurological findings. Acta Radiol [Stockh] 40:335–354

Mohr PD, Strang FA, Sambrook M, Boddie HG (1977) The clinical and surgical features of 40 patients with primary cerebellar ectopia (adult Chiari malformation). Quart J Med 181:85–96

Moreton RD (1943) Basilar invagination: so-called platybasia. Proc Mayo Clin 18:353

Newman PK, Terenty TR, Foster JB (1981) Some observations on the pathogenesis of syringomyelia. J Neurol Neurosurg Psychiatry 44:964–969

Nightingale S, Williams B (1987) Hindbrain hernia headache. Lancet 1:731–734

Paul KS, Lye RH, Strang FA, Dutton J (1983) Arnold Chiari malformation – review of 71 cases. J Neurosurg 58:183–187

Roth M (1986) Cranio-cervical growth collision: another explanation of the Arnold-Chiari malformation and of basilar impression. Neuroradiology 28:187–194

Saez RJ, Onofrio BM, Yangihara T (1976) Experience with Arnold-Chiari malformation 1960–1970. J Neurosurg 45:416–422

Salam MZ, Adams RD (1978) The Arnold-Chiari malformation. In: Vinken PJ, Bruyn GW (eds) Handbook of clinical neurology vol 32. Elsevier/North-Holland, Amsterdam, pp 99–110

Schady W, Metcalfe RA, Butler P (1987) The incidence of craniocervical bony anomalies in the adult Chiari malformation. J Neurol Sci 82:193–203

Schliep G (1978) Syringomyelia and syringobulbia. In: Vinken PJ, Bruyn GW (eds) Handbook of clinical neurology vol 32. Elsevier/North-Holland, Amsterdam, pp 255–327

Schmidt H, Sartor K, Heckl RW (1978) Bone malformations of the craniocervical region. In: Vinken PJ, Bruyn GW (eds) Handbook of clinical neurology vol 32. Elsevier/North-Holland, Amsterdam, pp 1–98

Sherman JL, Barkovich AJ, Citrin CM (1986) The MR appearances of syringomyelia: new observations. AJNR 7:985–995

Spillane JD, Pallis C, Jones AM (1957) Developmental abnormalities in the region of the foramen magnum. Brain 80:11

Taggert JK, Walker AE (1942) Congenital atresia of the foramens of Luschka and Magendie. Arch Neurol Psychiatry (Chic) 48:583–612

Tator CH, Meguro K, Rowed DW (1982) Favourable results with syringosuborachnoid shunts for treatment of syringomyelia. J Neurosurg 56:517–523

Wilkinson M (1978) The Klippel-Feil syndrome. In: Vinken PJ, Bruyn GW (eds) Handbook of clinical neurology vol 32. Elsevier/North-Holland, Amsterdam, pp 111–122

Williams B (1969) Hypothesis: the distending force in the production of "communicating syringomyelia". Lancet 2:189

Williams B (1970) Current concepts of syringomyelia. Br J Hosp Med 4:331
Williams B (1972) Combined cisternal and lumbar pressure recordings in the sitting position using
    differential manometry. J Neurol Neurosurg Psychiatry 35:142
Willams B (1977) Difficult labour as a cause of communicating syringomyelia. Lancet 2:51–53
Willams B (1986) Progress in syringomyelia. Neurol Res 8:130–145
Wolpert SM, Scott RM, Platenberg C, Runge VM (1988) The clinical significance of hindbrain
    herniation and deformity as shown on MR images of patients with Chiari II malformation.
    AJNR 9(6):1075–1080
Zimmerman CF, Roach ES, Troost BT (1986) See-saw nystagmus associated with the Chiari
    malformation. Arch Neurol 43(3):299–300

Chapter 13

Cervical Myelopathy due to Rheumatoid Arthritis

J.P.R. Dick

Cervical arthropathy, often with vertebral subluxation, is seen frequently in patients with rheumatoid arthritis (RA). Local pain is the commonest symptom; less commonly a myelopathy may develop though even quite gross disease may be clinically silent. In patients with acute or progressive myelopathy, surgical therapy is recommended and the currently accepted practice is to perform anterior decompression, with posterior spinal stabilization in addition, if indicated.

Introduction

RA can affect all synovial joints in the cervical spine, the interarticular facets of C1–2 and C2–3 being particularly vulnerable. Radiological changes are seen in up to 40% of inpatient series (Conlon et al. 1965) but a clinically overt myelopathy is uncommon despite the frequent occurrence of exaggerated deep tendon reflexes (Stevens et al. 1971). Only 2%–5% of patients with RA and cervical subluxation will develop a clinically overt myelopathy but, of these, half have a progressive course (Nakano et al. 1978; Marks and Sharp 1981). A variety of mechanisms have been suggested to account for the myelopathy.

History

Garrod (1890) commented on the increased deep tendon reflexes of some patients with RA and first drew attention to the cervical arthropathy. The first clear description of atlantoaxial subluxation causing death is given by Davis and Markley (1951) though earlier reports had referred to this complication in RA (Ely 1911). Subsequent large series published in the rheumatological and radiological literature have assessed the frequency of cervical arthropathy and clinical myelopathy (Sharp and Purser 1961; Conlon et al. 1965; Mathews 1969; Smith et al. 1972; Marks and Sharp 1981).

Anatomy

Abnormal anteroposterior movement of the atlas on the axis is usually termed atlantoaxial subluxation (AAS). This can be seen in normal children with nasopharyngeal inflammation (Watson Jones 1932) and in children with Down's syndrome. It is seen, to a minor degree, during normal adolescence (Sharp and Purser 1961). During flexion and extension of the head a fixed anatomical relationship is usually maintained between atlas and axis by the transverse and alar ligaments of the odontoid process. Rheumatoid involvement of these ligaments causes forward slip of the atlas on the axis in flexion. As a result the odontoid peg pushes backwards on to the spinal cord which is tethered anteriorly by the dentate ligament (Osborne et al. 1983). A pathological degree of separation between the arch of the atlas and the odontoid peg is defined as greater than 3 mm on a lateral radiograph of the cervical spine in flexion and this is seen in 25% of patients with RA (Conlon et al. 1965). However, as the spinal canal is widest at the craniocervical junction, only 13% of patients with AAS have neurological sequelae (Smith et al. 1972).

Myelopathy at this level may also arise from exuberant pannus formation around the odontoid peg (Stevens et al. 1986) or as a result of "cranial settling" in which there is a vertical and backward displacement of the odontoid peg into the foramen magnum (Menezes et al. 1985). Less commonly, myelopathy can develop as a result of vertebral artery compression. This occurs because the interfacetal joints are displaced posteriorly in neck extension and will compromise the vertebral artery as it enters the spinal canal. In head rotation a dominant vertebral artery may be compromised in much the same fashion (Robinson et al. 1986).

More frequently, myelopathy may be due to subaxial subluxations which are seen in 8% of patients with RA (Conlon et al. 1965). Unlike AAS the frequency of this radiological abnormality is correlated with age (Smith et al. 1972).

Pathology

The classical pathological changes of RA are seen at synovial joints in the cervical spine. Since the vertebral bodies are united by fibrocartilage, these changes are confined to the neurocentral and the interfacetal joints; in addition, there are synovial membranes anterior to the odontoid peg and anterior and posterior to the cruciate ligament. Pannus formation may occur at all three sites with consequent juxta-articular bone erosion and ligament damage. Subsequent vascularization and fibrinoid necrosis of the alar and cruciate ligaments increase ligamentous laxity and allow anterior dislocation; this process may be further exacerbated by the administration of steroids (Martel and Abel 1963). Vertical translocation of the dens into the cranial cavity occurs as a result of collapse of the lateral masses of the atlas. Of one series, 8% demonstrated "settling" of C1 on C2 (Mathews 1969); this increased to 33% at follow-up five years later (Mathews 1974).

Mechanism of Myelopathy

A small number of cases of active rheumatoid vasculitis in the cervical region have been pathologically confirmed (Ouyang et al. 1967; Markenson et al. 1979). However, most pathological studies suggest mechanical factors cause rheumatoid myelopathy.

On the basis of microscopic evidence, Hughes (1977) has suggested that intermittent compression of the anterior spinal artery causes central cord infarction two segments caudal to the level of vertebral compression. Both his study and that of Nakano et al. (1978) found irregular central areas of cord necrosis predominantly affecting the ventral horns. This picture is unlike that of venous infarction due to chronic cord compression in which the veins are thrombosed, laden with haemosiderin and maximum change occurs in the dorsolateral funiculus. Nakano et al. (1978) suggest that the major effect of intermittent mechanical trauma is on small sulcal and intraparenchymal arteries which run rostrocaudally and are perpendicular to anteroposterior compressive forces. Manz et al. (1983) examined pathologically four cases of rheumatoid myelopathy and demonstrated endarteritis obliterans of radicular and intraspinal arteries in three. Intimal fibrosis was striking and the authors felt that this reflected multiple minor episodes of arterial trauma rather than atherosclerotic disease as the origins of the parent main arteries were unaffected. Experimental studies in primates have shown that the combined effects of mechanical compression and anterior spinal artery ligation cause central cord necrosis similar in type to that seen in RA myelopathy. The notion of an ongoing mechanically-induced vascular myelopathy is further supported by recent MRI evidence showing that the spinal cord re-expands after decompression and posterior fixation (Zygmunt et al. 1988).

Presentation

Although striking AAS can occur in the absence of neck pain, such pain was the dominant feature in 19 of 31 patients in one series (Stevens et al. 1986). It is prominent during active disease, is present in the morning and is aggravated by head movement. It will first be felt in the suboccipital region and is referred over the cranium towards the temporal regions. This pain often radiates in a C2 distribution, so-called occipital neuralgia, and was present in 19 of 32 patients in Nakano et al.'s series (1978). Pain from other cervical segments is referred elsewhere; that from disease at C4 and C5 levels tends to be more severe than from C5 and C6 levels (Marks 1985) and is referred to the supraclavicular areas rather than to the shoulders.

An equally common presenting symptom is paraesthesia and numbness. This was seen in 23 of 31 patients in Marks and Sharp's series (1981), was more often seen in the hands than the feet and may have a glove and stocking distribution (Stevens et al. 1971; Marks and Sharp 1981; Stevens et al. 1986). As the myelopathy progresses the patient develops a mild spastic tetraparesis, worse in the upper limbs and a sensory level (Nakano et al. 1978). Marks and

Sharp (1981) point out that hand sensory symptoms initially may be unilateral leading to a diagnosis of mononeuropathy and subsequent delay in the appropriate diagnosis. Lhermitte's phenomenon and flexor spasms are not infrequent (Nakano et al. 1978; Marks and Sharp 1981; Stevens et al. 1986). Vertigo, diplopia and dysphagia associated with bulbar signs (trigeminal hypoaesthesia, Horner's syndrome and internuclear opthalmoplegia) may be seen in up to 20% of cases (Nakano et al. 1978). Their presence may be related to head position (Robinson et al. 1986).

Several authors point out the difficulty in assessing limb power due to pain or deformity; more reliable are exaggerated deep tendon reflexes, though the frequency with which they occur varies from 6% in rheumatological series (Conlon et al. 1965) to 66% (Stevens et al. 1971) in neurological series.

Examination of the neck is often limited by pain and should not be vigorous in patients with a symptomatic myelopathy. Sharp and Purser (1961) have shown that, in patients with AAS, posterior pressure on the forehead causes backward sliding of the head as subluxation is reduced. This is best appreciated by the index finger of the other hand placed on the spinous process of C2 and was seen in 16 of 36 patients with AAS in Stevens et al.'s series (1971).

Course

AAS is horizontal initially but after the passage of time will include a vertical element (Mathews 1974). Rarely this can cause brain stem compression and respiratory failure leading to death (Storey 1958). However, this outcome is unusual and radiological changes alone in the absence of clinical symptoms are not infrequent (Smith et al. 1972; Mathews 1974) and should not lead to unnecessary surgery. Nevertheless, significant symptomatic myelopathies do occur and it is said that of these 50% will progress (Crockard et al. 1986). Under these circumstances aggressive management is indicated as a brain stem death can occur. Ranawat et al. (1979) staged patients into three levels on clinical criteria:

I   Subjective paraesthesiae without objective signs
II Weakness and subjective paraesthesiae with only hyperreflexia
III Weakness and subjective paraesthesiae with objective evidence of weakness and long tract signs

Patients in Stage III require careful neurological evaluation with a view to surgical intervention. Meijers et al. (1984) point to certain "alarm signs" which should prompt careful assessment with a view to surgical intervention: these include severe neck pain, jumping legs, stone or marble sensations in the body and urinary problems.

Radiology

The radiological features of rheumatoid arthropathy in the neck include generalized and juxta-articular osteoporosis, narrowing of vertebral discs without osteophytosis, erosions at vertebral end plates and erosion and fusion of apophyseal joints (Marks and Sharp 1981). These are distinct from the changes seen in cervical spondylosis due to osteoarthritis though the two often coexist, particularly in older patients (Conlon et al. 1965). The commonest radiographic abnormality in RA is apophyseal joint erosion or blurring (usually at C2–C3) and this was seen in 35% of patients with rheumatoid arthritis (Conlon et al. 1965).

The second commonest abnormality, occurring in 20%–25% of all cases, was anterior subluxation of the atlas on the axis (Conlon et al. 1965). Of all patients with cervical arthropathy AAS is seen in 74%, subaxial dislocation in 41% and vertical subluxation in 24% (Redlund-Johnell 1984). AAS was correlated with the severity of joint changes in the hands but not with age (Smith et al. 1972) or with the presence of neck pain on head movement (Stevens et al. 1971).

Although the presence of AAS does not correlate with the presence or severity of cord symptoms or signs, greater mobility of AAS makes it more likely that the myelopathy will pursue an aggressive course (Stevens et al. 1986). The investigation of choice for assessing cord compromise at this level is CT myelography (Stevens et al. 1986). In this series 21 of 31 cases showed deformity of the spinal cord at the craniocervical junction with associated changes due to the rheumatoid process. MR imaging of this region can be equally revealing (Bundsuch et al. 1988) though there are few reports on its clinical usefulness (Zygmunt et al. 1988).

Subaxial subluxations also are seen in RA and when present are not infrequently the cause of neurological symptoms. This is probably due to the narrower spinal canal at this level. Of 31 cases of RA myelopathy 9 had cord atrophy due to subaxial disease alone (Stevens et al. 1986).

Management

In all patients with severe RA, plain radiographs of the cervical spine, particularly in flexion and extension, should be undertaken so that other medical personnel are aware of the potential for subluxation, particularly under anaesthesia. If the patient is asymptomatic regular follow-up with serial radiographs to detect the progression of any displacement is usually sufficient.

The indications for surgical intervention are relative in view of the risks of operating on patients with advanced RA who have a variety of additional clinical problems and who often have been on long-term steroids. They can be broadly summarized as increasing neck pain that is refractory to conservative measures, serial radiological evidence of increasing spinal instability or a deteriorating neurological condition.

A moulded custom-made firm collar maintaining the cervical spine in extension may be used if the neurological disability is slight or the patient's condition too poor for surgery; it should include the chin and occiput. A softer collar is usually insufficient. Myelopathy due to subaxial subluxations respond less well than do the myelopathies caused by degenerative spondylosis (Hamblen 1983). Marks and Sharp (1981) found that only 6 of 15 patients treated with collar alone showed substantial improvement. In patients without neurological signs, Smith et al. (1972) did not find that the use of a cervical collar was associated with improvement in neck pain and found there was a significant degree of non-compliance.

Light cervical traction in extension (1.8–2.2 kg) with skull calipers and a Halo or Stryker frame is routine preoperative practice by some authors (Hamblen 1983; Meijers et al. 1984); others, however, have noted acute neurological deterioration while on traction and have cautioned against its routine use (Crellin et al. 1970; Marks and Sharp 1981). Regular examination for evidence of neurological deterioration and careful radiological assessment in order to avoid spinal overdistraction is mandatory (Hamblen 1983). In addition, the elderly RA patient tolerates immobilization in bed and traction poorly. Traction therefore, should be performed for no more than a few days at the most, so as to avoid the complications of bed sores, thrombophlebitis and pneumonia.

Several surgical procedures for reducing and/or stabilizing AAS have been described. These initially consisted of a posterior fixation of the craniocervical junction by either atlantoaxial or occipitocervical bony fusion (Hamblen 1967; Ferlic et al. 1975; Ranawat et al. 1979). The major disadvantage of such attempts at bone fusion was the need for immobilization in traction for 6 to 12 weeks after surgery. Such series were associated with an average mortality of 25%, coupled with no functional improvement in a further 30% of patients. In addition, there was a low rate of successful fusion in the RA neck. Recognition of the need to achieve an immediate and lasting cervical fixation that would allow early postoperative ambulation led to the development of new metal fixation devices (Mitsui 1984; Ransford et al. 1986). These, together with improved preoperative assessment of the complex anatomy of the craniocervical junction by flexion-extension CT myelography have led to considerable improvements in the surgical results (Crockard et al. 1986; Stevens et al. 1986; Jackowski et al. 1987). Improved imaging has clearly identified those patients with a significant anterior compression that fails to reduce on neck extension. This may be caused either by an irreducibly subluxed odontoid peg, or by florid pannus. It is this group of patients who are most likely to deteriorate or show no improvement in their neurology following posterior fixation alone. In such instances an anterior transoral decompressive approach (Fang and Ong 1962) allows the total removal of both the odontoid peg and the periodontoid pannus. This has lead to a dramatic improvement in the outcome of surgical management of AAS. In several series not only has there been no postoperative mortality but there have also been substantial improvements in neurological and functional outcome (Crockard et al. 1986; Jackowski et al. 1987; Menezes and Van Gilder 1988).

References

Bundsuch C, Modic MT, Kearney F, Morris R, Deal C (1988) Rheumatoid arthritis of the cervical spine: surface coil MR imaging. AJR 151:181–187

Conlon PW, Isdale IC, Rose BS (1965) Rheumatoid arthritis of the cervical spine: an analysis of 333 cases. Ann Rheum 25:120–126

Crellin RQ, Maccabe JJ, Hamilton EBD (1970) Severe subluxation of the cervical spine in rheumatoid arthritis. J Bone Joint Surg 52B:244–251

Crockard HA, Pozo JL, Ransford AO, Stevens JM, Kendall BE, Essigman WK (1986) Transoral decompression and posterior fusion for rheumatoid atlanto-axial subluxation. J Bone Joint Surg 68B:350–356

Davis FW, Markley HE (1951) Rheumatoid arthritis with death from medullary compression. Ann Int Med 35:451

Ely LW (1911) Subluxation of the atlas; a report of two cases. Ann Surg 54:20–29

Fang HSY, Ong GB (1962) Direct approach to the upper cervical spine. J Bone Joint Surg (Am) 44:1588–1604

Ferlic DC, Clayton ML, Leidhoff JD (1975) Surgical treatment of the symptomatic unstable cervical spine in rheumatoid arthritis. J Bone Joint Surg (Am) 57:349–354

Garrod AE (1890) A treatise on rheumatism and rheumatoid arthritis. Griffin & Co, London

Hamblen DL (1967) Occipito-cervical fusion. Indications, technique and results. J Bone Joint Surg (Br) 49:33–45

Hamblen DL (1983) Surgical treatment of rheumatoid arthritis; the cervical spine. In: Harris NH (ed) Postgraduate textbook of clinical orthopaedics. Wright and sons, Bristol, UK, pp 487–497

Hughes JT (1977) Spinal cord involvement by C4/5 vertebral subluxation in rheumatoid arthritis: a description of 2 cases examined at necropsy. Ann Neurol 1:575–582

Jackowski A, Crockard HA, Ransford AO (1987) Transoral odontoidectomy and posterior stabilization in rheumatoid arthritis: an analysis of 34 patients with symptomatic atlanto-axial subluxation. J Neurol Neurosurg Psychiatry 50:1093–1094

Manz HJ, Luessenhop AJ, Robertson DM (1983) Cervical myelopathy due to atlantoaxial and subaxial subluxation in rheumatoid arthritis. Arch Pathol Lab Med 107:94–98

Markenson JA, McDougal JS, Tsairis P, Lockshin MD, Christian CL (1979) Rheumatoid meningitis: a localized immune process. Ann Intern Med 90:786–789

Marks JS (1985) Rheumatoid neck. Br J Hosp Med 33:96–100

Marks JS, Sharp J (1981) Rheumatoid cervical myelopathy. Q J Med 199:307–319

Martel W, Abel MR (1963) Fatal atlanto-axial luxation in rheumatoid arthritis. Arthritis Rheum 6:224–231

Mathews JA (1969) Atlanto-axial subluxation in rheumatoid arthritis. Ann Rheum Dis 28:260

Mathews JA (1974) Atlanto-axial subluxation in rheumatoid arthritis: a 5 year follow-up study. Ann Rheum Dis 33:526

Meijers KAE, Cats A, Kremer HPH, Luyendijk W, Onvlee GJ, Thomeer RTWM (1984) Cervical myelopathy in rheumatoid arthritis. Clin Exp Rheumatol 2:239–245

Menezes AH, VanGilder JC (1988) Transoral-transpharyngeal approach to the anterior cranio-cervical junction: ten year experience with 72 patients. J Neurosurg 69:895–903

Menezes AH, Van Gilder JC, Clark CR, El-Khoury G (1985) Odontoid upward migration in rheumatoid arthritis: an analysis of 45 patients with "cranial settling". J Neurosurg 63:500–509

Mitsui H (1984) A new operation for atlanto-axial arthrodesis. J Surg (Br) 66B:422–425

Nakano KK, Schoene WC, Baker RA, Dawson DM (1978) The cervical myelopathy associated with rheumatoid arthritis: an analysis of 32 patients with 2 post mortem cases. Ann Neurol 3:144–151

Ouyang R, Mitchell DM, Rozdilsky B (1967) Central nervous system involvement in rheumatoid disease: report of a case. Neurology 17:1099–1105

Osborne D, Triolo P, Dubois P, Drayer B, Heinz E (1983) Assessment of the cranio-cervical junction and atlanto-axial relations using metrizamide-enhanced CT in flexion and extension. AJNR 4:843–845

Ranawat CS, O'Leary P, Pellicci PM, Tsairis P, Marchisello P, Dorr L (1979) Cervical spine fusion in rheumatoid arthritis. J Bone Joint Surg 61A:1002–1010

Ransford AO, Crockard HA, Pozo JL, Thomas NP, Nelson IW (1986) Cranio-cervical instability treated by a contoured loop. J Bone Joint Surg 68B:173–177

Redlund-Johnell I (1984) Dislocations of the cervical spine in rheumatoid arthritis. Thesis, Lund University, Sweden

Robinson BP, Seeger JF, Zak SM (1986) Rheumatoid arthritis and positional vertebrobasilar insufficiency: case report. J Neurosurg 65:111–114

Sharp J, Purser DW (1961) Spontaneous atlanto-axial dislocation in ankylosing spondylitis and rheumatoid arthritis. Ann Rheum Dis 20:47

Smith PH, Benn RT, Sharp J (1972) Natural history of rheumatoid cervical luxations. Ann Rheum Dis 31:431–439

Stevens JC, Cartiledge NEF, Saunders M, Appleby A, Hall M, Shaw DA (1971) Atlanto-axial subluxation and cervical myelopathy in rheumatoid arthritis. Q J Med 40:391–408

Stevens JM, Kendall BE, Crockard HA (1986) The spinal cord in rheumatoid arthritis with clinical myelopathy: a computed myelographic study. J Neurol Neurosurg Psychiatry 49:140–151

Storey G (1958) Changes in the cervical spine in rheumatoid arthritis with compression of the cord. Ann Phys Med 4:216

Swinson DR, Hamilton EBD, Mathews JA, Yates DAH (1972) Vertical subluxation of the axis in rheumatoid arthritis. Ann Rheum Dis 31:359–363

Watson Jones R (1932) Spontaneous hyperaemic dislocation of the atlas. Proc Roy Soc Med 25:586

Zygmunt S, Saveland H, Brattstrom H, Ljunggren B, Larsson EM, Wollheim F (1988) Reduction of periodontoid pannus following posterior occipito-cervical fusion visualized by magnetic resonance imaging. Br J Neurosurg 2:315–320

Chapter 14

Meningitic Disorders and Myelopathies

E.M.R. Critchley

The spinal cord is that part of the central nervous system lying within the vertebral canal. It extends as an oval tube from the medulla oblongata at the foramen magnum to the L1–2 interspace or the upper part of the L2 vertebra. Its enveloping membranes are confluent with those covering the surface of the brain. The pia mater is intimately adherent to the cord with fine septa penetrating into the parenchyma. The arachnoid mater covers the cord more loosely, extending laterally over the dorsal ganglia and emergent roots, and downwards over the nerves of the cauda equina where it is attached to the sacrum at S2. CSF, secreted in the main by the choroid plexuses within the ventricular system of the brain, is contained within the transparent arachnoid membrane. Externally, the dura mater forms a tougher, opaque membrane over the surface of the brain and spinal cord. At spinal level it is tethered laterally by the dentate ligaments and ensheathes the arachnoid, pia, spinal cord and upper part of the cauda equina before ending at S2–3.

Any inflammatory, irritative or infiltrative disorder of the leptomeninges (pia mater and arachnoid) will cause a meningitic reaction – meningitis – with thickening of the meninges and exudation of cells and protein into the CSF of the subarachnoid space. Almost invariably, the meningeal reaction also involves the dura and spreads into the substance of the brain and spinal cord producing local inflammatory, infiltrative or arteritic changes. Viral diseases, predominantly but not invariably, invade the brain producing an encephalitis. Some secondary changes occur elsewhere but the pyogenic reaction is minimal. Where a bacterial infection clearly involves the substance of the brain, terms such as encephalomyelitis or myeloencephalitis are used; but even where there has been little encephalitic reaction, a bacterial meningitic infection will result in systemic changes such as pyrexia and leucocytosis; cerebral irritation with headache, epilepsy, cranial nerve palsies or photophobia; as well as cerebrospinal and spinal manifestations. There are two valid reasons that explain the undue emphasis usually given to the spinal component of meningitis: the clinical recognition of its presence by means of tests which depend essentially upon the presence of muscle spasm over the irritated meninges, and the use of a lumbar puncture needle, penetrating the lower subarachnoid space, in diagnosis, and sometimes therapeutically, in the management of meningitis.

Most spinal infections result from haematogenous spread. The meninges may be invaded directly as happens with disseminated miliary tuberculosis, via the choroid plexus with bacteria entering the CSF directly, or as a result of septic emboli lodging in the smaller arteries causing mycotic aneurysms to develop and rupture. Ascending vascular spread via the venous plexuses of blood vessels around the cord is a rare but well-documented cause of infection. Next most common after blood-borne infection is direct spread from local sites of infection such as bone, the sinuses and middle ear. In the case of certain viral infections neural spread from the nasopharynx and other infected tissues may also occur. Lastly, direct penetration of the meninges can occur aided by dysraphism, fractures or the introduction of contaminants – bacteria, chemicals, or the development of dermoids – via a lumbar puncture needle. Repeated episodes of meningitis raise questions of additional factors such as dural tears with CSF leakage, dermal sinuses, unhealed fractures, midline deformities and immunodeficient states.

An acute epidural abscess is likely to be the result of a blood-borne infection but at least 50% of chronic abscesses and granulomas develop from contiguous infection from neighbouring bones. Most epidural abscesses are caused by staphylococci but brucella, typhoid and gram-negative infections due to *E. coli*, pseudomonas or proteus may also present with the formation of an epidural abscess. Such abscesses are mostly seen over several segments of the thoracic spine. Partial compression of the cord may result, accompanied by excessive secretion of protein into the CSF to give Froin's syndrome with a thick, yellow, gelatinous and proteinaceous spinal fluid; but such classical signs suggest delayed diagnosis.

Subdural infection usually arises via the paranasal sinuses where the adherent dura becomes infected and the infection spreads on to its inner more vascular layer. Once the dura has been penetrated, the leptomeninges offer little resistance and fungal infections in particular spread locally to produce a combination of chronic meningitis, thrombophlebitis, microabscesses and granulomata.

The CSF offers an excellent culture medium for many organisms but the innate vascularity of the meninges enables a rapid blood-borne cellular response to develop. Where the infection is bacterial, the resultant pyogenic exudation shows a predominantly polymorphonuclear pleocytosis; if the infection is viral a lymphocytic pleocytosis is more usual. These cellular changes are accompanied by a seepage of protein into the CSF rendering it more sticky and eventually impeding flow. If the meningitis becomes chronic, as may happen with subacute or partially treated infections, fibroblasts proliferate and adhesions develop blocking the basal cisterns, sealing off the foramina of Lushka and Magendie, or matting together the roots of the cauda equina. Later complications include the development of hydrocephalus, arachnoid cysts at various levels, and a progressive spinal arachnoiditis. Spinal arachnoiditis occurs particularly as a response to the injection of toxic chemicals. Radioopaque contrast media have been especially inculpated in the past but the combination of aetiological factors required is far from clear with the suggestion that there should be some evidence of infection as well as irritation. Thus certain non-infective causes of chronic meningitis such as neoplasia, sarcoidosis, Behçet's and chronic benign lymphocytic meningitis (Mollaret's meningitis), are associated with a low incidence of arachnoiditis whereas chronic infections with tuberculosis, brucellosis and fungi frequently cause widespread arachnoid reactions.

Meningitis may be overlooked and obscured by other disease manifestations in the very young and very old. At the extremes of life the differential diagnosis of unexplained pyrexia, failure to thrive or inanition require an examination of the CSF. Chronic infections may present insidiously in all age groups, but especially in the immunocompromised individual. Nonetheless, most forms of meningitis present with a tetrad of headache, fever, increasing drowsiness and meningeal irritation. Headache is almost invariable and usually severe, continuous and increasing in intensity, especially at the back of the head and neck. Its presence may be indicated in young children and in those too ill to complain by other accompanying features such as photophobia, vomiting and papilloedema. Even taking these characteristics into account it is a lesser diagnostic feature than meningeal irritability.

The neck is the most mobile part of the spinal column and any muscular spasm in response to irritation due to meningitis, raised intracranial pressure or blood in the CSF is best seen as nuchal rigidity developing within a few hours. In its extreme form, nuchal rigidity encompasses the whole length of the spine with opisthotonus due to extreme hyperextension of the back. However, nuchal rigidity can be missed in the early stages, with overwhelming infection, or in the presence of disc pathology. Neck rigidity essentially occurs in the sagittal plane and can be elicited by placing a hand behind the head and trying to flex the neck passively. The presence of rigidity primarily in the sagittal plane is helpful in separating meningeal irritation from limited movements due to cervical spondylosis or to meningism occurring as a result of swollen neck glands or throat infections in children. A useful test in a child or young person is to see whether they can flex their head to touch their knees, or to "kiss the knees".

There are more formal tests. Kernig's test is useful in children and young adults. Extension of the knee with the hip flexed produces spasm and pain in the hamstrings. In the elderly, Brudzinski's set of signs of meningeal irritation is obtained more readily. Firstly, there may be spontaneous flexion of the knees and hips with attempted flexion of the neck, and secondly, extension of the knee with the hip flexed results in flexion of the other knee, or occasionally in extension.

Investigation of Acute Meningitis

Whenever possible a CT or ultrasound scan should be performed before a lumbar puncture. If the patient is drowsy, has had fits, or there is any suspicion of raised intracranial pressure a CT scan is mandatory. Even so, unless the meningitis is part of a septicaemia and the diagnosis can be obtained by blood culture, or in the course of an endemic a pathognomonic rash of meningococcal meningitis has been observed, examination of the CSF is required in order to make an accurate diagnosis and enable the clinician to contend with an unusual organism, an unusual strain, antibiotic resistance or antibiotic hypersensitivity necessitating a change in treatment as the meningitis progresses (Addy 1987). A CT scan should alert the clinician to the presence of a cerebral abscess, which may have ruptured to produce meningitis, to raised intracranial pressure from cerebral oedema complicating purulent bacterial infections or in the later stages to hydrocephalus, arachnoid cysts or secondary abscess formation. Drowsiness and coma, altered conscious levels due to fits, shock and disseminated intravascular coagulation may all develop and require urgent action.

It is accepted practice to start therapy with broad spectrum antibiotics whilst awaiting the outcome of CSF examination and to modify the treatment once the organism is known. The problem is how to minimize the risks of obtaining CSF in the presence of the complications mentioned. If there is any suspicion of raised intracranial pressure, the clinician may either elect to give a bolus of mannitol 2 g/kg intravenously before the CSF is examined or to obtain CSF from the cerebral ventricles. In the event of hydrocephalus a needle or catheter can be introduced into the ventricles via an open or bulging fontanelle or, in older children and adults, via burr holes. The catheter can then be used to withdraw CSF for examination, to relieve the increase in intracranial pressure and to continue to monitor intracranial pressure. If there is raised intracranial pressure but slit-like ventricles the clinician will have to decide between treating empirically with antibiotics or inserting a subarachnoid screw to monitor intra-cranial pressure before beginning treatment (Brown and Steer 1986; Newton 1987).

Neonatal meningitis, resulting from intrapartum infection with *E. coli*, group B streptococci or *Listeria*, carries a mortality of 20%–50%. Later infections up to three months after delivery are usually from exogenous contaminants such as *Staphylococcus aureus*, pseudomonas and *Klebsiella* with a lesser mortality of 10%–20%. In childhood the prevalent organisms are *Neisseria meningitis* and *Haemophilus influenzae* and in the elderly, *Streptococcus pneumoniae* and *E. coli*. A detailed discussion of the management of meningitis is outside the scope of this book and can be found in Critchley (1988) or Wood and Anderson (1988).

Tuberculous Infections

Tuberculous (TB) infection of the CNS may take on many protean forms but it is essential to recognize that the onset of TB meningitis may be as acute as any other type of bacterial or viral infection. The difference often lies in the subsequent progress. Instead of reaching a plateau or showing regression, the infection may fulminate and the patient becomes increasingly stuporose. Meningeal involvement is always secondary to TB infection elsewhere and may develop on a background of myalgia, anorexia, generalized malaise, low grade fever and intermittent headache. The onset of meningeal signs can be accom-panied by headache, nerve palsies and drowsiness. If unsuccessfully treated a third phase follows with progressive neurological defects, coma and decerebra-tion. Infants can present with full fontanelles and vomiting, children with abdominal pain and fits, and adults with focal features – an apparent stroke, a painful or paralysed eye, acute hydrocephalus or acute cerebral oedema (Tandon and Pathak 1973). Acute TB meningitis used to be the scourge of children under six years of age in developing countries. Even after the intro-duction of effective antibiotics, there was a 35% mortality with much attendant morbidity. Despite a perceptible shift from younger children to older children and young adults as the major risk group the mortality still remains unaccept-ably high.

Inflammation, exudation, giant cell proliferation and caseation are features of a fully developed TB meningitis; but many patients begin with a serous meningitis related to the haematogenous dissemination of miliary tuberculosis secondary to the breakdown of a silent Ghon focus in the lungs or gastro-intestinal tract. In about 75% of these patients the chest X-ray will show miliary tubercles with enlarged mediastinal lymph nodes. Very occasionally tubercles may be seen with the ophthalmoscope in the choroidal layer of the eye appearing as rounded, white patches about half the size of the optic disc. Miliary tubercles are secreted via the choroid plexus and become scattered over the leptomeninges. At first the CSF is clear and in all respects normal, but changes rapidly within one or two days into an opalescent fluid capable of forming a fine, fibrinous clot on standing. The white cell count rises to 100–200/mm^3, initially with a slight preponderance of polymorphs over lymphocytes but the ratio is soon reversed. The protein content may exceed 15 g/l and the sugar fall below 40% of the blood sugar level. The cornerstone of successful management is early diagnosis: any delay in the onset of treatment weighs on the prognosis. Rather than await the identification of acid-fast bacilli or the outcome of cultures and guinea-pig inoculation tests, therapy should be started on clinical suspicion and backed up by a thorough search for organisms in the lumbar CSF and even ventricular fluid.

Meningitis may be associated with any form of underlying systemic tuber-culosis (Rich 1952) and its various forms described with reference to the main pathological characteristics e.g. focal plaques with caseation, acute inflam-matory caseous meningitis or proliferative meningitis. TB as a disease is highly dependent upon the state of resistance of the host, the presence of infection elsewhere, the state of nutrition, and the immune responses. The onset of meningitis may be protracted over several months. The patient may have no discernible fever but complain of malaise, apathy, listlessness, anorexia, weight loss, occasional vomiting and focal symptoms. The complications of a chronic, slowly progressive meningitis include the development of arachnoiditis, sub-dural empyemata, and perivascular arteritic inflammatory changes involving infarction and granuloma formation within the spinal cord.

Caseous changes may remain focal at any site within the nervous system with the production of tuberculomata. A further breakdown in resistance may present with meningitis after a long latent period. Similarly, tuberculous spinal osteomyelitis secondary to haematogenous spread may involve one or more vertebral bodies and discs with minimal symptoms until an acute paraplegia develops secondary to vertebral collapse or direct extension leads to epidural granuloma or abscess formation, or even to meningitis. The differential diag-nosis of a progressive paraplegia in the presence of TB includes: (1) vertebral collapse, (2) cord compression secondary to an epidural abscess or granuloma, (3) cord ischaemia and infarction secondary to arteritis or thrombophlebitis in the neighbourhood of a tuberculous infection, (4) an expanding subdural empyema, or (5) arachnoiditis or a high CSF protein resulting in a spinal block.

Neurobrucellosis

The intraspinal manifestations of brucellosis mimic closely those of TB and fungal infections. Systemic brucellosis primarily involves the whole of the reticuloendothelial system with secondary involvement of bone. Organisms enter and proliferate within the cytoplasm of macrophages, thus the acute stage may be followed by a protracted, subclinical or relapsing illness. Non-specific symptoms such as headache, back pain and low grade fever can persist for months or years. In the acute stages meningism can arise from tender, enlarged cervical lymph nodes and occasionally there may be an acute serous meningitis which responds readily to tetracycline.

Four main intraspinal manifestations of brucellosis can occur with chronic infection, often presenting in combination.

Spinal Brucellosis or Spondylitis

Infection of a disc is most liable to occur in the lumbosacral or lower thoracic spine with spread to the adjacent vertebral bodies. Local tenderness and pain are common and the spine may become deformed with sciatica and radicular pains resulting from root compression. Vertebral erosion may lead to collapse with compression of the cord or cauda equina and the development of paraplegia. Alternatively, local spread can affect the meninges with epidural abscess formation also producing compression.

Chronic Lymphocytic Meningitis

The lymphocytic meningitis closely resembles that of TB with normal or reduced sugar levels and a greatly raised protein. Chronic meningitis may also affect the brain – meningoencephalitis, or the cord – meningomyelitis. Cerebral oedema or basal adhesions may result in a raised intracranial pressure with papilloedema and headache. Similarly, the high protein and arachnoid adhesions may result in a spinal block with paraplegia.

Radiculopathy

A Guillain-Barré like syndrome is described with radiculopathy, peripheral neuropathy and autonomic manifestations.

Myelopathy

The cord itself may be involved with demyelination, e.g. progressive ataxic quadriparesis (Al Deeb et al. 1989), acute transverse myelopathy, infarction or other vascular manifestations. In AIDS or other immune-deficient states, brucellosis may appear as an opportunistic infection.

The presence of chronic infection may be confirmed by a raised ESR and standard brucella agglutination tests. Identification of the organism can be difficult but may be achieved from blood or marrow culture or CSF. The accepted treatment of neurobrucellosis is one or more six-week course of oral tetracycline 2–3 g daily or co-trimoxazole b.d. with intramuscular streptomycin 1 g daily, gentamicin 6 mg/kg or rifampicin, but eradication cannot be guaranteed.

Sarcoidosis

About 5% of patients with sarcoidosis develop symptomatic nervous system disease, sometimes in isolation and sometimes in a setting of extraneural sarcoidosis. The percentage is higher if ocular manifestations – uveitis, conjunctivitis, scleral scarring and choroidoretinitis – are also included. The majority of neurological manifestations, amounting to 75% of the total, are peripheral, typically involving the facial nerve, singly, bilaterally or in Heerfordt's triad of uveoparotid fever. Other cranial nerves may be affected singly or as a cranial polyneuritis. Peripheral manifestations may develop unevenly with the evolution of mononeuritis multiplex or produce a combination of neuropathy and radiculopathy as in the Guillain-Barré syndrome.

Twenty-five per cent of neurosarcoidosis involves the CNS. Disease manifestations are seen relatively early in the course of the systemic illness, notably with the development of diabetes insipidus or other neuroendocrine dysfunction. The predominant lesion is a basal granulomatous meningitis blocking the basal cisterns and invading the parenchyma, infiltrating and compressing structures at the base of the brain. Leptomeningeal granulomata may be patchy rather than continuous. Their presence may account for the development of cranial nerve palsies and for symptomatic spinal cord sarcoidosis. Thus brain stem and spinal neurosarcoidosis can frequently masquerade as multiple sclerosis or transient ischaemic attacks in vertebrobasilar territory. A low grade or subclinical lymphocytic meningitis possibly occurs more frequently than a granulomatous meningitis; thus at least 75% of patients with neurosarcoidosis, perhaps presenting with a hypothalamic granuloma, will be shown to have a raised spinal fluid protein and a lymphocytic pleocytosis.

The pathology of the spinal lesions is little different from that of the more overt lesions at the base of the brain, but if they arise in isolation they can present much diagnostic difficulty. Isolated intra- or extramedullary granulomas in the cervical cord, or less commonly in the thoracic and lumbar cord, can present similarly to ependymomas or gliomas at the same site. Compression of the cord can develop from within, from without or from multiple parenchymatous granulomata associated with adhesive arachnoiditis. Granulomatous vasculitis and local infiltration can produce primary segmental demyelination, axonal degeneration, multiple small infarcts and, ultimately, necrosis of the cord. A common clinical presentation is of progressive paraplegia, especially at the thoracic level. The myelographic appearance is that of cord compression, but unless the diagnosis appears certain from the presence of other systemic manifestations it is advisable to confirm the sarcoid lesion by biopsy before treating with high-dose steroids. An improvement may be confirmed radiographically but a careful follow-up is required to exclude yeast, tubercle or fungal infection which may mimic neurosarcoidosis or be alighted as opportunistic infections by prolonged treatment with corticosteroids.

Neurosyphilis

Early Presentations

Spirochaetal invasion of the meninges can occur in the primary and secondary stages and at any time before the onset of the tertiary stage. The result is usually a clinically silent lymphocytic meningeal reaction in which a positive diagnosis from the CSF is only possible in 10%–15% of cases. Subsequently the lymphocytosis disappears and the fluid returns to normal. Later however, a brisk symptomatic meningeal reaction can occur, occasionally associated with optic neuritis, or cranial and spinal nerve lesions. The CSF is abnormal with positive treponemal reactions, a raised protein and a prolific cytosis with up to 1000/µl lymphocytes, polymorphs and plasma cells. A reduction of the CSF sugar content can make the differential diagnosis from TB meningitis dependent on the treponemal tests. If untreated at this stage the meningitis may continue to develop with granulomatous involvement of the meninges, adhesions and endarteritis.

Congenital Syphilis

Before two years of age, neurological signs are rare. However, hydrocephalus can develop secondarily to an acute or subacute meningitis. Later onset congenital syphilis has the same spectrum as the adult variety of the disease. A high proportion of meningeal and vascular forms are noted, cervical pachymeningitis is described but congenital tabes is extremely rare.

Meningovascular Syphilis

Meningovascular syphilis assaults the brain or spinal cord or both together. The essential lesion is an arteritis, sometimes with intermittent symptoms as in so-called cerebral congestive attacks. Fits and hemiplegia may be more permanent or there can be a relentless progression of symptoms. Arteritis of the meninges causes widespread, diffuse thickening of the pia arachnoid. Pachymeningitis cervicalis hypertrophica differs from cervical spondylosis in that the brunt of the thickening involves the pia arachnoid rather than dura and ligamentum flavum. A painful radiculopathy of the upper limbs may develop from root compression with a less marked spastic weakness of the legs. In addition, meningovascular syphilis involving the cervical region may produce tabetic amyotrophy or amyotrophic meningomyelitis resembling motor neurone disease (ALS). The features in common are an asymmetric wasting of the shoulder girdles and upper limbs with spasticity of the lower limbs, but distinct differences exist in that an appreciable proportion of patients have Argyll-Robertson pupils, impaired vibration sense in the lower limbs and loss of sphincter control.

   In meningovascular syphilis the cellular and protein changes in the CSF are less marked than in the earlier acute symptomatic meningitis but there is infiltration of the Virchow-Robin spaces by lymphocytes and plasma cells, an obliterative endarteritis and spinal arachnoiditis. The end result of a diffuse syphilitic spinal arachnoiditis can be: root symptoms with small gummata along the nerve roots, arachnoid cysts, vascular occlusion, and a slow strangulation of the cord under a swollen pia arachnoid with obliteration of small penetrating arteries thereby producing a concentric peripheral rim of demyelination and infarction – a syphilitic halo (Hughes 1978).

At the beginning of the century, spinal meningovascular syphilis was a major cause of transverse myelitis. The syndromes tended to be subacute or chronically progressive and invariably involved a combination of leptomeningeal exudation with granulomata, and a pan- or endarteritis. Erb's syphilitic paraplegia is a progressive form of meningomyelitis of the thoracic region with radicular pains, intense spasticity, some loss of vibration and position sense and severe sphincter impairment. Other manifestations may be thrombosis of major arteries such as the anterior spinal artery, infarction of a lateral branch of the anterior spinal artery causing a hemitransection akin to the Brown-Séquard syndrome, or multiple scattered lesions that bear a macroscopic resemblance to multiple sclerosis – so-called syphilitic sclerosis.

Tabes Dorsalis

Two to five per cent of patients with syphilis ultimately develop tabes or taboparesis 10, 15, 20 or more years after the primary infection. Tabes dorsalis is regarded as a parenchymatous affliction of the cord but this is not strictly true. There is a meningeal cellular reaction and vascular changes are rarely absent. Concentric lesions occur round the dorsal roots which appear pinkish and gelatinous. As a result, retrograde degeneration affects Lissauer's tracts and the posterior columns of the spinal cord. The cord shrinks and appears flattened in its antero–posterior diameter.

Most clinical manifestations which develop slowly in the fullness of time depend on this insidious sensory degeneration. Irritative sensory changes account for: (1) lightening pains or "screws" in the legs and trunk occurring as clusters of lancinating agony which can respond to carbamazepine 100 mg t.d.s., (2) laryngeal, gastric, rectal or bladder crises with pain concentrated upon a viscus, (3) areas of skin hyperaesthesia which gradually become hypo-anaesthetic. These involve the nose and upper lip (Duchenne's tabetic mask), the breast plate area of the trunk, ulnar borders of the forearms and the fronts of the shins. Sensory loss mainly affects the lower limbs with (1) Romberg's sign of ataxia dependent on eye closure, (2) hyporeflexia, areflexia, and sluggish or absent plantar responses, (3) muscle hypotonia, (4) a sensation of walking on cotton wool, (5) impaired and delayed responses to Achilles tendon pressure, (6) neuropathic arthropathies producing Charcot's joints, and (7) trophic skin ulceration over pressure points.

Visceral sensory impairment can result in constipation, impotence, paralytic ileus or bladder retention, cysts and overflow. Clumsiness and pseudoathetosis may be present in the upper limbs. Involvement of sympathetic afferents may account for bilateral ptosis with compensatory puckering of the brows and synechial degeneration of the iris with adhesions causing the irregularity of the Argyll-Robertson pupil. Ependymitis and gliosis, affecting the oculomotor fibres in the pretectal region dorsal to the Edinger Westphal nucleus, prevent the response to light but spare the ventral fibres which subserve accommodation (Harriman 1976). Treatment of tabes dorsalis is essentially symptomatic and does not affect the progression of the disease.

Neoplastic Meningomyelitis

The comparative frequency of neoplastic meningitis contrasts with the occasional finding of solitary leukaemic or lymphomatous deposits lodged within the meninges and with the exceedingly rare event of haematogenous metastases thriving within the spinal cord. Diffuse or multifocal infiltration of the leptomeninges by tumour cells can envelop the whole spinal cord, nerve roots and basal cisterns of the brain, with or without associated intraparenchymal lesions (Olsen et al. 1974). Apart from primary neuroectodermal tumours and haematopoietic malignancies, the other tumours that commonly lead to meningeal spread include primary lesions in the lung, breast, gastrointestinal tract and malignant melanoma (Moseley et al. 1989). In a series of 216 patients with malignant melanoma, leptomeningeal infiltration was seen in 24% of cases, thus occurring in 44% of patients with CNS metastatic disease (Patel et al. 1978). In a separate clinicopathological study, leptomeningeal metastases were seen at necropsy in 70% of those with CNS disease (Amer et al. 1978). Although the proportion of patients developing neoplastic meningitis from primary lesions elsewhere is much smaller than with malignant melanoma, the generalization can be made that neoplastic meningitis develops insidiously and some patients remain asymptomatic. Others develop root pains, sensory loss or paraparesis, and the progression can be potentially lethal, compressing, strangling or necrosing the cord.

Neoplastic meningitis may be apparent from myelography, CT scanning or MRI, and the CSF findings may mimic those of TB meningitis. Examination for mitotic cells in the CSF can be most helpful in the diagnosis and management of malignant disease even in the absence of a definite neoplastic meningitis. Unfortunately, conventional CSF cytological methods are frequently unsatisfactory with a reported rate of detection as low as 20% in some series (Bigner and Johston 1981). A frequent fault is to report malignant cells as lymphocytes. However, with the addition of monoclonal antibody immunocytology to conventional techniques, cytological accuracy is enhanced and the type of malignant cell can also be determined (Moseley et al. 1989).

Cord lesions secondary to neoplasia are uncommon. Intraparenchymal infiltration by leukaemic cells leading to a myelopathy and radiculopathy is recorded (Norris 1979) but of greater interest is the possibility of changes due to the remote effects of carcinoma. Acute or subacute necrotizing myelopathies with progressive glial involvement, a reactive astrocytosis and eventual necrosis may cause death from respiratory insufficiency. The other condition believed to be a remote effect of carcinoma is amyotrophic myelopathy. The neurological effects of this syndrome are usually indistinguishable from motor neurone disease (ALS) but in some patients fewer anterior horn cells are destroyed and there appears to be a cellular reaction verging on frank infiltration of the spared ventral horns and CNS ganglia (suggesting a definite similarity to poliomyelitis). The course is relatively benign (Norris 1979). Historically, the first association between malignancy and ALS involved gastric neoplasms but of the recorded cases over 80% arise from bronchial endothelium and reticulo-endothelial tissue. Some improvement in the amyotrophy can follow successful removal of the neoplasm.

Tropical Myeloneuropathies

Slow viruses, treponemal infections, plant toxins and nutritional factors have long featured in the presumed aetiology of tropical myelopathies. The homogeneity of the various subtypes has been questioned and there may be several aetiopathologies.

Lathyrism is perhaps the best understood. The disease is endemic in Central India and has occurred in outbreaks throughout the Mediterranean littoral. Flour, made by grinding the chickling pea (*Lathyrus sativus*), contains a toxin -B,N-oxalylaminoalanine (BOAA) which causes marked spasticity in the legs with cramps and secondary wasting (Spencer et al. 1986). Extensive corticospinal degeneration of both ventral and lateral tracts occurs with lesser involvement of the dorsal columns.

Tropical ataxic neuropathy (TAN) is a sensory ataxia due to symmetrical dorsal column lesions often associated with optic atrophy, deafness and a polyneuropathy. Outbreaks occur in Mozambique during periods of drought when the usual process of detoxicating the cyanogenic glycosides contained in cassava roots by soaking thoroughly then sun-drying, cannot be performed. The children at risk are those with malnutrition or malabsorption of methionine and other sulphur-containing aminoacids as the excess dietary cyanide is inadequately converted to thiocyanate (Cliff et al. 1985).

A neurotropic retrovirus, identical with or cross-reacting with human T-lymphotropic virus type 1 (HTLV-1), may explain the aetiology of at least 60%–75% of cases of tropical spastic paraparesis (TSP) found in the Caribbean and sub-Saharan Africa and of patients with Japanese myelopathy (HAM). Positive but low titres of HTLV-1 antigens have also been identified in patients diagnosed as having clinically definite multiple sclerosis (MS) in both Florida and Japan but not in MS patients elsewhere.

Tropical spastic paraparesis (TSP) usually affects women more than men, commonly begins in the fourth decade (30–40 years) and is slowly progressive over a decade. No race is immune. Early cases are often asymptomatic with increased reflexes and a spastic gait. Low back pain, constipation and bladder symptoms become noticed, with impotence in men. Eventually there is a frank paraplegia with some weakness of the arms. The spinal lesions bear a resemblance to AIDS myelopathy and to the degenerative changes of subacute combined degeneration of the cord but do not respond to vitamin B12. Axonal degeneration and myelin loss are best seen in the lumbar region but extend upwards to the brain stem involving predominantly the pyramidal tracts with lesser changes in other spinal tracts and peripheral nerves, mild gliosis and scattered spongiform changes. Somatosensory and visual evoked potentials are abnormal in about 50%. The CSF is usually normal though there can be a chronic meningomyelitis with perivascular infiltration and hyaline arteriolar thickening. Where this is so, oligoclonal bands and lymphoctyes containing HTLV-1 virions can be identified. Whereas the incidence of TSP and HTLV-1 antigenicity have not fallen, the proportion with treponemal seropositivity has declined with the eradication of yaws (Rodgers-Johnson et al. 1986).

Japanese HTLV-1 associated myelopathy (HAM) shows more obvious sensory loss with extensive demyelination of both the corticospinal tracts and dorsal columns. The meningovascular changes are more prominent with up to 2000 lymphocytes/μl. Although no overt case of adult T-cell leukaemia has been identified with HAM, 39% in some series have had blood transfusions and adult T-cell leukaemic cells have been found in the peripheral blood and CSF (Roman 1987). A further complication has been the finding of an altered antibody response to Epstein-Barr associated antigens (Itoyama et al. 1988).

AIDS-related Myelopathies

AIDS-related myelopathies (ARDS myelopathies) are fairly common. They start insidiously and may remain asymptomatic for some time. However, Denning et al. (1987) reported the occurrence of a symptomatic transient myelopathy developing at the time of seroconversion, presumably associated with primary HIV infection. The myelopathy improved over six weeks with some residual signs. The more typical AIDS myelopathy is a vacuolar myelopathy, pathologically resembling subacute combined degeneration of the spinal cord and found post mortem in 20 out of 89 patients dying from AIDS (Petito et al. 1985). The vacuoles are surrounded by a thin myelin sheath and appear to arise from swelling within myelin sheaths. The lower thoracic cord appears grey, slightly expanded and shows particular involvement of the posterior and lateral columns. One-third of the patients are asymptomatic but others develop a monoparesis or paraparesis with spasticity, ataxia and incontinence. Spinal cord dysfunction occurring as a complication of HIV infection may occur during latent HIV infection (Jakobsen et al. 1989) and has distinctive features. The most common complaints are of weakness of the legs and incontinence. Ambulation is often difficult, and the weakness is frequently attributed inappropriately to general debility from supervening infections or malnutrition rather than to spinal cord dysfunction (Berger 1987). Physical examination reveals spastic paraparesis with hyperreflexia and extensor plantar responses. The gait is typically spastic-ataxic. Sensory examination often displays greater impairment of the sensations of position and vibration than of light touch, temperature and pin-prick, but this is not invariable. There may be a concomitant peripheral neuropathy. These clinical findings are important as they rule out potentially treatable disorders that may result in myelopathy, including other viral infections associated with AIDS. Myelopathies caused by these viruses often assume a more fulminant tempo than the subacute course of HIV myelopathy (Berger 1987).

AIDS patients secondarily infected by herpes simplex type 2 viruses may develop a progressive thoracic myelopathy (Britton et al. 1985) or an acute ascending necrotizing myelopathy (Wiley et al. 1987). The patients initially complain of radicular and back pain and HSV type 2 viruses have been isolated from spinal root ganglia and spinal cord, suggesting a direct invasion of the cord by the virus from spinal ganglia. Likewise cytomegalovirus infection in AIDS has lead to progressive segmental thoracic myelopathy with necrosis of the anterior spinal artery (Tyler et al. 1986).

In the presence of AIDS, syphilitic infections may realight and take on a new form unique to AIDS; thus Lowenstein et al. (1987) have described acute syphilitic transverse myelitis with lesions shown by angiography, CT and MRI.

Acute Transverse Myelopathy

Myelopathy refers to pathology of the substance of the cord. The term, acute transverse myelopathy, is a useful anatomical formulation for disease syndromes involving the cord bilaterally, at or up to a horizontal segmental level which may lie in the sacral, lumbar, thoracic or cervical portion of the cord. The term also implies a monophasic illness with the onset of symptoms and signs developing over a period of 2 hours to 14 days and resulting in a diagnostic triad of: complete sensory loss below the level of involvement, an initially flaccid paraparesis or quadriparesis, and severe impairment of sphincter function.

Myelopathies may occur as part of a more widespread disease process. Where this is so, spinal cord involvement may accompany or be overshadowed by other manifestations such as encephalitis, peripheral neuropathy or polyradiculopathy. However, rapidly developing transverse lesions of the spinal cord, occurring as the sole manifestation of a disease process, often present a difficult diagnostic and therapeutic problem.

The probable diagnosis of acute transverse myelopathy is made more likely if there is a preceding history of an exanthema, vaccination or an upper respiratory tract infection. The alternative diagnosis of MS may be suggested if the patient has had previous neurological symptoms. With recurrent episodes, recurring at exactly the same level each time, a third diagnosis, namely a spinal arteriovenous malformation, is also possible. However, the immediate differential diagnosis is the exclusion of cord compression either from an intrinsic tumour or from an extradural tumour or abscess. Unless these conditions can be excluded beyond reasonable doubt, the definitive test is lumbar myelography. Unfortunately, examination of the spinal fluid without myelography provides little useful information.

Initially the cord lesion is limited longitudinally to a few segments and the full thickness of the cord is not usually involved. The lesion is not necessarily stable but may progress rostrally spreading as an ascending myelitis. Radiographic support for the diagnosis of acute transverse myelitis comes from the finding of a spinal cord of normal calibre; but this is not invariably so. With the rapid development of transverse myelopathy, oedematous swelling of the cord may trap and compress radicular veins within the cord causing further congestion so that the clinical level in effect marks the upper boundary of this drainage. Where swelling has occurred an attempt may be made to establish the nature of the lesions by MR imaging. But if this is not possible or the findings remain uncertain, surgical decompression and biopsy may be the only way to exclude other intrinsic lesions. Decompression rarely has an adverse effect on the course of the disease and has been used in the past to establish whether the disease has progressed to necrosis or if recovery is still possible.

Acute transverse myelopathy as an isolated event remains a relatively rare but probably underdiagnosed condition. Berman et al. (1981) found 62 patients who fulfilled the necessary diagnostic criteria in Israel over a 20-year period from 1955–1975; thus giving an incidence of 1.34 per million. Transverse myelitis (or myelopathy) is often classified as a demyelinative condition developing as a result of secondary non-specific hypersensitivity phenomena similar pathologically to the lesions of acute disseminated encephalomyopathy. In this form it may be indistinguishable from spinal mutliple sclerosis; thus Lipton and Teasdall in 1973 reported a follow-up study of 34 patients: 7 of whom were diagnosed 5 to 42 years later as having multiple sclerosis. Nowadays the proportion developing multiple sclerosis can be further reduced by means of visual, auditory and upper limb somatosensory evoked potentials, by MR imaging or CT scanning of the brain or by MR imaging of the spinal cord.

Viral Aetiology

In recognizing that acute transverse myelography is essentially an anatomical formulation we recognize that there may be many disparate causes and that the natural history of one form may not coincide with another. Between 20% – 40% of cases have a probable viral origin (Tyler et al. 1986) and represent the most typical picture of transverse myelitis. The diagnosis of a viral infection is never straightforward. In a classical paper (Wells 1971) investigated 19 patients from the Cardiff area of South Wales who had developed an acute neurological disorder with predominant spinal and radicular symptoms following an upper respiratory infection during the winter of 1969–1970. Serological tests showed that the infection was probably due to influenza A virus in 8 cases and to other viruses (including adenovirus and herpes zoster) in 6, while in 5 cases the studies were negative. It was not possible to isolate a virus or to culture it from the blood in any case. The interval between the onset of the febrile illness and the development of neurological complications varied from 1 to 112 days, and it was indeed so variable that it was difficult to draw any valid conclusions whether the neurological state resulted from direct viral invasion or from an autoimmune or hypersensitivity process, though the latter seemed more probable. It is also possible that some symbiosis between viruses can occur; thus Boiardi et al. (1986) reported the recurrence of herpes zoster myelitis in combination with a Coxsackie infection; and cases of transverse myelitis have been reported in the past during epidemics of poliomyelitis (Foley and Beresford 1974).

Transverse myelitis can develop over hours or days. The sequence of events is usually similar. Both sexes are equally affected and there is little variation with age. The most common site of affliction is the upper or mid-thoracic cord. There may be an acute pyrexia and radiculopathy or back pain localized over a few spinal segments, soon followed by symptoms of spinal cord transection. A low grade temperature may persist for several days. Bilateral paraesthesiae start in the feet and ascend with numbness and sensory impairment until a discrete sensory level is reached. Sphincter dysfunction occurs with urinary retention and loss of bowel control. There follows a progressive flaccid weakness of the lower limbs and abdominal muscles. With high dorsal lesions assisted ventilation is required. The paresis may remain flaccid if the spinal cord starts to necrose. More often the initial flaccid weakness gives way to an increasingly spastic paraplegia.

The CSF can be normal, or mildly abnormal with a pleocytosis and a slightly raised protein. Occasionally it is frankly xanthochromic with high levels of protein often exceeding 10 g/l and up to 200 lymphocytes. Such abnormal findings usually occur when the onset is apoplectic. A clinical state of spinal shock develops, as seen after traumatic transection, and the cord becomes oedematous. The presence of an acute spinal block may be confirmed by myelography, with or without CT, but the differential diagnosis is more clearly revealed by MRI which may give an abnormal signal over the full extent of the lesion.

With milder degrees of myelopathy, not affecting the full thickness of the cord, various patterns of sensory loss may be seen. Thus vibration and joint position sensation may be spared suggesting that there has been segmental occlusion of the anterior spinal artery. Occlusion of the anterior spinal artery mainly involves anterior horn cells and corticospinal tracts; spinothalamic sensation is lost at the beginning but tends to recover and dorsal column sensation is spared. It may also be difficult to differentiate transverse myelopathy from an acute ascending polyradiculopathy unless an ascending sensory level is present on the trunk thereby indicating that the spinal cord is affected. As with acute disseminated encephalomyelitis, the pathology of the cord can vary from patchy perivenous demyelination to a severe necrotizing, haemorrhagic form. The cord may appear oedematous and hyperaemic with perivascular cuffing, arteritis and yet more extensive vascular involvement, and there may be an inflammatory cellular exudation involving the leptomeninges.

There is a tendency to compare the natural history of acute transverse myelopathy with that of an isolated spinal plaque of MS with recovery within approximately six weeks. Such a supposition can be very misleading. Full recovery is not invariable: Lipton and Teasdall (1973) reported a mortality of 14.5%, a reasonable recovery may occur in just over 33% often spread over three or more months, with residual deficits in about 25% (Berman et al. 1981; Lancet 1986); 23% progress to the Foix-Alajouanine syndrome (Foix and Alajouanine 1926) of subacute necrosis of the spinal cord (Berman et al. 1981).

After the initial stage the majority of patients pass to a stable plateau phase lasting days or weeks before proceeding imperceptibly into a phase of recovery. Improvement may take place over several months, often with a mild residual disability which fails to clear. Those who fail to make a good recovery may develop osteomalacia with necrotic softening and cavitation of the whole extent of the cord below the lesion. Once this occurs further recovery is unlikely. A small number of patients make a delayed but complete functional recovery apart from the persistence of hyperreflexia and extensor plantar responses.

Three mechanisms have been postulated to explain the viral pathogenesis of acute transverse myelopathy:

1. Viral invasion of the spinal cord – the mechanism which most probably explains myelopathy in AIDS

Table 14.1.   Viruses which cause myelitis in humans

DNA viruses	
Enveloped:	Herpes viruses (simplex, simiae, varicella-zoster), Epstein-Barr and cytomegalovirus
	Pox viruses: vaccinia and variola
Non-enveloped:	Hepatitis B
RNA viruses	
Non-enveloped:	Picornaviruses: Coxsackie, ECHO, polio
	Other enteroviruses: hepatitis A, encephalomyocarditis virus
Enveloped:	Togaviruses: arborviruses, tick-borne encephalitis, rubella
	Retroviruses: HTLV-1, HTLV-111 (HIV)
	Orthomyxoviruses: influenza
	Paramyxoviruses: measles, mumps
	Bunyaviruses: Californian encephalitis
	Arenaviruses: lymphocytic choriomeningitis
	Rhabdoviruses: rabies

(After Tyler et al. 1986.)

2. A toxic myelopathy – extremely hard to prove or disprove
3. A delayed hypersensitivity reaction – this is the most probable explanation of myelopathy following vaccination (Bitzen 1987)

Of the neurotropic viruses, the DNA viruses are more prone to cause myelopathy than the RNA viruses. Table 14.1 shows those included in causing myelitis in humans.

Herpes Viruses

These are most commonly incriminated in sporadic cases. Broadbent (1866) described muscle wasting with zoster infections. As the intercostal muscles are most frequently involved, wasting may be difficult to quantify clinically. Zoster myelopathy can lead to dysfunction of the bladder and anus (Jellinek and Tulloch 1976). The authors emphasize that severe sphincter disturbances, e.g. retention, loss of sensation, or incontinence are the result of bilateral lesions; thus hemisection of the spinal cord does not cause sphincter problems. Recovery is usually complete and the segmental distribution of any rash does not necessarily coincide with the level of myelopathy. Retention may occur with thoracic or lumbar lesions, and sacral involvement may be accompanied by sensory loss and a flaccid detrusor paralysis. Herpes zoster infections can be unpredictable, remaining dormant until another viral infection reduces the body's resistance; and myelopathy can be a feature of symptomatic herpes zoster infections, e.g. developing at the site of trauma, a metastatic deposit or a prolapsed intervertebral disc.

Acute necrotizing myelitis has been a frequent complication of herpes simiae infection in laboratory workers, less commonly with herpes simplex infection. It is particularly prone to occur in immune-compromised individuals. Clinically a rapidly progressive myelitis with necrotizing arteritis is found with Cowdray type A inclusions or HSV 2 antigens within the spinal cord (Wiley et al. 1987). Some cases have followed a viraemia provoking a severe inflammatory response to the viral infection and in others there is evidence of virus dissemination from intra-axonal spread into the spinal cord from the dorsal root ganglia.

Other Viruses

Immunosuppression in the recipients of renal transplants can lead to disseminated cytomegalovirus infection with acute transverse myelopathy (Spitzer et al. 1987). Rubella myelitis has been reported in conjunction with encephalitis in children and confirmed by MR imaging (Bitzen 1987). Rubella virus specific IgM has been detected in serum and spinal fluid using ELISA Rubazyme M. Likewise the Epstein-Barr virus has been identified by the direct fluorescent antibody test.

A syndrome primarily involving the bladder with acute but transient urinary retention can arise from sacral myeloradiculitis (Vanneste et al. 1980; Herbaut et al. 1987). It may be associated with anogenital herpes simplex infections, but non-herpetic causes include ECHO, cytomegaloviruses and Epstein-Barr viral infections. The differential diagnosis includes multiple sclerosis and disc protrusions.

Following Vaccination

Myelopathy may complicate smallpox vaccination (Shyamalan and Singh 1964), pertussis immunization, and rabies vaccination. The incidence of postvaccinal encephalomyelitis was between 1 in 5000 and 1 in 2 000 000 vaccinations. Postvaccinal encephalomyelitis was rare in infancy but more liable to occur with primary vaccination between the ages of 4–16 than with secondary vaccination. After an incubation period of 8–15 days the onset is abrupt or explosive with encephalitic symptoms. A flaccid paralysis from transverse myelitis was more frequently observed than hemiplegia. Survivors are said to make a complete recovery but Miller (1953) recognized numerous mild residual deficits.

Neuroparalytic accidents used to occur in 1 in 1000 to 1 in 4000 patients treated with anti-rabies vaccines. An acute disseminated encephalomyelitic reaction would occur because all three anti-rabies vaccines – Pasteur, Semple and even duck embryo vaccines – contain myelin (Behan and Currie 1978). Until vaccines were grown on duck embryos or tissue culture, patients received a lengthy course of repeated inoculations with an emulsion of animal nervous tissues containing dead or attenuated rabies virus. A monophasic illness would develop suddenly after an incubation period of 1–3 months and run a downhill course with a mortality of 30%. The condition could be almost indistinguishable from MS with dense plaques of demyelination scattered asymmetrically throughout the neuraxis (Matthews and Miller 1972). At other times the clinical picture resembled the Guillain-Barré syndrome with an ascending myelitis, transverse myelitis usually in the thoracic or lumbar segments, or a polyradiculitis with facial nerve involvement (Adaros and Held 1971; Toro et al. 1977). In no case are Negri bodies present.

Parasitic Infections

Schistosomiasis has been the most frequently reported cause of an acute tropical myelopathy (Kerr et al. 1987; Suchet et al. 1987) The eggs of *S. haematobium* and *S. mansoni* may lodge as emboli in the blood vessels of the cord and in infested areas there is probably much asymptomatic or unrecognized spinal cord involvement. However, symptoms may result from:

1. Vascular syndromes, e.g. anterior spinal artery occlusion
2. Granulomata around spinal roots or the cauda equina
3. Multiple small granulomata within the cord surrounding one or more eggs
4. Larger granulomata microscopically resembling gliomata

The lower lumbar and sacral regions of the spinal cord are most likely to be infected and widening of the conus has been reported radiologically (Kerr et al. 1987). Patients may present with wasting, fasciculation, back pain and distal weakness. The condition has been successfully treated with praziquantel, either given with steroids or in conjunction with oxamniquine and niridazole.

Another reported tropical cause of myelopathy is larva migrans (Weng et al. 1987). The diagnosis can be made on the clinical course of the disease and the finding of eosinophilia, serum IgE, raised CSF IgG and IgA and the presence of larvae in the CSF.

Collagen Vascular Disease

Spinal cord damage in collagen vascular diseases can occur as a result of thrombosed arteries or veins, or from microscopic haemorrhages. A true myelopathy can also result from a vasculopathy with proliferative changes involving small blood vessels. Transverse myelitis can occur in mixed connective tissue disease in the presence of antibodies to ribonucleoprotein (anti-RNP) (Pedersen et al. 1987) or, more commonly, in systemic lupus erythematosus (SLE). In SLE the vascular changes may be associated with demyelination or with areas of gliosis with associated perivascular collections of mononuclear cells and deposits of immune complexes and reactive (antineuronal) antibodies, also present in the CSF and plasma (Siebold et al. 1982; Kaye et al. 1987). Some cases, particularly in childhood, may be related to immune deficiency syndromes (Kaye et al. 1987).

Transverse myelitis may occasionally be the first manifestation of lupus erythematosus (Siekert and Clark 1955; Granger 1960) but the total number of reported cases does not exceed 40. The spinal cord is most vulnerable to damage in the event of an exacerbation of the underlying disease (Andrews et al. 1970). The most common neurological level is mid-thoracic in 60% (Hachen and Chantraine 1979–1980) and an abnormal signal may be obtained over a wide area by MR imaging (Kenik et al. 1987). In the vast majority of patients the paraplegia is complete and irreversible and multiple zones of myelomalacia in both grey and white matter with fibrinoid degeneration of arterioles may be present post mortem. Myelopathy at cervical (20%) or lumbar (20%) levels tends to be less severe with only partial motor and sensory loss (Piper 1953; Andrianakos et al. 1975).

In 3 of the 40 patients reported in the literature (April and VanSonnenberg 1976), systemic lupus sclerosis was combined with Devic's syndrome of neuro-myelitis optica. Demyelination of white matter in SLE is a relatively rare finding. However, demyelinating plaques in MS display an outer ring of immune complexes and the overlapping condition of lupus sclerosis is well described where the levels of immunoglobulins in the CSF are particularly high.

The results of treatment of SLE myelopathy with high dosage corticosteroids have been disappointing. A slow recovery occurred in only 3 paraplegic patients and in 1 quadriplegic patient from a total of 26 (Andrianakos et al. 1975). Anecdotally, chloroquine has been successful in the treatment of one patient (Granger 1960). Slovick (1986) advocated the use of plasma exchange and immunosuppression and reported the successful treatment of one patient.

Transverse Myelopathy Related to Acute Disseminated Encephalomyelitis

Myelopathy occurring in conjunction with the Guillain-Barré syndrome of allergic, postinfective peripheral neuropathy or polyradiculopathy, confirms the hypothesis that many forms of transverse myelopathy can arise as a result of a cell-mediated response. The violence of this response may vary from perivenous demyelination to a severe necrotizing myelopathy. The clinical diagnosis of an accompanying myelopathy may not be easy but is suggested by the development of extensor plantar responses and severe sphincter disturbances.

In Devic's disease bilateral retrobulbar or optic neuritis with massive demyelination of the optic nerves may be followed after a few months by similar massive demyelination of the spinal cord. Thereafter the disease may be self-limiting or run a progressive downward course (Walton 1977). Demyelinating lesions, often with destruction of axis cylinders, are seen elsewhere in the neuraxis and there is a distinct tendency to necrosis and cavity formation within the spinal cord. Many remain unconvinced that Devic's disease is a distinct pathological entity (Hughes 1978).

In subacute myelo-optico-neuropathy (SMON) diarrhoea and abdominal pain are followed by the acute or subacute onset of an ascending sensory neuropathy spreading over the lower half of the body, accompanied in two-thirds of those affected by an ataxic gait. Half the patients also develop motor weakness in the lower limbs. Myelopathy or neuropathy with or without optic atrophy occurs in 26.2% of non-Japanese patients (Thomas 1984). The disease was originally thought to be a viral disorder but clioquinol toxicity is now incriminated as the causal agent. Yagi et al. (1978) found that the neurotoxicity of clioquinol depends on decomposition of the conjugated form and chelation with iron and other metals. When a concentration of free clioquinol in serum of 20 µg/ml has been maintained for several days (Tamura 1975) the drug is taken up in chelated form by neural tissue where it produces destructive peroxidases (Yagi et al. 1978). The simultaneous ingestion of drugs containing aluminium, calcium, magnesium, copper and bismuth will produce different chelates. Different combinations can affect the clinical severity of the disorder (Okada et al. 1984).

Myelopathy can also result from toxicity from other drugs: heavy metal poisoning, arsphenamine, paraquin, orthocresyl phosphate; drugs injected into the subarachnoid space, e.g. penicillin; or contrast agents used in aortography.

An allergic myelopathy can develop from scorpion stings, hymenoptera stings and spider bites (Rosenberg and Coull 1982). The venom of some scorpion species contains powerful neurotoxins capable of producing paralysis of the hind limbs and respiratory muscles of laboratory animals. Such findings fuel speculation that myelopathy in man may result from a direct neurotoxic effect as an alternative to a secondary immune-mediated response.

Ischaemic myelopathy is a recognized complication of anterior spinal artery occlusion, circulatory arrest as from clamping of the aorta, or Stokes-Adams attacks. Myelopathy following burns, heat stroke or trauma could be due to similar anoxic changes as a consequence of ischaemia, disseminated intravascular coagulopathy or electrolyte imbalance (Delgado et al. 1985). Alternatively, there may be an allergic response to the release of altered proteins into the circulation producing an autoimmune reaction within the spinal cord.

Opiates

Myelopathy has been described among heroin addicts. The circumstances of drug addiction, particularly when intravenous drugs are taken, favour both sepsis and thromboembolism. These factors require exclusion before a direct toxic effect on the spinal cord is accepted (Hughes 1978). Ell et al. (1981) list hypotension, toxic or hypersensitivity reactions, reactions to contaminants or to the heroin itself, vasculitis, embolism and hyperextension injury among the factors which may be involved and suggest that the most usual causative factor is an adulterant taken with the heroin. In favour of a hypersensitivity reaction is the fact that some cases have occurred after a period of abstinence (Ell et al. 1981). The chances of recovery are uniformly poor.

Treatment of Myelopathies

In many ways the least satisfactory aspect of acute transverse myelopathy is its treatment and the prevention of complications. A proportion of all types of myelopathy can improve spontaneously but an attempt should be made to determine the underlying pathology and treat accordingly. Where specific agents can be given, e.g. acyclovir for herpes simplex or zoster, or praziquantel for myelopathy following schistosomiasis, there can be a reasonable expectation of improvement. Corticosteroids are potentially indicated where the cause of the myelopathy is unknown, where there is a possibility of a collagen disease, or an allergic reactive state (i.e. a hypersensitivity reaction). The results of steroid therapy remain uncertain and their efficacy has yet to be established. Early treatment with methylprednisolone has not been evaluated and should be tried as early as possible in the disease unless there is a clear alternative form of treatment available.

If the cord appears swollen it is advisable to perform a diagnostic decompression and biopsy and to follow this with dexamethasone. Acyclovir and similar drugs may be used in AIDS myelopathies where viruses other than HIV are implicated. Antibiotics, if necessary covered by steroids, should be used in myelopathy with meningovascular syphilis. In other situations, as with collagen vascular disease, Slovick's suggestion (1986) of a combination of plasma exchange and immunosuppression should be considered.

Spinal Multiple Sclerosis

Multiple sclerosis is a disease of the CNS and lesions are characteristically distributed in time and space. In established disease it is rare for the spinal cord not to be involved. Among the manifestations recorded in patients with MS examined at autopsy, 98% will have developed paresis of the lower limbs, spasticity and hyperreflexia, 82% will have had urinary disturbances and 65% paraesthesiae such as episodes of numbness or a positive Lhermitte's phenomenon. The occurrence of MS limited to the spinal cord is probably rare but plaques seen only in the spinal cord are found occasionally in patients at autopsy. However, lesions of the spinal cord are the presenting feature in at least one-third of patients with MS (Shibasaki et al. 1981). In many it may be possible to confirm the diagnosis by finding evidence of silent lesions elsewhere, e.g. by visual evoked potentials or MR imaging. The finding of a lesion elsewhere merely increases the probability that the spinal cord manifestation is due to MS; it never constitutes absolute proof. The diagnosis of spinal MS depends upon the clinical presentation, the finding of confirmatory evidence and exclusion of alternative diagnoses, and increasingly upon supportive evidence from oligoclonal banding in the CSF, somatosensory evoked potentials and MR imaging of the cervical cord. At present none of these sophisticated investigations provide absolute proof of the diagnosis.

Among the highly characteristic presenting manifestations are:

1. Intermittent weakness of a leg occurring either on exertion with dragging of the foot after prolonged activity or as a paroxysmal symptom with sudden loss of power causing unexpected falls, locking of the knees or collapse of the legs.

2. About 10% of patients presenting with acute transverse myelopathy are found to have MS (Poser 1984). This may take one of three characteristic

forms: as a partial Brown-Séquard syndrome, as a spastic paraplegia with negative myelography, or as numbness below the waist with sphincter disturbance and loss of vaginal sensation often improving spontaneously before myelography is possible.

3. As a chronic myelopathy or progressive spastic paraparesis. This may be the presenting form of the condition in middle age and in the elderly (Noseworthy et al. 1983). The differential diagnosis may include cord compression, cervical spondylosis or familial or sporadic forms of spastic paraparesis.

4. Paroxysmal phenomena such as Lhermitte's sign or unilateral spasms of limbs which are often painful with the limb "kicking out" or adopting a brief tetanic posture.

5. Isolated bladder disturbances, e.g. retention, urgency, or hesitancy of micturition; impairment of sex functions or, rarely, bowel dysfunction. Usually MS can only be diagnosed by exclusion.

6. Uncertain or bizarre paraesthesiae, hemianaesthesia or intermittent weakness or clumsiness. Some of these symptoms may have an allergic basis or even suggest hysteria. It is often wiser to regard them as due to an allergic neuritis unless there is positive proof of MS.

MR imaging of the cervical spinal cord to identify plaques is possible but difficult. Longitudinal (sagittal or coronal) cuts are more likely to be of value than axial cuts because of the longitudinal arrangement of plaques as seen post mortem. The cervical spinal cord is small compared to the brain stem or cerebrum and requires high imaging resolution but the signal to noise ratio can be improved by the use of surface coils (Maravilla et al. 1984). The thoracic and lumbar cord is almost impossible to image because of its smaller size and the presence of respiratory and cardiac movement artefact.

The differentiation of progressive spastic paraplegia due to MS from familial spastic paraparesis depends upon finding lesions at MR imaging, or delayed visual evoked potentials. A relative lymphocytosis in the CSF with a raised IgG, oligoclonal bands, or the presence of HLA DR2 antigen increases the likelihood of MS. Somatosensory evoked potentials from upper or lower limbs can be abnormal with either condition and although it is often worth trying the response to steroids over 4–6 weeks, this is an unreliable factor in making a differential diagnosis.

References

Adaros HL, Held JR (1971) Guillain-Barré syndrome associated with immunization against rabies: epidemiological aspects. In: Rowland LP (ed) Immunological disorders of the nervous system. Williams and Wilkins Co, Baltimore, pp 178–186

Addy DP (1987) When to do a lumbar puncture. Arch Dis Child 62:873–875

Al Deeb SM, Yaqub BA, Sharif HS, Phadke JG (1989) Neuro-brucellosis: clinical characteristics, diagnosis and outcome. Neurology 39:498–501

Amer MH, Al-Sarraf M, Baker LH, Vaitkevicius UK (1978) Malignant melanoma and central nervous system metastases. Incidence, diagnosis, treatment and survival. Cancer 42:660–668

Andrews JM, Cancilla PA, Kunin J (1970) Progressive spinal cord signs in a patient with disseminated lupus erythematosus. Bull Los Angeles Neurol Soc 35:78–85

Andrianakos AA, Duffy J, Suzuki M, Sharp JT (1975) Transverse myelopathy in systemic lupus erythematosus: report of 3 cases and a review of the literature. Ann Intern Med 83:616–625

April RS, VanSonnenberg E (1976) A case of neuromyelitis optica (Devic's syndrome) in systemic lupus erythematosus: clinicopathologic report and a review of the literature. Neurology 26:1066–1070

Behan PO, Currie S (1978) Clinical neurovirology. Saunders, London.

Berger JR (1987) Neurologic complications of human immunodeficiency virus infection. Postgrad Med 81:72–79

Berman M, Feldman S, Alter M, Zilker N, Kahama E (1981) Acute transverse myelitis: incidence and etiologic considerations. Neurology 31:966–971

Bigner SH, Johnston WW (1981) Cytopathology of cerebrospinal fluid. Acta Cytol 25:461–479

Bitzen M (1987) Rubella myelitis and encephalitis in childhood: report of 2 cases with magnetic resonance imaging. Neuropaediatrics 18:84–87

Boiardi A, Ferrante P, Porta E, Sghirlanzoni A, Bussone G (1986) Herpes zoster myelitis: nervous system complications. Ital J Neurol Sci 7:617–622

Britton CB, Masa-Tejada R, Fenoglio CM, Hays AP, Carvey GC, Miller JR (1985) A new complication of AIDS: thoracic myelitis caused by herpes simplex virus. Neurology 35:1071–1074

Broadbent WW (1866) Zoster infections of the nervous system. Br Med J i:460

Brown K, Steer C (1986) Strategies in the management of children with acute encephalitis. In: Gordon N, McKinlay I (eds) Neurologically sick children, treatment and management. Blackwell, Oxford, pp 219–293

Cliff J, Lundqvist P, Martensson J, Rosling H, Sorbo B (1985) Association of high cyanide and low sulphur intake in cassava-induced spastic paraparesis. Lancet 2:1211–1212

Critchley EMR (1988) Neurological emergencies. Saunders, London

Delgado G, Tundu T, Gallago J, Villenerva JA (1985) Spinal cord lesions in heat stroke. J Neurol Neurosurg Psychiatry 48:1065–1067

Denning DW, Anderson J, Rudge P, Smith H (1987) Acute myelopathy associated with primary infection with human immunodeficiency virus. Br Med J 294:143–144

Ell JJ, Uttley D, Silver JR (1981) Acute myelopathy in association with heroin addiction. J Neurol Neurosurg Psychiatry 44:448–450

Foix C, Alajouanine T (1926) La myelite necrotique subaigue. Rev Neurol 2:1–42

Foley KM, Beresford HR (1974) Acute poliomyelitis beginning as transverse myelopathy. Arch Neurol 30:182–183

Granger DP (1960) Transverse myelitis with recovery: the only manifestation of systemic lupus erythematosus. Neurology 10:325–329

Hachen H, Chantraine A (1979–80) Spinal involvement in systemic lupus erythematosus. Paraplegia 17:337–346

Harriman DGF (1976) Infective diseases of the central nervous system. In: Blackwood W, Corseilles JAN (eds) Greenfield's neuropathology. Arnold, London, pp 238–268

Herbaut AG, Voordecker P, Monseu G, Germeau F (1987) Benign transient urinary retention. J Neurol Neurosurg Psychiatry 50:354–355

Hughes JT (1978) Pathology of the spinal cord, 2nd edn. Lloyd-Luke, London

Itoyama Y, Minato S, Goto I, Okochi K. Yamamoto N (1988) Elevated serum antibody titers to Epstein-Barr virus in HTLV-1 associated myelopathy. Neurology 38:1650–1653

Jakobsen J, Smith T, Gaub J, Helweg-Larsen S, Trojaborg W (1989) Progressive neurological dysfunction during latent HIV infection. Br Med J 299:225–228

Jellinek EH, Tulloch WS (1976) Herpes zoster with dysfunction of bladder and anus. Lancet 2:1219–1222

Kaye EM, Butler IJ, Conley S (1987) Myelopathy in neonatal and infantile lupus erythematosus. J Neurol Neurosurg Psychiatry 50:923–926

Kenik JG, Krohn K, Kelly RB, Bierman M, Hammeke MD (1987) Transverse myelitis and optic neuritis in systemic lupus erythematosus: a case report with magnetic resonance imaging findings. Arthritis Rheum 30:947–950

Kerr RSC, Marks SM, Sheldon PWE, Teddy PJ (1987) *Schistosomiasis mansoni* in the spinal cord: a correlation between operative and radiological findings. J Neurol Neurosurg Psychiatry 50:822–823

Lancet (1986) Acute transverse myelopathy. Lancet 1:20–21 (leading article)

Lipton HL, Teasdall RD (1973) Acute transverse myelitis in adults: a follow-up study. Arch Neurol 28:252–257

Lowenstein DH, Mills C, Simon RP (1987) Acute syphilitic transverse myelitis: unusual presentation of meningovascular syphilis. Genitourinary Med 63:333–338

Maravilla KR, Wemret JC, Suss R, Nunnally R (1984) Magnetic resonance demonstration of multiple sclerosis plaques in the cervical cord. Am J Neuroradiol 5:685–689

Matthews WB, Miller H (1972) Diseases of the nervous system. Blackwell, Oxford

Miller HG (1953) Prognosis of neurologic illness following vaccination against smallpox. Arch Neurol 69:695–706

Moseley RP, Davies AG, Bourne SP, et al. (1989) Neoplastic meningitis in malignant melanoma: diagnosis with monoclonal antibodies. J Neurol Neurosurg Psychiatry 52:881–886

Newton RW (1987) Intracranial pressure and its monitoring in childhood: a review. J R Soc Med 80:566–570

Norris FH (1979) Neurological manifestations of systemic disease. In: Vinken PJ, Bruyn GW (eds) Handbook of clinical neurology, vol 38. North Holland, Amsterdam, pp 669–677

Noseworthy J, Paty DW, Wonnacott J, Feasby T, Ebergs G (1983) Multiple sclerosis after the age of 50. Neurology 33:1537–1544

Okada H, Aoki K, Ohno Y, Kitazawa S, Ohtani M (1984) Effects of metal containing drugs taken simultaneously with clioquinol upon clinical features of SMON. J Toxicol Sci 9:371–404

Olsen M, Chernik N, Posner J (1974) Infiltration of the leptomeninges by systemic cancer. A clinical and pathological study. Arch Neurol 30:122–137

Patel JK, Didolkar MS, Pickren JW, Moore RH (1978) Metastatic pattern of malignant melanoma. A study of 216 autopsy cases. Am J Surg 135:807–810

Pedersen C, Bonen H, Boesen F (1987) Transverse myelitis in mixed connective tissue disease. Clin Rheumatol 6:290–292

Petito CK, Navie BA, Cho ES, Jordan BD, George DC, Price RW (1985) Vacuolar myelopathy pathologically resembling subacute combined degeneration in patients with acquired immune deficiency syndrome. N Engl J Med 312:878–879

Piper PG (1953) Disseminated lupus erythematosus with involvement of the spinal cord. JAMA 153:215–217

Poser CM (1984) Taxonomy and diagnostic parameters in multiple sclerosis. Ann NY Acad Sci 436:233–245

Rich AR (1952) The pathogenesis of tuberculosis. Thomas, Springfield, Illinois

Rodgers-Johnson P, Morgan O StC, Zaninovic V, et al. (1986) Treponematosis and tropical spastic paraplegia. Lancet 1:809

Roman GC (1987) Retrovirus associated myelopathies. Arch Neurol 44:659–663

Rosenberg NL, Coull BM (1982) Myelopathy after scorpion sting. Arch Neurol 39:127

Shibasaki H, McDonald WI, Kuroiwa Y (1981) Racial modification of clinical picture of multiple sclerosis: comparison between British and Japanese patients. J Neurol Sci 49:253–271

Shyamalan NC, Singh SS (1964) Transverse myelitis after vaccination. Br Med J i:434–435

Siebold JR, Buckingham RD, Medsger JA, Kelly RA (1982) Cerebrospinal immune complexes in systemic lupus erythematosus involving the central nervous system. Semin Arthritis Rheum 12:68–76

Siekert RG, Clark EC (1955) Neurologic signs and symptoms as early manifestations of systemic lupus erythematosus. Neurology 5:84–88

Slovick DI (1986) Treatment of acute myelopathy in systemic lupus erythematosus with plasma exchange and immunosuppression. J Neurol Neurosurg Psychiatry 49:103–105

Spencer PS, Roy DN, Ludolph A, Hugon J, Dwived MP, Schaumburg HH (1986) Lathyrism: evidence for the role of the neuroexcitatory aminoacid BOAA. Lancet 2:1066–1067

Spitzer PG, Tarsy D, Eliopoulos GM (1987) Acute transverse myelitis during disseminated cytomegalovirus infection in a renal transplant recipient. Transplantation 44:151–153

Suchet I, Klein C, Horwitz T, Lalla S, Doodha M (1987) Spinal cord schistosomiasis: a case report and review of the literature. Paraplegia 25:491–496

Tamura Z (1975) Clinical chemistry of clioquinol. Jpn J Med Sci Biol 28:(suppl) 68–77

Tandon PN, Pathak SN (1973) Tuberculosis of the central nervous system. In: Spillane JD (ed) Tropical neurology, Oxford University Press, Oxford, pp 37–51

Thomas PK (1984) Neurotoxicity of halogenated hydroxyquinolones: non-Japanese cases. Acta Neurol Scand 70:(suppl 100) 155–158

Toro G, Vergara I, Roman G (1977) Neuroparalytic accidents of antirabies vaccination with suckling mouse brain vaccine. Arch Neurol 34:694–700

Tyler KL, Gross RA, Cascino GD (1986) Unusual viral causes of transverse myelitis: hepatitis A virus and cytomegalovirus. Neurology 36:855–858

Vanneste JAL, Karthaus PPM, Davies G (1980) Acute urinary retention due to sacral myeloradiculitis. J Neurol Neurosurg Psychiatry 43:954–956

Walton JN (1977) Brain's diseases of the nervous system. Churchill Livingstone, London
Wells CEC (1971) Neurological complications of so-called "influenza": a winter study in south-east Wales. Br Med J i:369–373
Weng C, Huang CY, Chan PH, Preston P, Chen PY (1987) Transverse myelitis associated with larva migrans: finding of larvae in cerebrospinal fluid. Lancet 1:423
Wiley CA, Van Patten PD, Carpenter PM, Powell HC, Thal LJ (1987) Acute ascending necrotizing myelopathy caused by herpes simplex virus type 2. Neurology 37:1791–1794
Wood M, Anderson M (1988) Neurological infections. Saunders, London
Yagi K, Ohishi S, Ohtsuka K (1978) Effects of clioquinol on the cultured retinal nerve cells. Reports of SMON research commission, 94–96. (in Japanese, quoted by Okada et al. 1984)

Chapter 16

Three Tropical Spinal Cord Syndromes

C.U. Velmurugendran

Spinal Arachnoiditis

Under a variety of titles – spinal arachnoiditis, chronic spinal meningitis, meningitis serosa circumscripta spinalis, spinal complications of TB meningitis, intraspinal tuberculous granuloma – different authors have described a spectrum of conditions which, though resulting from different aetiological agents, have a common pathological basis, namely a primary or secondary inflammatory reaction of the spinal leptomeninges. Although spinal arachnoiditis seems to be disappearing in the Western World, it is still common in tropical countries such as India. Ramamurthi (1961) found that "arachnoiditis" was the commonest cause of spinal cord compression in patients admitted to the Department of Neurosurgery at Madras where, out of a total of 123 operated cases of spinal cord compression, 43 were due to arachnoiditis, followed by 28 with neurofibromas. Compression due to Pott's tuberculous deformity of the spine was not included in this series. Mani et al. (1969) examined 170 cases of spastic paraplegia in Bangalore and found that, after a condition which they described as South India paraplegia, arachnoiditis formed the second largest group.

In 1909 Horsley described the clinical features and operative findings in two patients with "chronic spinal meningitis" and mentioned that he had seen 21 similar patients over a period of two years. He observed that the condition was probably commoner than spinal cord tumour and that many cases of acute myelitis may in fact be cases of spinal meningitis. Howell (1936) reported that "arachnoiditis" was not uncommon and could be diagnosed by assessment of clinical features, CSF examination and myelographic studies. He mentioned trauma and infection as the two main causative factors. Elkington (1951) analysed the clinical and operative findings in 41 cases, initially calling the entity meningitis serosa circumscripta and later spinal arachnoiditis. He commented on the avascular nature of the arachnoid membrane and questioned its capability of manifesting inflammatory changes except in association with similar changes in the other meninges. Ransome and Monteiro (1947) appear to have been the first to draw attention to the tuberculous aetiology of extensive spinal "arachnoiditis" occurring as an unusual variety of TB meningitis. Bucy and Oberhill (1950), Dibble and Cascino (1956), Arseni and Samit (1960), Jenkins and Hill (1963), and Parsons and Pallis (1965) have all described radiculomyelopathy resulting from spinal meningeal inflammation under the term intraspinal tuberculomas. The pathology of these cases was one of extensive spinal leptomeningitis and hence the term "tuberculomas" may not be suitable in so far as it is suggestive of a space-occupying lesion within the cord.

In India, patients with chronic spinal meningitides are to be seen in all parts of the country. Singh et al. (1959) published a clinical report of two cases of spinal meningitis of probable tuberculous aetiology. The few others that have been published by Carbrall (1961) from Sri Lanka, Ramamurthi (1961) and Arjundas (1961) from South India deal with a mixed group of conditions such as cases due to specific and non-specific infections, prolapsed intervertebral disc, tumour or trauma as well as a large "idiopathic" group. All these appear to result, as Elkington (1951) pointed out, from one common denominator of fibrosis with or without inflammation and thickening of arachnoid membranes with a series of blockages of CSF pathways.

Aetiopathology

Infective Agents

Tuberculosis

This seems to be the commonest cause of spinal meningitis in India today. It originates in three ways:

1. A tuberculous lesion starting primarily in the spinal structures, as the first expression of TB of the nervous system
2. Secondary extension downwards of an already established intracranial TB basal meningitis
3. Secondary extension from caries of the vertebrae

The Primary Spinal Variety. This comprised 20 of 70 cases reported by Wadia and Dastur (1969) forming the largest group among the aetiological agents. The clinical features frequently resembled ascending myelitis. CSF analysis pointed to a subarachnoid block; the patients died in coma from what was seen at autopsy to be a secondary spread of tuberculosis to the basal meninges from the spinal canal. At autopsy the spinal meningeal exudate was described "as if a yellow jelly had been poured into the subarachnoid space and allowed to set". They found the tubercle bacilli in the basal meninges. Others such as Bucy and Oberhill (1950) and Arseni and Samit (1960) described a much slower clinical form which can be clinically indistinguishable from a spinal cord tumour. The diagnosis in all their cases was made after operation and biopsy from which TB bacilli were cultured. Dastur and Wadia (1969) believed that the meningitis was initiated by a flare up of a local parenchymatous focus on the surface of the spinal cord, just as a Rich focus may break down to produce a tuberculous basal meningitis.

Secondary Involvement of the Spinal Meninges. Spread from a tuberculous basal meningitis to the spinal cord is commoner and more often recognised extensor plantar responses. Acute retention of urine may accompany or precede the paralytic symptoms. Loss of sensation up to a segmental level on the trunk is often found. Thus the clinical presentation may at times resemble an acute or subacute transverse myelitis confined to a single level of the cord. When the root pains, sensory level, motor disturbance and areflexia do not indicate a single level, a multifocal radiculomyelopathy is likely. In this situation it is not uncommon to see a patient with severe root pain in the upper limbs and a sensory loss down to D10, who also complains of severe sciatica accompanied by bilateral foot drop, absent ankle jerks and extensor plantar responses. In the ascending variety, severe sciatica is followed by an ascending weakness which initially affects the lumbosacral roots. In extreme cases, there is a hypotonic, areflexic weakness of all four limbs with respiratory and bladder paralysis. Such cases are readily mistaken for the Guillain-Barré syndrome. The majority of patients with the more acute forms of the condition have past or present evidence of tuberculosis. In some of these patients, meningitis developing in the spinal meninges soon spreads intracranially to cause drowsiness, confusion, neck stiffness and other clinical signs of basal meningitis. Spinal extension of TB basal meningitis usually appears within weeks in an inadequately treated case, but has also been seen in fully treated but resistant cases. If the condition is caused by syphilis, other parameters of luetic disease such as Argyll-Robertson pupils may be found. A past history of spinal anaesthesia may give a clue to the diagnosis of pyogenic arachnoiditis.

Chronic Form

In this form the clinical features are indistinguishable from a spinal cord compression due to a tumour. The disease may progress slowly over months or years, and remain unrecognized unless the clinical features point to a multifocal disease. In practice the condition may remain unsuspected until myelography or a laminectomy is performed.

Investigations

Lumbar Puncture

In the acute form of the disease the lumbar puncture may show evidence of either a partial or a complete subarachnoid block. The Queckenstedt test may be positive, the fluid xanthochromic and protein in excess of 0.1 g/l. All but 2 of 24 patients examined by Wadia and Dastur (1969) had a raised protein. The cellular response is mostly lymphocytic. The sugar content of the CSF was reduced only in some cases with a tuberculous aetiology. The CSF VDRL may be positive in the syphilitic cases. A rising CSF protein in a patient under treatment for TB meningitis should alert the physician to the possibility of a developing subarachnoid block which may or may not be followed by paralysis. The CSF should be stained, cultured and inoculated into laboratory animals to identify if possible the infective agent. A dry tap may be obtained at times.

In the chronic and localized form the CSF may be normal. There is very little increase in cell content but the protein is often raised. When the CSF protein is very high or is xanthochromic in a patient presenting with a disc prolapse, coincident arachnoiditis must be suspected. Systemic tuberculosis or cryptococcal infection may be diagnosed from a chest X-ray or suspected from the presence of a raised erythrocyte sedimentation rate.

Myelography

The contrast medium is usually introduced through the lumbar route though occasionally a cisternal puncture is required if there is a dry lumbar tap, or to determine the upper extent of an established block. The principal diagnostic features of arachnoiditis seen by myelography are:

1. On screening the dye column moves very slowly with filling defects and fragmentation
2. There is often a total block with a ragged edge or one extending obliquely over two or more vertebral levels
3. The dye column, with or without a block, may show
   a) multiple small filling defects
   b) candle guttering extending for many segments of the spinal canal
   c) in the region of the cauda equina, the presence of exudate around the roots may give an appearance of "a bundle of faggot sticks", tapering to a "rat's tail"
   d) in a few cases multiple small round clear areas or a single large one may point to cyst formation

Most often the level of myelographic block does not correlate well with the clinical level. The absence of correlation is seen more often with the acute form of this disease.

Differential Diagnosis

The acute form has to be differentiated from the Guillain-Barré syndrome, in which root pain and pyramidal tract signs are rare, bladder disturbance occasional, and segmental sensory loss up to a definite anatomical level rarely found; whereas all these are the hallmarks of an acute spinal radiculomyelopathy. Features of Froin's syndrome are accompanied by a cellular response, not seen in the albumino-cytological dissociation characteristic of Guillain-Barré syndrome. Once clinically suspected, the myelogram usually enables the distinction to be made.

In the absence of severe root pains, the differentiation from acute transverse and ascending myelitis and acute spinal meningitis may be difficult. Careful screening of the myelogram for subtle signs such as irregularities of the column of contrast or the presence of filling defects may be required. The differential diagnosis between subacute and chronic compression of other aetiologies and spinal meningitis is not always easy even after myelography. In borderline cases, where doubt still exists, a diagnostic surgical procedure may be justified since the prognosis is completely changed by appropriate treatment. At times it is only the bioposy report that settles the diagnosis.

Pathology

Tuberculosis

The following description is common to all three varieties of TB spinal meningitis. Exudate surrounds the cord forming a thick collar which is often more dense over the posterior than anterior surface. The meninges appear thick, opaque and lustreless. Tubercles with a caseating centre may be seen within the exudate. The dura is often adherent and cannot be separated from the structures enclosed within it. In most autopsy specimens there is considerable atrophy of the spinal cord.

The exudate surrounds but does not infiltrate the roots, posterior root ganglia or the cord. In addition to the presence of tubercles, the other common histological change is an obliterative endarteritis. This may affect small vessels and occasionally produce periarteritis and subintimal fibrosis in medium-sized vessels. As the granulomatous reaction becomes chronic, mucous and arachnoid cysts develop.

The spinal cord may show a border zone of rarefaction and spongeosis of the cord, demyelination and axonal degeneration of the pyramidal tracts, degeneration of anterior horn cells, evidence of arteritis and, occasionally, an intramedullary tuberculoma.

The differentiation of cryptococcal arachnoiditis from tuberculous can be difficult though PAS staining of biopsy sections can help.

Atlantoaxial Dislocation

The atlas and axis function as a single unit by means of a single median and two lateral joints. Stability is maintained by the interlocking of the anterior arch of the atlas with the odontoid process of the axis, which is firmly kept in position by the transverse ligament. Dislocation occurs when stability is disturbed by congenital or acquired disease (Werne 1957). Wadia (1960) has emphasized the unusually high incidence of the congenital variety in India and this was borne out by subsequent case reports throughout the country (Bharucha and Dastur 1964; Srinivasan et al. 1967; Singh et al. 1969).

Clinical Features

There are three main groups of symptoms:

1. Cervical pain and stiffness

2. Transitory attacks
3. Progressive neurological disturbances

Cervical Symptoms

Pain and stiffness are not as prominent as in acquired dislocation. However, limitation of neck movements especially on lateral rotation is seen in half the patients.

Transitory Attacks

Transitory attacks of paralysis arising from the upper cervical cord or the lowermost part of the medulla form a very characteristic part of the symptomatology of chronic atlantoaxial dislocation, whether congenital or acquired. Twenty-one out of 52 patients reported by Wadia (1960, 1967) gave a history of paralytic attacks. Attacks of paralysis of the limbs, paraesthesiae below the neck, unconsciousness and, more rarely, blurring of vision were precipitated by exaggerated flexion, extension or rotation of the neck. Most episodes lasted from a few minutes to half an hour. The frequency varied from a single episode to a large number over many years.

Neurological Signs and Symptoms

The predominant manifestation was involvement of the pyramidal tracts, presenting often in an asymmetrical fashion in all four limbs. Spasticity, exaggerated deep tendon reflexes, and extensor plantar responses were consistently seen but the abdominal reflexes were more often preserved than absent. Urinary symptoms were uncommon even in severe paralysis. The posterior column signs were less evident than pyramidal signs. Vibration sense was symmetrically impaired or lost as far as the clavicles in most patients. Disturbed spinothalamic sensation and cerebellar dysfunction were found only occasionally. Localized muscle wasting and weakness of the shoulder or hand muscles with fasciculation were seen in 15 out of 52 patients in Wadia's series. Horner's syndrome was present in 3 patients. Cranial nerve palsies were rare. None were found by Wadia (1967). However, Bharucha and Dastur (1964) mention a slightly higher frequency of "bulbar" signs and ataxia, especially in cases where there was associated occipitalization.

The course of the disease can be slowly progressive. Males are more often affected than females and the disease may be associated with a variety of congenital anomalies.

Investigations

Confirmation of the diagnosis is established by good radiology. Ideally, the radiological examination should include:

1. X-rays of the skull and cervical spine (lateral view in flexion and extension) and open mouth view of the atlantoaxial joint
2. Lateral cervical tomography in flexion and extension; AP tomography and myelography are undertaken when further elucidation is required. Teleradiological visualization of neck movements is extremely useful
3. CT scan of the craniovertebral junction

There are two main measurements:

1. In lateral flexion, in an adult, a maximum distance between the odontoid and the anterior arch of the atlas should not exceed 3 mm. In a child about 4.5 mm is permissible. A distance greater than this is an indication of atlantoaxial dislocation. Though the distance may vary from 5 to 12 mm, in most cases it is between 7 and 9 mm. When the odontoid is separated from the body of the axis or is absent, this measurement can not be used. In this situation the distance between the inferior rim of the anterior arch of the atlas and the remaining attached part of the odontoid or the anterior superior edge of the body of the axis is considered. Normally, no gap exists. These patients also have a clearly visible forward dislocation of the atlas, varying between 7 and 12 mm in flexion.

2. The spinal canal is measured in a lateral X-ray of the cervical spine from the posterior surface of the odontoid to the nearest bony projection on the posterior rim of the foramen magnum or the occipitalized atlas. This varies between 19 and 32 mm. Neurological signs are likely to arise when the diameter of the spinal canal is narrowest on flexion. Wadia (1967) found that 30 of his 52 patients had a diameter of less than 10 mm. If there is no change in the measurements between flexion and extension of the neck, the dislocation is designated as "fixed". If the dislocation is easily corrected by straightening the neck, it is designated a "gliding" dislocation.

Classification

Group 1. There is a combination of occipitalization of the atlas, fusion of C2 to C3 vertebrae, dislocation backward of the odontoid process and compression of the spinal cord. The odontoid may be normal, long or short.

Group 2. There is no occipitalization of the atlas. The basic anomaly is the maldevelopment of the odontoid process.

Group 3. There is no occipitalization and the odontoid is normal in shape without any separation. In flexion the dislocation is clearly seen with the odontoid dislocated backwards and not upwards.

The main points of differentiation between the 3 groups are:

1. In groups 1 and 2, patients are much younger than in group 3
2. A short neck and low hairline are commonest in group 1, seen occasionally in group 2 and not at all in group 3
3. Cervical symptoms are seen especially in group 1 and neck movements are free in groups 2 and 3
4. Associated dysplastic facies are most frequently present in group 1

CSF examination is usually normal but occasionally the protein may be as high as 0.8–0.9 g/l.

Mechanism of Dislocation

The probable reasons for dislocation at the atlantoaxial joint are: maldevelopment or malfunctioning of the transverse ligaments; maldevelopment of the odontoid process; maldevelopment of the lateral articulating facets between the atlas and the axis; and occipitalization of the axis.

Differential Diagnosis

When all the clinical features are present the diagnosis is straightforward and can be confirmed by radiology. But when the presentation is atypical, differentiation from other compressive lesions such as tumours may be difficult and only careful radiology and myelography will settle the matter.

Differentiation from other anomalies of the craniovertebral junction can be made clinically and radiologically. In basilar invagination, transitory attacks have rarely been described. On the other hand, lower cranial nerve palsies, cerebellar signs, signs of involvement of the spinothalamic tract, and signs of raised intracranial pressure are seen more often. These clinical features are rare in atlantoaxial dislocation.

Prognosis and Treatment

The prognosis is intimately connected with surgical treatment. Wadia (1967) advises surgical treatment for all patients with neurological signs, however slight, except for those over 60 years who are in poor general health and have little neurological disturbance. He advocates reduction of the dislocation either spontaneously or by use of skull traction. The lateral atlantoaxial joints are then fused by an anterior approach. For those who do not benefit substantially, a later posterior decompression and sectioning of dural bands is recommended. Surgery may arrest the deterioration and some patients may actually improve.

Motor System Disease in India

In motor system, or motor neurone, disease degeneration occurs involving the anterior horn cells or pyramidal tracts or both. The incidence of motor system disease in India varies from 3% to 5% (Wadia 1972; Gourie-Devi et al. 1984). At the Institute of Neurology in Madras about 50 cases of motor system disease present annually and account for 1%–2% of admissions. The main types of motor system disease encountered are:

1. Classical motor neurone disease (ALS)
2. Werdnig-Hoffman disease and its variants

ugelberg-Welander disease and its variants
. Chronic spinal muscular atrophies
5. Madras pattern of motor neurone disease
6. Monomelic type of motor neurone disease
7. Postpoliomyelitis progressive muscular atrophy

The clinical features of motor neurone disease (ALS) are basically similar to those seen elsewhere except for the fact that the onset of the disease is early, often in the second decade, and progression very gradual. There is a male preponderance. Though consanguinous marriages are common in India, a familial incidence of the disease is rare.

Werdnig-Hoffman disease and its variants are encountered. Bharucha and Bhandari (1987) found 14 cases with muscular atrophy and a very benign course among their series of floppy children. Survival was up to 9 years. Wadia (1972) described two benign variants of the disease in patients aged 4 to 5 years. He also described a recessive form of juvenile spinal muscular atrophy, or Kugelberg-Welander disease.

Chronic Spinal Muscular Atrophies

A group of chronic spinal muscular atrophies have been described by Sayeed et al. (1975, 1976) with involvement of anterior horn cells and lower cranial nerves, but not involving pyramidal tracts. These patients showed a typical electromyographic picture of anterior horn cell disease with normal nerve conduction velocities. The histological studies of the muscles showed group fibre atrophy and normal architecture of the nerves. The plasma citrate level was elevated and pyruvate levels were normal. The slow progression and biochemical findings suggest that they should be classified as a separate group. In 1987, Desai described a similar group of patients and noted the high incidence of skeletal abnormalities such as kyphoscoliosis and pes cavus.

The Madras Pattern of Motor Neurone Disease

This was first described by Jagannathan and Kumaresan in 1987. The clinical features include:

1. Young age of onset
2. Absence of a family history
3. Progressive but benign course with no mortality (2 patients have been followed for over 15 years)
4. Persistent but asymmetrical limb involvement for many years in more than half the cases
5. Lower cranial nerve involvement in two-thirds of patients with impairment of hearing in a third
6. Sparing of cognitive function, sensory system and other parts of the neuraxis

The Madras form of MND can be easily distinguished from Facio Londe disease by the absence of genetic inheritance and the slow progression. A similar illness has been seen in aborigines living in Groote Eylandt in Australia (Gajdusek 1987). There is a slow progression with the onset in adolescence or sometimes in early life, leading to severe amyotrophy with a normal life expectancy. Non-familial spinal segmental muscular atrophy in 32 juvenile and young subjects has been described by Virmani and Mohan (1985). These cases showed atrophy which was restricted to the proximal segment of an arm or leg with gradual progression. They were non-endemic. Cases with pyramidal and autonomic involvement have been described from Delhi, Chandigarh and Trivandrum (Virmani 1975; Gourie-Devi and Suresh 1988).

Monomelic Type of MND

The essential clinical features are unilateral atrophy/weakness of intrinsic muscles of the hand and forearm flexors with sparing of the brachioradialis, and involvement of anterior and posterior crural and quadriceps muscles. Bilateral involvement is rare. The absence of bulbar, pyramidal and autonomic nervous system involvement and the absence of any electromyographic evidence of neurogenic involvement of clinically unaffected muscles are characteristic features (Virmani and Mohan 1985). These also serve to differentiate the condition from cases reported by Japanese workers with pyramidal involvement in the ipsilateral upper and lower limbs and EMG evidence of neurogenic involvement of the contralateral upper extremities. Due consideration needs to be given to exclude late onset progression of poliomyelitis, vascular insufficiency, syphilitic arteritis and exposure to toxins leading to anterior horn cell disease. The EMG and histopathological features of monomelic amyotrophy are consistent with chronic anterior horn cell disease.

Postpoliomyelitis Progressive Muscular Atrophy

Intranuclear inclusion bodies have been found in anterior horn cells and hypoglossal nuclei in cases of amyotrophic lateral sclerosis. Similar observations were made in sporadic cases by Schochet et al. (1969). Anterior horn cell wasting with or without encephalomyelitis has been attributed to Coxsackie B virus infection. A higher incidence of motor neurone disease than expected by chance has been observed in cases with a history of old poliomyelitis (Zilka 1962). Some patients with spinal muscular atrophy may show an elevated antibody titre to poliovirus, suggesting that the spinal muscular atrophy represents the consequence of the poliovirus assuming a slow virus pattern.

References

Arachnoiditis

Arjundas G (1961) Intraspinal compressions. Neurology (Bombay) 9:164
Arseni CC, Samit DC (1960) Intraspinal tuberculous granulomas. Brain 83:285–292
Bucy PC, Oberhill HR (1950) Intradural spinal granulomas. J Neurosurg 7:1
Carbrall SA (1961) Spinal arachnoiditis and archanoid cysts. Neurology (Bombay) 9:91

Dastur DK, Wadia NH (1969) Spinal meningitis with radiculopathy: part 2 – pathology and pathogenesis. J Neurol Sci 8:261–297
Dibble JB, Cascino J (1956) Tuberculoma of the spinal cord. JAMA 162:461
Elkington J StC (1951) Arachnoiditis. In: Feiling A (ed) Modern trends in neurology, vol 1. Butterworths, London, pp 149–161
Horsley V (1909) Chronic spinal meningitis. Br Med J i:513
Howell CMH (1936) Arachnoiditis. Proc R Soc Med 30:33
Jenkins RB, Hill C (1963) Intradural spinal tuberculoma with genito-urinary symptoms. Arch Neurol Sci 9:179
Mani KS, Mani AJ, Mongomery RD (1969) A spastic paraplegia syndrome in South India. J Neurol Sci 9:179–199
Parsons M, Pallis CA (1965) Intradural spinal tuberculomas. Neurology (Minneap) 15:1018–1022
Ramamurthi B (1961) Intraspinal arachnoiditis. Indian J Med Sci 15:776–781
Ransome GA, Monteiro ES (1947) A rare form of tuberculous meningitis. Br Med J i:413
Siddiqui NA (1968) Spinal arachnoiditis. Neurology (India) 16:131–134
Singh A, Jolly SS, Goyal AC (1959) Spinal tuberculous meningitis. Neurology (Bombay) 7:74
Wadia NH, Dastur DK (196.) Spinal meningitis with radiculomyelopathy: part 1, clinical and radiological features. J Neurol Sci 8:239–260

Atlantoaxial Dislocation

Bharucha EP, Dastur HM (1964) Craniovertebral anomalies. Brain 87:469–480
Singh S, Dutta AK, Gupta S (1969) Craniovertebral anomalies with neurological deficit. J Assoc Physicians India 17:469–473
Srinivasan K, Balasubramaniam V, Ramamurthi B (1967) Craniovertebral anomalies. Neurology (India) 15:42
Wadia NH (1960) Chronic progressive myelopathy complicating atlanto-axial dislocation due to congenital abnormality. Neurology (Bombay) 8:81
Wadia NH (1967) Myelopathy complicating atlanto-axial dislocation. (A study of 28 cases.) Brain 90:449–472
Werne S (1957) Studies in spontaneous atlas dislocation. Acta Orthop Scand suppl 23, pp 1–150

Motor System Diseases

Arjundas G, Sayeed ZA, Velmurugendran CU (1974) Motor system disease. In: Progress in clinical medicine in India, pp 293–300
Bharucha EP, Bhandari SN (1987) Motor neurone disease in India. In: Gourie-Devi M (ed) Motor neurone disease. Oxford IBH, New Delhi, pp 165–170
Desai AD (1987) Chronic spinal muscular atrophies in India. In: Gourie-Devi M (ed) Motor neurone disease. Oxford IBH, New Delhi, pp 195–212
Gajdusek DC (1987) Past, present and future in motor neurone disease. In: Gourie-Devi M (ed) Motor neurone disease. Oxford IBH, New Delhi, pp 243–248
Gourie-Devi M, Suresh TG (1988) Madras pattern of motor neuron disease in South India. J Neurol Neurosurg Psychiatry 51:773–777
Gourie-Devi M, Suresh TG, Shankar SK (1984) Monomelic amyotrophy. Arch Neurol 41:388–394
Jagannathan K, Kumaresan G (1987) Madras pattern of motor neurone disease. In: Gourie-Devi M (ed) Motor neurone disease. Oxford IBH, New Delhi, pp 191–193
Sayeed ZA, Velmurugendran CU, Arjundas G, Mascareen M, Valmikinathan K (1975) Anterior horn cell disease seen in South India. J Neurol Sci 26:489–498
Sayeed ZA, Mascareen M, Arjundas G, Valmikinathan K (1976) Plasma lactate in anterior horn cell disease. J Neurol Sci 29:1–17
Schochet SS Jr, Hardman JM, Ladewig PP, Earle KM (1969) Intraneuronal conglomerates in sporadic motor neuron disease. A light and electron microscopic study. Arch Neurol 20:548–553
Virmani V (1975) Pattern of motor neurone disease in North India. J Assoc Physicians India 23:695–701
Virmani V, Mohan PK (1985) Nonfamilial spinal segmental muscular atrophy. Acta Neurol Scand 72:336–340
Wadia RS (1972) Diseases of the anterior horn cell. J Assoc Physicians India 20:416–422
Zilka K (1962) Motor neurone disease following poliomyelitis. Proc R Soc Med 55:1028–1035

Chapter 17

The Conus Medullaris and Sphincter Control

M. Swash

The anal and urinary sphincters are responsive to filling of the anorectum and urinary bladder respectively. The normal storage and voiding functions of these organ systems reflect their pressure/volume relationships, and the ability of the detrusor mechanisms to overcome the passive and active resistance to the passage of faeces and urine offered by the anal canal and urethra. In both systems voiding may occur in response to the activity of the smooth muscle of the anorectum and colon, and of the urinary bladder, or it may be assisted by the additional contraction of the abdominal wall. In both systems, voiding depends on the orderly relationship between detrusor mechanisms and relaxation of the smooth and striated muscular sphincters that guard the exits of the bladder and anal canal. In this review, the anatomical arrangements responsible for continence and voiding will be described, and the role of the conus region of the spinal cord will be considered in relation to disorders of its function.

Innervation of the Anorectum

The rectal mucosa receives sensory innervation from non-myelinated, beaded nerve fibres terminating in free axonal swellings. This type of innervation resembles that found elsewhere in the gut (Duthie and Gairns 1960). More distally, from a region 10–15 cm above the anal valves to the hairy skin of the anal canal itself the innervation of the mucosa is richer, consisting of free and specialized nerve endings. The latter consist of Meissner corpuscles, Golgi-Mazzoni bodies, Krause end-bulbs, genital corpuscles, and other less well-classified endings. Pacinian corpuscles are also found in the deeper layers of the anal canal close to the internal anal sphincter. Pacinian corpuscles are found in large number in the mesentery of the gut, including that of the rectum. Duthie and Gairns (1960) pointed out that the innervation of the lower rectum and anal canal resembled that of the skin elsewhere in the body, a feature that is perhaps not surprising in view of the developmental origin of the anal canal from the ectodermal anal pit. Free and encapsulated nerve endings are probably more numerous in the region of the anal valves than more distally (Duthie and Gairns 1960; Gould 1960). Duthie and Gairns (1960) noted that touch, pin-prick and thermal stimuli were all readily perceived in the anal canal in a zone corresponding to the distribution of this extensive sensory innervation, an observation that has since been confirmed by others (Roe et al. 1986; Rogers et al. 1988). However, it must be noted that there is no immediate physiological basis for temperature sensation in the rectum or upper anal canal and this sensory experience appears to be relatively limited to the lower part of the anal canal.

The rectum contains motor and sensory neurones of the enteric nervous system in its myenteric and submucosal plexuses. These have the same function in the regulation of contraction of the smooth muscle components of the rectal wall as in other parts of the gut (Furness and Costa 1987; Gershon 1990). No detailed studies are available of the anatomy and function of the rectal enteric nervous system, and there is no information as to whether the interstitial cells of Cajal, the pacemaker cells for smooth muscle cell activity elsewhere in the gut, are present in the rectum (Thuneberg 1982). It is assumed that there is some regulation of the activity of the enteric nervous system of the rectum from its parasympathetic and sympathetic input, as there is in other parts of the gut.

In the human the internal anal sphincter (IAS) is relatively sparsely innervated. It is virtually devoid of ganglia of the enteric nervous system, perhaps simply because there is no further enteric tissue caudad to the IAS to which enteric ganglia could project, rather than from some particular specialization of the IAS with respect to other gut smooth muscle. Ultrastructural studies of the IAS disclose the presence of sparse, unmyelinated nerve fibres, some containing dense-core vesicles that come into close apposition to smooth muscle cells without making synaptic contact with this syncitium of cells (Swash et al. 1986). Visceral innervation to the IAS is derived from the same projections of the autonomic nervous system as the rectum.

Afferent projections from the rectum consist of thinly myelinated, slowly-conducting parasympathetic and sympathetic nerve fibres that enter the dorsal horn of the spinal cord through the posterior roots, and either project rostrally through the spinal cord to the hypothalamus or participate in segmental reflex pathways. The sensory innervation of the anal canal, unlike that of the rectum, is of somatic origin; the afferent projections from sensory receptors in the anal canal enter the dorsal horn through thickly myelinated, fast-conducting fibres and project rostrally to the thalamus and sensory cortex in the posterior columns of the cord. Visceral sensations from the rectum also reach consciousness, probably as a result of projections from the hypothalamus rather than from direct projections of the visceral nervous system itself. The efferent projections of the autonomic nervous system to the rectum and anal canal are also derived both from the sympathetic and parasympathetic nervous systems.

Parasympathetic nerve fibres reach the rectum in the sacral nerves. These fibres arise in the intermediolateral cell columns of the sacral spinal cord at the S2–4 levels. They emerge from the cord with the ventral spinal nerve roots and give rise to the pelvic nerve plexus. Their second order neurones lie in this plexus or in the walls of the anorectum. Sympathetic innervation to the anorectum is derived from the thoracolumbar chain of ganglia, and is carried in the hypogastric nerves. Stimulation of the sympathetic nerve fibres in the hypogastric nerves in the human has yielded controversial results. Carlstedt et al. (1988) found that the IAS contracted in response to pelvic sympathetic nerve stimulation, but others have recorded sphincter relaxation in similar experiments (Shepherd and Wright 1968; Lubowski et al. 1987). These differences may relate to different experimental conditions, such as depth of anaesthesia, or to differences in the resting state of the muscle. For example, there is doubt also as to whether the parasympathetic innervation of the IAS contributes to its resting tone (Frenckner and Ihre 1976; Meunier and Mollard 1977). The resting anal pressure, representing tonic contraction of the IAS, decreases during high but not during low spinal anaesthesia, indicating a tonic effect of excitatory sympathetic activity, but no effect of any tonic parasympathetic activity on the sphincter muscle (Burnstock 1990). On the other hand, damage to the sacral outflow seems to cause a lower resting anal tone, suggesting that resting parasympathetic tone may play a role in the maintenance of IAS contraction. Burnstock and colleagues (1990) have concluded that, in general, smooth muscle sphincters are controlled independently from non-sphincteric smooth muscle. Stimulation of the parasympathetic nerves supplying the internal anal sphincter muscle inhibits the spontaneous resting tone of this muscle, by an effect mediated by non-adrenergic, non-cholinergic nerves (NANC) (Burnstock 1990). The neurotransmitter for this effect is likely to be purinergic. The possible role of neuropeptides in increasing or decreasing resting anal tone is uncertain, but neuropeptide Y is thought to be active at this location. Acetylcholine contracts the internal anal sphincter. Whatever the role of the visceral innervation, it is certainly less important than that of the enteric nervous system, as shown by the large relaxation of the IAS that occurs in response to dilatation of a balloon in the rectum – the recto-anal reflex.

The identification of the receptors subserving the sensation of rectal distension has proved difficult. Although it was for long thought that these receptors must be located in the wall of the rectum, experiments in patients after rectal excision and colo-anal anastomosis showed that this sensation was often preserved postoperatively, suggesting that the receptors for this sensation must lie outside the rectum and presumably, therefore, must be located in the pelvic floor musculature or in the pelvic fascia. The muscles of the pelvic floor contain muscle spindles as well as Pacinian corpuscles, and it is possible that this sensation of rectal filling is mediated by these receptors, together with the "sampling" function of the anorectal mucosal receptors themselves.

Innervation of the Bladder

The bladder receives parasympathetic innervation that induces contraction of the smooth muscle of the detrusor. This is partly acetylcholinergic, but the response of the detrusor muscle to pelvic (parasympathetic) nerve stimulation is only partially blocked by atropine (Langley and Anderson 1895), a phenomenon now recognized as due to the presence of a NANC transmitter acting at this site (Moss and Burnstock 1985). This NANC transmitter is ATP (Burnstock 1990). There is thus a clear implication that acetylcholine and ATP may be co-transmitters in the bladder wall, and perhaps also in the intrinsic neurones of the bladder wall (Burnstock 1990). Speakman et al. (1989) have confirmed the presence of this NANC component of neurotransmission in the trigonal area of the human bladder and have shown that this is probably purinergic. Such responses are virtually absent from the dome of the bladder.

The sympathetic innervation to the bladder is derived from the hypogastric nerves and these nerve endings contain both noradrenaline and neuropeptide Y (Crowe and Burnstock 1989). In addition, substance P and calcitonin gene-related peptide have been located in the abundant sensory-motor nerves of the trigone region of the bladder, and vasoactive intestinal peptide and leu-encephalin have been located in parasympathetic nerves, and also in the intrinsic ganglia (Burnstock 1990). Both 5-hydroxytryptamine and prostaglandins have also been shown to be capable of eliciting contractile responses in the bladder wall musculature; the latter may form part of the normal response to noxious stimuli in the bladder, e.g. infection. The degree of homology of the neurotransmitters found in the intrinsic innervation of the bladder with that of the enteric nervous system is uncertain but is unlikely to be close in view of the differing embryological origins of these two tissues. However, it has recently become apparent that the intrinsic neurones and ganglia of the bladder wall and urethra (Burnstock 1990) contain circuitry that supports integrative activity of the bladder smooth muscle, and that may also subserve a sensory function.

The innervation of the urethra differs from that of the body of the bladder. Its adrenergic nerves are excitatory, inducing powerful contractile responses, and there is an additional innervation from cholinergic fibres, together with a non-purinergic NANC component (Ito and Kimoto 1985; Burnstock 1990). The latter may serve to relax the urethral smooth muscle.

Innervation of Pelvic Floor Muscles

The innervation of the pelvic floor muscles is derived from the S2, S3 and S4 sacral segments. The afferent and efferent nerve fibres providing sensory and motor innervation to these muscles travel in the pelvic nerves and in the pudendal nerves. The pelvic nerves enter the levator ani and puborectalis (PR) muscles from their peritoneal surface (Stelzner 1960; Duthie and Gairns 1960), and the pudendal nerves innervate the external anal sphincter (EAS) muscle through its inferior rectal branches that approach the muscle through Alcock's canal and the ischiorectal fossa. Perineal branches of the pudendal nerves pass forward through the perineum to innervate the periurethral striated urinary sphincter muscles, and thus to control urinary continence. The direct pelvic route for the somatic innervation of the PR muscle has been shown by two related electrophysiological investigations (Percy et al. 1981; Snooks and Swash 1986), and this is strong evidence for a separate developmental origin for the EAS and PR muscles (see above).

The external urethral sphincter muscle (EUS) may be a site in which there is a functional interaction between somatic efferent innervation and the autonomic nervous system, since close proximity relationships between the striated muscle fibres of this muscle and nor-adrenergic and VIP-ergic nerves have been observed (Crowe et al. 1989). The conventional somatic innervation of the EUS is derived from the paired perineal branches of the pudendal nerves and the intrinsic component of the striated urethral sphincter muscle,

located in the urethral wall itself, seems to be derived, like the innervation of
the puborectalis muscle, from direct somatic innervation given off from pelvic
branches of the sacral plexus (S3 and S4) (Snooks and Swash 1986).

Central Connections of the Sphincter Innervation

The motor nerve fibres innervating the EUS, EAS and PR muscles, but
probably not those innervating the levator ani muscle, arise in the ventral grey
matter of the sacral cord. The lower motor neurones innervating these muscles
lie in the S2 and S3 segments, forming a discrete motor nucleus named after
Onuf, who described it in 1899 (Onuf 1900). These neurones differ from other
somatic efferent motor neurones in that they are smaller and more densely
packed, and show architectonic features resembling parasympathetic neurones,
which lie nearby in the lateral cell columns of the sacral cord. Other characteristics that suggest a functional interrelationship with parasympathetic
neurones include the presence of direct afferent connections with paraventricular hypothalamic neurones, and a rich peptidergic input. Leu-encephalin,
VIP and somatostatin are found in and around the Onuf nucleus, but not on
the adjacent somatic efferent neurones (Roppolo et al. 1985). In addition,
clinicopathological studies have shown that these neurones are lost in primary
autonomic failure, and in Shy-Drager syndrome (Sung et al. 1979), but not in
amyotrophic lateral sclerosis or spinal muscular atrophy (Mannen et al. 1977).
The Onuf nucleus cells have connections mainly orientated in the rostrocaudal
plane, a feature that may be related to the tonic output of the cells of this
nucleus, since a similar anatomical pattern is found in the cells of the phrenic
nucleus in the cervical spinal cord (Kuzuhara et al. 1980). Lateral dendritic
branches probably establish connections with the parasympathetic neurones in
the adjacent cell columns of the lateral grey matter, with primary afferents
from the pudendal nerves and with descending fibres from brain stem and
cortical centres.

   The upper motor neurones for the voluntary sphincter muscles lie close to
those innervating the lower limb muscles in the parasagittal motor cortex,
adjacent to the sensory representation of the genitalia and perineum in the
sensory cortex. Corticospinal fibres project from the motor cortex direct to the
motor cells of the contralateral Onuf nucleus; some fibres recross in the sacral
cord to project to the ipsilateral nucleus, so that there is bilateral cortical input to
the two halves of this nucleus, and so to the two sides of the somatic sphincter
muscles in the anorectum (Nakagawa 1980). Using transcutaneous electrical
stimulation of the motor pathways in alert human subjects at the level of the
cortex and cauda equina, Merton et al. (1982) showed that these upper motor
neurone pathways form a fast-conducting oligosynaptic pathway. This pathway
consists of a narrow strip of fibres in the lateral corticospinal tract in which the
efferent fibres are situated medial to the afferent fibres (Nathan and Smith
1953). The frontal lobes are important in defaecation, straining and micturition
(Andrews and Nathan 1964) and direct projections from the paraventricular
hypothalamic nuclei and from the pontine reticular formation may also be
important in the central integration of visceral and somatic muscle func-

tion required for defaecation and micturition, and for continence (Swash and Mathers 1989). In dogs, defaecatory behaviour can be induced by distension of the rectum, and this reflex response was shown by Fukuda and Fukai (1986) to be dependent on reflex straining centres in the pons and medulla.

De Groat and Kawatani (1985) have constructed a diagram of the central reflex connections and encephalinergic mechanisms that regulate micturition in the cat. It is reasonable to suppose that a similar system of neuronal connections is involved in the control of defaecation. In their micturition model (Fig. 17.1) micturition is initiated by a supraspinal reflex pathway passing through a "micturition centre" in the brain stem. This pathway is excited by input from small unmyelinated afferents originating in tension receptors in the bladder wall, that project to the brain stem centre. A spinal reflex mechanism, that becomes evident in spinal man, is inhibited in the intact nervous system. De Groat (1990) has suggested that the micturition reflex is inhibited by descending brain stem activity, directed onto the Onuf nucleus in the sacral cord, and it is likely that defaecation is similarly inhibited by this pathway. The descending pathway that initiates voiding therefore acts as a switch, burning off the tonic activity of the sphincter muscles that maintains continence in the resting state. The diagram clearly indicates the importance of the functional interrelationship between the autonomic and somatic components of the sphincter mechanisms.

Conus Medullaris and Cauda Equina Disorders

The separation of cauda equina and conus lesions in clinical practice is difficult, mainly because the clinical features of lesions at these two sites overlap. Pure lesions of the conus medullaris are rare and perhaps occur most frequently in multiple sclerosis. However in *multiple sclerosis*, lesions of the conus are usually accompanied by lesions elsewhere in the central nervous system. *Vascular disorders*, e.g. spinal cord infarction, rarely involve the conus medullaris in isolation, and intermittent claudication of the cauda equina produces symptoms and signs that are, at least in part, due to a combination of ischaemia both of the cauda equina and of the conus medullaris. *Trauma* to the lumbosacral spine, similarly, is more likely to produce either a combination syndrome or a pure cauda equina lesion because of the vulnerability of the spinal roots to traumatic damage as they exit from the spinal canal through the intervertebral foramina. *Intrinsic tumours* of the conus medullaris, especially astrocytomas and ependymomas, selectively damage the conus medullaris, and produce the best demonstration of the typical features of this syndrome. Unfortunately, because there are few abnormalities on conventional neurological examination in the early stages of the disorder, the diagnosis is often missed until the syndrome is relatively advanced.

The typical features of a conus lesion, illustrated by the slowly progressive course of a patient with an *intrinsic tumour* in this region, derive from damage to the middle and lower sacral segments (Brodal 1981). The clinical signs, largely confined to the pelvic floor, may be missed by the inexperienced examiner, since routine neurological examination of the legs, and even of the lateral buttocks, may reveal no abnormality, and the plantar responses may be

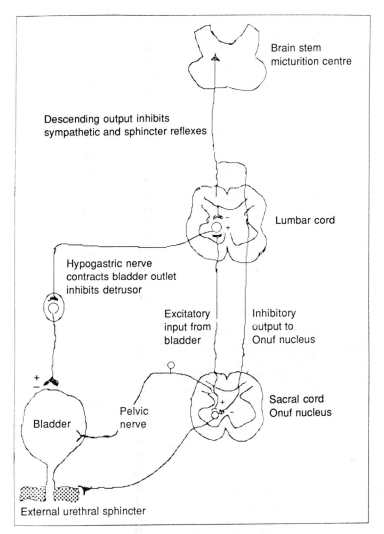

Brain stem micturition centre

Descending output inhibits sympathetic and sphincter reflexes

Lumbar cord

Hypogastric nerve contracts bladder outlet inhibits detrusor

Excitatory input from bladder

Inhibitory output to Onuf nucleus

Bladder

Pelvic nerve

Sacral cord Onuf nucleus

External urethral sphincter

Fig. 17.1. Diagram to show the reciprocal excitatory and inhibitory innervation of detrusor and striated urethral sphincter muscles in the control of urine storage and of micturition. Note that the descending projection from the pontine micturition centre to the Onuf nucleus at the S2 level in the conus medullaris is inhibitory to the striated sphincter, thus acting as a "switching off" mechanism in relation to the normal continuous activity of that muscle. (Diagram from work of De Groat 1985, 1990.)

flexor. There is weakness and loss of tone in the pelvic floor musculature, including the muscles of the perineum and perianal region. The anal reflex is absent, and there is loss of sensation in the perianal and perivulval or scrotal region. This sensory disturbance may extend onto the posterior aspect of the upper thigh if it extends rostral to the S2 level. This is "saddle anaesthesia". In low conus lesions, the S1 segment is not involved and, therefore, the ankle jerks are normal, a finding accounting for most instances of failure to make the diagnosis. The preganglionic parasympathetic connections in the cord are inter-rupted leading to paralysis of the bladder detrusor, retention of urine and, sometimes, especially in women, to the development of incontinence with overflow. There is no reflex contraction of the bladder as occurs with cord transection syndromes at higher levels, in which the inhibitory outflow from the pontine micturition centres to the Onuf nucleus is interrupted, leading to an "automatic bladder". There is also incontinence of faeces, with a patulous anus, together with impaired motility of the descending colon and rectum, due to the preganglionic parasympathetic lesion, resulting in impaction of faeces. In men there is failure of penile erection and ejaculation, although seminal emission can occur since the sympathetic innervation of the seminal vesicles and ductus deferens is intact. In some patients with progressive conus lesions, and rarely in acute demyelination of the conus region, priapism occurs, and there are often various components of the complete syndrome developing separately during the course of the onset of the syndrome. If the lesion extends rostrally a few segments, there may be associated wasting of the gluteal and posterior thigh muscles but this feature is often absent or difficult to recognize. Both plantar responses are flexor unless the lesion extends rostrally to about the level of S1. The spine itself is normal. In intrinsic lesions of this type there is usually a greal deal of spontaneous pain in the perineal area, that has a characteristic spinothalamic persistence. This pain may be burning or lancinat-ing and is often made worse by movement or by defaecation. It persists despite rest, and may be debilitating, being unrelieved by analgesics, except perhaps to some extent by carbamazepine or Dolobid. When the conus lesion is due to *extrinsic compression*, usually by a *central disc prolapse*, or by a *spinal fracture*, the onset is abrupt, with pain, incontinence, numbness in the perineum, and severe low back pain. The prognosis for functional recovery, even with urgent surgical decompression, is poor. *Secondary tumours* in this region usually present with local pain from bony invasion before features of cauda equina or conus involvement develop. Other localized tumours, e.g. *chordoma*, may be large before they involve the conus or cauda equina roots, so that a major and wide excision is required with a difficult postoperative course.

Lesions restricted to the *cauda equina* are usually painful, with pain experi-enced in the distribution of the affected nerve roots. Most cauda equina lesions, except central disc prolapse syndromes, involve the whole cauda equina, for example, chronic adhesive arachnoiditis syndromes, so producing pain radiating down the backs of both legs, perhaps asymmetrically, toward the soles of the feet, as well in the buttocks. Sensory loss is often extensive affecting the L5 and S1–5 distributions, and there is extensive wasting of the buttocks, posterior thighs and lateral lower leg muscles, with foot drop and absent ankle jerks but preserved knee jerks. The plantar responses, if elicit-able, are flexor. There is painful restriction of straight leg raising depending on the degree of mechanical tethering of the affected nerve roots. The bladder and bowel are paralysed, and there is denervation of the perineal muscles resembling that seen in conus lesions.

Sacral spinal dysraphism may be associated with conus and cauda equina lesions, and despite the congenital nature of the disorder the clinical features may progress, probably because the cord is tethered at its insertion into the abnormal sacral spinal sac, leading to repeated stretch injury during move-ment. The patient usually shows loss of spinal height as part of the malformation, and there is an abnormal gibbus at the site of the dysraphism. If the lesion extends to the lumbar cord the plantar responses will be extensor (provided that there is sufficient muscle acting around the foot to allow the reflex to be tested). Saddle sensory loss is usually present and this may have extended in distribution as part of the clinical progression of the syndrome before presentation.

In *multiple sclerosis* incontinence of urine (Miller et al. 1965) and faeces (Swash et al. 1987) is common, and there may also be constipation (Glick et al. 1982) or urinary retention. These apparently conflicting features are the expected result of conus involvement but proof that they result from a single lesion in this site is invariably lacking (Mathers et al. 1990). Indeed, most patients with multiple sclerosis have multiple lesions in different parts of the nervous system and the pathways for bladder and bowel control are so long and extend through so many vulnerable parts of the nervous system that it is hardly surprising that bladder and bowel dysfunction form so conspicuous a part of the clinical features of the disease. Many patients with multiple sclerosis and incontinence have electrophysiological evidence of lower motor neurone lesion involving the striated sphincter muscles (Miller et al. 1965; Glick et al. 1982). There is evidence that this may often be associated with childbirth, thus relating denervation of these muscles to damage to the pelvic floor innervation of the type found in the common variety of stress incontinence that is so common in women who have borne children (Swash 1990), rather than demyelination-induced damage to the central component of the lower motor neurone pathways in the cord.

Pure efferent lesions of the bladder innervation in the pelvis, and pure afferent lesions in the cord, such as tabes dorsalis, also lead to a large flaccid bladder without reflex micturition. These conditions can be diagnosed by the absence of the other features of cauda equina or conus lesion. However, infiltrative lesions in the pelvis can also involve the somatic innervation of the perineum, and may thus mimic in all respects the features of a conus lesion. Most infiltrative lesions in the pelvis are asymmetrical, a finding that is also a feature of cauda equina disease, but which is less marked in conus lesions. A finding of extensor plantar response, only present if the conus lesion is rostral to the S1/L5 level, is also important in raising the suspicion of a conus lesion. The advent of CT and MR scanning in the investigation of suspected pelvic infiltration, and its parallel use in patients investigated by myelography, has made this otherwise difficult clinical diagnosis much more secure.

Investigation and Diagnosis

Modern imaging techniques have greatly enhanced the capability of the clinician in the diagnosis of these difficult problems, and in the planning of appropriate medical, surgical and oncological therapies. However although relatively non-invasive, the technology of modern medical imaging is expensive and furthermore it cannot provide a guide to functional assessment of the pelvic floor or viscera. There is therefore a place in clinical investigation for functional tests of bladder and bowel, and for neurophysiological assessment of the striated pelvic floor musculature and its central connections.

Cystometry and Anal Manometry

These tests are useful in assessing functional capacity, but a description of their methodologies is beyond the scope of this chapter. Modern reviews are available elsewhere (Drife et al. 1990; Henry and Swash 1991). They are useful in providing objective measurement of the processes of storage and voiding of urine and of faeces, for example of measuring flow rate during micturition as an index of detrusor function, in measuring maximal tolerated storage volumes of urine or faeces as an index of the integrity of the central neural processes subserving the relation between storage and initiation of the micturition response, in imaging the processes of micturition or defaecation, and in assessing the first perceived volume of urine or faeces as a measure of sensory function. These assessments can be carried out simultaneously with electromyography of the external urinary and anal sphincter muscles in order to provide timing of the relationship of detrusor activity and relaxation of the voluntary, striated sphincter musculature. These tests measure the functional competence of the pelvic sphincters, and of the smooth muscle of the bowel and anorectum.

Electrophysiological Tests of the Lower Motor Neurone Pathway to the Pelvic Floor Muscles

Motor conduction in the terminal part of the pudendal nerves can be studied using commercially available surface electrodes mounted on a disposable examination glove. The pudendal nerve is stimulated transrectally at the level of the sciatic notch by bipolar electrodes located at the tip of the examiner's index finger, and the evoked motor response recorded from the external anal sphincter muscle by surface electrodes mounted at the base of the finger attachment (Kiff and Swash 1984). A catheter-mounted, bipolar ring electrode placed in the urethra at the level of the striated urinary sphincter muscle allows simultaneous recording of the perineal nerve terminal motor latency (Snooks and Swash 1984). Transcutaneous electrical or magnetic stimulation over the lumbar spine at two levels (T12 and L5) can be used to detect cauda equina lesions by measuring the latency of the motor response to the striated urinary or anal sphincter muscles (Swash and Snooks 1986; Chokroverty et al. 1989).

EMG, or single fibre EMG, has been used extensively in clinical research and in routine clinical management for assessing the presence of chronic partial denervation (reinnervation) in the striated pelvic floor sphincter muscles (Neill and Swash 1980; Fowler et al. 1984; Henry and Swash 1991). Polyphasic motor unit potentials are found when the lower motor neurone is damaged at any site, whether distally in the pelvis, or in the cauda equina or conus medullaris. The nerve conduction studies can more precisely localize the abnormality to these levels.

Sensory pathways in the nervous system relevant to the problem of conus lesions can be assessed using somatosensory evoked potentials following stimulation of the skin of the anus, the dorsal nerve of the penis or clitoris, and of the lower urinary tract (Mathers and Swash 1990). However, these methods are not often used in routine clinical practice. Attempts to use measurements of short- or long-latency components of the cutaneous anal reflex in clinical diagnosis have not proved reliable because of the complexity of the response and the variability in the latency of the various components recorded (Swash 1982; Vodusek et al. 1983).

References

Andrews J, Nathan P (1964) Lesions of the anterior frontal lobes and disturbances of micturition and defaecation. Brain 87:233–262

Brodal A (1981) Neurological anatomy in relation to clinical medicine, 3rd edn. Oxford University Press, p 779

Burnstock G (1990) Innervation of bladder and bowel. In: Bock G, Whelan J (eds) Neurobiology of incontinence. CIBA Foundation symposium 151. Wiley, Chichester, pp 2–43

Carlstedt A, Nordgren S, Fasth S, Appelgren L, Hulten L (1988) Sympathetic influence on the internal anal sphincter and rectum in man. Int J Colorectal Dis 3:90–95

Chokroverty S, Sachdeo R, Dilullo J, Duvoisin RC (1989) Magnetic stimulation in the diagnosis of lumbosacral radiculopathy. J Neurol Neurosurg Psychiatry 52:767–772

Crowe R, Burnstock G (1989) A histochemical and immunohistochemical study of the autonomic innervation of the lower urinary tract of the female pig. Is the pig a good model for the human bladder and urethra? J Urol 141:414–422

Crowe R, Burnstock G, Light JK (1989) Adrenergic innervation of the striated muscle of the intrinsic external urethral sphincter from patients with lower motor spinal cord lesion. J Urol 141:47–49

De Groat WC (1990) Central neural control of the lower urinary tract. In: Bock G, Whelan J (eds) Neurobiology of incontinence. CIBA Foundation symposium 151. Wiley, Chichester, pp 27–56

De Groat WC, Kawatani M (1985) Neural control of the urinary bladder: possible relationship between peptidergic inhibitory mechanisms and detrusor instability. Neurourol Urodyn 4:285–300

Drife JO, Hilton P, Stanton SL (eds) (1990) Micturition. Springer-Verlag, London

Duthie HL, Gairns FW (1960) Sensory nerve endings and sensation in the anal region of man. Br J Surg 47:585–590

Fowler CJ, Kirby RS, Harrison WJG, Milroy ELJ, Turner-Warwick R (1984) Individual motor unit analysis in the diagnosis of disorders of urethral sphincter innervation. J Neurol Neurosurg Psychiatry 47:637–641

Frenckner B, Ihre T (1976) Influence of autonomic nerves on the internal anal sphincter of man. Gut 17:306–312

Fukuda H, Fukai K (1986) Location of the reflex centre for straining elicited by activation of pelvic afferent fibres of decerebrate dogs. Brain Res 380:287–296

Furness JB, Costa M (1987) The enteric nervous system. Churchill Livingstone, Edinburgh

Gershon MD (1990) The enteric nervous system: neurotransmitters and neuromodulators. Curr Opin Neurol Neurosurg 3:517–522

Glick ME, Meshkinpour H, Haldeman S, Bhatia NN, Bradley WE (1982) Colonic dysfunction in multiple sclerosis. Gastroenterology 83:1002–1007

Gould RP (1960) Sensory innervation of the anal canal. Nature 187:337–338

Henry MM, Swash M (1991) Coloproctology and the pelvic floor, 2nd edn. Butterworth-Heinemann, London

Ito Y, Kimoto Y (1985) The neural and non-neural mechanisms involved in urethral activity in rabbits. J Physiol (Lond) 367:57–72

Kiff ES, Swash M (1984) Slowed motor conduction in the pudendal nerves in idiopathic (neurogenic) anorectal incontinence. Br J Surg 71:614–616

Kuzuhara S, Kanazawa I, Nakanishi T (1980) Topographical localization of the Onuf's nuclear neurons innervating the rectal and vesical striated sphincter muscles: a retrograde fluorescent double labelling study in cat and dog. Neurosci Lett 16:125

Langley JN, Anderson HK (1895) The innervation of the pelvic and adjoining viscera. IV: the internal generative organs. J Physiol (Lond) 19:122–130

Lubowski DZ, Nicholls RJ, Swash M, Jordan MJ (1987) Neural control of internal anal sphincter function. Br J Surg 74:668–670

Mannen T, Iwata AR, Toyokura Y, et al. (1977) Preservation of a certain motoneuron group of the sacral cord in amyotrophic lateral sclerosis: its clinical significance. J Neurol Neurosurg Psychiatry 40:464–469

Mathers SE, Swash M (1990) The neurology of sphincter control mechanisms. In: Kennard C (ed) Recent advances in clinical neurology 6. Churchill Livingstone, Edinburgh, pp 157–186

Mathers SE, Ingram DA, Swash M (1990) Electrophysiology of motor pathways for sphincter control in multiple sclerosis. J Neurol Neurosurg Psychiatry 53:955–960

Merton PA, Morton HB, Hill DK, et al. (1982) Scope for a technique for electrical stimulation of human brain, spinal cord and muscle. Lancet 2:597–600

Meunier P, Mollard P (1977) Control of the internal anal sphincter (manometric study with human subjects). Pflugers Archivs 370:233–239

Miller H, Simpson CA, Yeates WK (1965) Bladder dysfunction in multiple sclerosis. Br Med J i:1265

Moss HE, Burnstock G (1985) A comparative study of electrical field stimulation of the guinea pig, ferret and marmoset bladder. Eur J Pharmacol 114:311–316

Nakagawa S (1980) Onuf's nucleus of the sacral cord in the South American monkey (Saimiri); its location and bilateral cortical input from area 4. Brain Res 191:337–344

Nathan PW, Smith MC (1953) Spinal pathways subserving defaecation. J Neurol Neurosurg Psychiatry 16:245–256

Neill ME, Swash M (1980) Increased motor unit fibre density in the external anal sphincter muscle in anorectal incontinence: a single fibre EMG study. J Neurol Neurosurg Psychiatry 43:343–347

Onuf (Onufrowicz) B (1900) On the arrangement and function of the cell groups of the sacral region of the spinal cord in man. Arch Neurol Psychopathol 3:387–412

Percy JP, Neill ME, Swash M, Parks AG (1981) Electrophysiological study of motor nerve supply of pelvic floor. Lancet 1:16–17

Roe AM, Bartolo DCC, Mortensen NJM (1986) A new method for assessment of anal sensation in various anorectal disorders. Br J Surg 73:310–312

Rogers J, Henry MM, Misiewicz JJ (1988) Combined sensory and motor deficit in primary neuropathic faecal incontinence. Gut 29:5–9

Roppolo JR, Nadelhaft I, De Groat WC (1985) The organization of pudendal motoneurons and primary afferent projections in the spinal cord of the rhesus monkey revealed by horseradish peroxidase. J Comp Neurol 234:475–488

Shepherd JJ, Wright PG (1968) The response of the internal anal sphincter in man to stimulation of the presacral nerve. Am J Digestive Dis 13:421–427

Snooks SJ, Swash M (1984) Perineal nerve and transcutaneous spinal stimulation: new methods for investigation of the urethral striated sphincter musculature. Br J Urol 56:407–411

Snooks SJ, Swash M (1986) The innervation of the muscles of continence. Ann R Coll Surg Engl 68:406–409

Speakman MJ, Walmsley D, Brading AF (1989) An in vitro pharmacological study of the human trigone – a site of non-adrenergic, non-cholinergic neurotransmission. Br J Urol 61:304–309

Stelzner F (1960) Uber die Anatomie des analen Sphincterorgans wie sie der Chirurg sieht. Z Anat Entwicklung 121:525–535

Sung JH, Mastri AR, Segal E (1979) Pathology of the Shy-Drager syndrome. J Neuropathol Exp Neurol 38:353–367

Swash M (1982) Early and late components in the human anal reflex. J Neurol Neurosurg Psychiatry 45:767–769

Swash M (1990) The neurogenic hypothesis of stress incontinence. In: Bock G, Whelan J (eds) Neurobiology of incontinence. CIBA Foundation symposium 151. Wiley, Chichester, pp 156–169

Swash M, Mathers S (1989) Sphincter disorders and the nervous system. In: Aminoff M (ed) Neurology and general medicine. Churchill Livingstone, New York, pp 449–470

Swash M, Snooks SJ (1986) Slowed motor conduction in lumbo-sacral nerve roots in cauda equina lesions; a new diagnostic technique. J Neurol Neurosurg Psychiatry 46:808–816

Swash M, Gray A, Lubowski DZ, Nicholls RJ (1986) Ultrastructural changes in internal anal sphincter in neurogenic faecal incontinence. Gut 29:1692–1698

Swash M, Snooks SJ, Chalmers DHK (1987) Parity as a factor in incontinence in multiple sclerosis. Arch Neurol 44:504–508

Thuneberg L (1982) Interstitial cells of Cajal: intestinal pacemaker? Adv Anat Embryol Cell Biol 71:1–130

Vodusek DB, Janko M, Lokar J (1983) Direct and reflex responses in perineal muscles on electrical stimulation. J Neurol Neurosurg Psychiatry 46:67–71

Chapter 18

Spinal Vascular Disease

M.J. Aminoff

Vascular disorders of the spinal cord are a rare but important cause of disability. They merit consideration particularly because disability can often be prevented by a rational approach to the treatment of certain of these disorders.

Vascular Anatomy

Three sorts of artery enter the spinal canal with the anterior and posterior nerve roots. The radicular arteries supply just the nerve roots, whereas the radiculopial arteries also feed the pial-leptomeningeal arterial plexus. Only the radiculomedullary arteries contribute to the blood supply of the spinal cord, and these are present only at certain segmental levels.

The spinal cord is supplied by the anterior and posterior spinal arteries. The posterior spinal arteries are paired vessels that arise intracranially from the vertebral arteries. They interconnect with an anastomotic arterial plexus and, as they descend the length of the spinal cord, are fed at different levels by a variable number of posterior radiculomedullary vessels.

The anterior spinal artery, which also arises from the intracranial vertebral arteries, is a single vessel that descends the length of the spinal cord overlying the anterior longitudinal fissure. It is supplied by a variable number of vessels, usually between four and seven, as it descends. For descriptive purposes, the supply to the anterior spinal artery is best considered in three longitudinal territories. In the cervical and upper thoracic region, the anterior spinal artery receives contributions from usually three or more segmental vessels, including one vessel arising from the costocervical trunk. In the midthoracic region (between T4 and T8) the anterior spinal artery is often fed by only a single vessel, and it has its smallest diameter in this region, sometimes being discontinuous. In the region below T8, the anterior spinal artery receives its blood supply mainly from a single large vessel, the artery of Adamkiewicz, which commonly arises from a segmental vessel between about T9 and L2 on the left side.

Branches of the anterior and posterior spinal arteries form a fine plexus around the cord from which radially-oriented branches are given off. Blood flow through these vessels supplies much of the white matter and the posterior horns of grey matter. The largest branches of the anterior spinal artery are the central or sulcocommissural arteries, which arise (in varying number) at each segmental level in the anterior longitudinal fissure and turn to one or other side of the cord. The central arteries are larger and more numerous in the cervical and lumbar cord than in the thoracic. Blood passes through them to supply the grey matter (except the posterior horns) and the innermost portion of the white matter.

An anterior median group of intrinsic veins drains the capillaries of the grey and white commissures, the medial cell columns of the anterior horns, and the anterior funiculi, emptying through the central veins into the anterior median spinal vein which runs in the anterior longitudinal fissure. The rest of the cord drains through radial veins to the coronal plexus of venous channels that runs longitudinally over the posterior and lateral surfaces of the cord. The superficial veins around the cord drain by the medullary veins which accompany the nerve roots to the intervertebral foramina, where radicular veins draining the nerve roots and communications from the anterior and posterior epidural and paravertebral plexuses also converge.

Ischaemic Myelopathies

An ischaemic myelopathy may occur when space-occupying lesions cause vascular compression, may contribute to post-traumatic cord dysfunction, and may occur as a sequel to irradiation. Thus, neoplastic or granulomatous epidural or extravertebral lesions may cause a rapidly progressive paraparesis by obstruction of an entering artery. In some instances there may be an apparent discrepancy between the level of the lesion and the clinical deficit. For example, a sensory disturbance may extend for several segments above the level of a cord lesion, because the territory supplied by a radicular vessel contributing to the cord circulation extends beyond the vessel's level of origin. Again, wasting of the intrinsic muscles of the hand in patients with a foramen magnum lesion may occur if the anterior spinal artery is compressed (Symonds and Meadows 1937; Henson and Parsons 1967).

Pathology may involve the aorta and those of its branches (i.e., the intercostal, lumbar or vertebral arteries) supplying the spinal circulation. Pathological involvement of the spinal arteries and their branches may also occur. When this leads to cord infarction, treatment is symptomatic. Care of the skin, bladder and bowels is important, as is active rehabilitation of the patient.

Disorders of Vessels Supplying the Spinal Circulation

Paraplegia may follow occlusion of the abdominal aorta when the blood supply to the artery of Adamkiewicz is interrupted, and sometimes occurs despite a seemingly normal peripheral circulation (Cook 1959). An ischaemic myelopathy may similarly occur with dissecting or non-dissecting aortic aneurysms (Goodin

1989), inflammatory aortitis (Goodin 1989), and infective and non-infective emboli involving the aorta (Dickson et al. 1984; Syrjanen et al. 1986), and after aortic surgery (Ross 1985; Shaw 1986; Skillman 1986). The most critical aortic region encompasses the site of origin of the artery of Adamkiewicz, and thus is between the eighth thoracic and second lumbar segments. Abdominal aortography may also cause an acute ischaemic myelopathy (Killen and Foster 1960), the occurrence of which probably depends on such factors as the concentration of and duration of exposure to the contrast agent, the injection pressure, and injury to the artery of Adamkiewicz. Cervical myelopathy may result from imaging studies such as mediastinal angiography (DiChiro and Wener 1973), aortography (Brust et al. 1959), and injection of contrast material into the thyrocervical trunk during cerebral angiography, as well as from vertebral artery thrombosis (Boudin et al. 1966).

Adult-type coarctation of the aorta may cause ischaemia and hypotension of segments of the cord supplied from the aorta below the narrowed segment, leading to weakness and sensory disturbances in the legs, and a sphincter disturbance. Neurogenic intermittent claudication (Chapter 11) may also occur, due to diversion of blood away from the cord by retrograde flow in the anterior spinal artery to bypass the narrowed aortic segment (Kendall and Andrew 1972). In classical coarctation, a collateral circulation involving the anterior spinal artery may be visualized radiologically or at autopsy, lying usually between the C6 and T4 segments. Flow is from enlarged vertebral, thyrocervical and costocervical spinal arteries, via a distended anterior spinal artery, to dilated radicular branches of the intercostal vessels below the coarctation, thereby bypassing the stenosed aortic segment. A cervicothoracic myelopathy may result, relating either to cord compression by the enlarged collateral vessels or to a steal phenomenon (Herron et al. 1958; Weenink and Smilde 1964). Aneurysmal distension of the anterior spinal artery or a segmental feeder may occur, and subsequent rupture will then lead to subarachnoid haemorrhage (Wyburn-Mason 1943; Blackwood 1958). Treatment is of the underlying coarctation.

Marked hypotension, regardless of aetiology, may cause an ischaemic myelopathy. Some authors have reported an especial vulnerability of the watershed regions between the three longitudinal territories of the anterior spinal artery, or of the midthoracic region, where the anterior spinal artery is usually supplied by only a single, small feeder. The regional extent of such vulnerable areas is unclear, and whether they are truly at increased risk of ischaemic damage is uncertain (Goodin 1989). In any given segment of the cord, a reduction in blood flow sometimes involves predominantly the central area between the territories of the anterior and posterior spinal arteries, with particular involvement of grey matter (Zulch 1962; Kepes 1965; Garland et al. 1966).

Acute ischaemic total transverse myelopathy is characterized by the rapid development of a flaccid areflexic paraplegia or quadriplegia, with analgesia and anaesthesia below the lesion, and urinary and faecal retention. Severe back pain may occur initially at the level of the lesion. The CSF is usually normal, but in the acute phase sometimes exhibits a mild pleocytosis and increased protein concentration. With occlusion of the named spinal arteries, certain distinctive clinical features may be found.

Disease of the Spinal Arteries

Occlusion of the spinal arteries or their intramedullary branches may result from thrombus, atherosclerosis (Gruner and Lapresle 1962), or an inflammatory process such as syphilis (Williamson 1894; Spiller 1909), polyarteritis nodosa (Roger et al. 1955), systemic lupus erythematosus (Andrianakos et al. 1975), Sjögren's syndrome (Alexander et al. 1981), rheumatoid arthritis (Watson et al. 1977), and sarcoidosis (Matthews 1965). Cardiogenic emboli are rare causes of spinal artery occlusion (Madow and Alpers 1949; Wolman and Bradshaw 1967), as also are embolic fragments of nucleus pulposus (see p. 285). Rapid decompression of divers may lead to nitrogen embolism (the "bends"), and a similar disorder may follow rapid exposure to high altitude, with haemorrhagic or ischaemic necrosis of the cord, especially in the thoracic region, and resulting paraplegia. A transverse myelitis or Brown-Séquard syndrome has been reported as a sequel to injection of heroin or quinine adulterant, and may relate to a vasculitis, hypersensitivity reaction, hypotension or embolization (Richter and Rosenberg 1968; Krause 1983).

The territory supplied by the anterior spinal artery is more vulnerable to ischaemia than that supplied by the posterior spinal circulation. This is because there are fewer vessels feeding the anterior than the posterior spinal arteries, and because the anterior spinal artery is a single – sometimes discontinuous – vessel whereas the posterior spinal arteries are in reality an anastomotic network.

Anterior Spinal Artery Occlusion. This results in infarction of the anterior two-thirds of the cord. Many cases attributed to occlusion of the anterior spinal artery are probably due to occlusion of a major radicular feeder or the vessel from which such a feeder originates (Garland et al. 1966). Sudden back pain, sometimes having a girdle or radicular distribution, may occur at the onset, and a flaccid paraplegia or quadriplegia then develops over several minutes or hours, depending on the involved level of the cord, accompanied by retention of urine. Pyramidal signs ultimately develop below the level of the lesion as "spinal shock" wears off, while wasting occurs of muscles supplied from the infarcted region. Typically, pain and temperature appreciation are impaired, with relative sparing of light touch and proprioceptive sensation. A Brown-Séquard syndrome may result from occlusion of a central or sulcocommissural artery, which supplies only one side of the cord, or from occlusion of one anterior spinal artery when this vessel is duplicated (Wells 1966). Swelling of the cord may be visualized by imaging studies. There is a poor prognosis for recovery except when definite improvement occurs within the first 48 hours.

The Posterior Spinal Artery Syndrome. This is characterized clinically by impaired vibration and joint position sense below the level of the lesion due to ipsilateral posterior column involvement, with segmental anaesthesia and areflexia. A pyramidal deficit may also be present if the lateral funiculus is affected, but is usually transient and mild compared to the sensory disturbance. Because of the many feeders to these vessels, infarction in the territory of the posterior spinal arteries is rare, but described (Gruner and Lapresle 1962; Garland et al. 1966; Hughes 1970).

Ischaemia Affecting Predominantly the Anterior Horns. This causes a lower motor neurone deficit, sometimes combined with minor pyramidal signs but with sensory sparing. This presentation may simulate progressive spinal muscular atrophy or amyotrophic lateral sclerosis but sphincter dysfunction is an occasional accompaniment, and autopsy reveals haemorrhagic necrosis in the anterior horns (Gruner and Lapresle 1962; Jellinger and Neumayer 1962). The clinical disorder usually has an insidious onset and a gradually progressive course, but occasionally it begins abruptly (Jellinger and Neumayer 1962; Herrick and Mills 1971). Cases have been ascribed to spinal arteriosclerosis (Skinhoj 1954; Gruner and Lapresle 1962), and to aortic disease or surgery (Beattie el al. 1953; Kepes 1965; Herrick and Mills 1971). The selective grey matter involvement probably results from its increased vulnerability to hypoxia (Gelfan and Tarlov 1955) or to its location in the watershed area between the anterior and posterior spinal circulations.

Venous Infarction of the Cord

Venous infarction of the cord is rare except in the context of an associated arteriovenous malformation (AVM). When it does occur, spinal venous stasis and thrombosis are usually associated with malignant disease, sepsis, vertebral disorders, or a generalized thrombotic syndrome. Sudden pain in the back is followed within a few hours or so by weakness and sensory loss that develop in the legs, accompanied by urinary and faecal retention. Progression commonly occurs over the next few days, leading to a clinical picture of cord transection, and often ultimately to a fatal outcome from pulmonary embolism or the underlying disease associated with the infarction. The CSF is often normal, but a pleocytosis and increased protein concentration are not uncommon. Imaging studies may reveal a swollen cord. Postmortem examination reveals distended, thrombosed spinal veins, and there may be haemorrhagic necrosis of the cord itself, especially centrally.

Intervertebral Disc Embolism

A number of cases of nucleus pulposus embolism of the spinal cord have been recognized. There is a preponderance of women among the reported cases, and ages have ranged between 15 and 77 years (Bots et al. 1981). Presentation is typically with acute pain in the back or neck, followed after a few minutes by rapidly progressive limb weakness and sensory impairment, usually to all modalities. The neurological deficit is fully established within a few hours. The cervical cord is the region affected most often, but involvement may initially be in the lumbosacral area (Jurcovic and Eiben 1970). Death eventually follows, usually due to infective complications. The correct diagnosis is generally not made until autopsy, when emboli histochemically identical to the fibrocartilage of the nucleus pulposus are found in the spinal arteries or veins, and sometimes in the vertebral marrow interstitial spaces and sinusoids (Srigley et al. 1981). The manner in which such material enters the vascular system is not known. It may be that fragments of nucleus pulposus enter the arterial circulation through a tear in an adjacent radicular artery after lateral rupture of degen-

erated disc material, that an increase in disc pressure is responsible for inject-
ing disc material into small blood vessels (which are said to be present in
degenerate but unruptured annulus fibrosus), or that anomalous vascularity next
to or within the vertebral disc is responsible (Naiman et al. 1961; Hayes et al.
1978). Material may also be extruded directly into an overlying venous sinus.

Neurogenic Intermittent Claudication

Neurogenic intermittent claudication has been used to designate symptoms that
develop after a predictable amount of exercise and disappear with rest, and
that result from disorders of the spinal cord and cauda equina.

Intermittent Claudication of the Cauda Equina

Pain, numbness and paraesthesias that develop with exercise and are relieved
by rest characterize this syndrome, which is more common in men than women.
Symptoms may begin in the feet and spread up to involve the buttocks, or
conversely begin proximally and spread down the legs. Similar symptoms
typically occur with the adoption of certain postures. Clinical examination is
usually normal unless performed while the patient is symptomatic, when there
may be motor and sensory abnormalities. Imaging studies are diagnostic in
showing compression of the cauda equina (Blau and Logue 1961; Wilson 1969),
as by a central disc protrusion. Treatment is surgical.

Sagittal narrowing of the lumbar spinal canal, with compression of nerve
roots at one or more levels, predisposes to the disorder. Reported associations
include developmental or spondylotic narrowing of the vertebral canal, spina
bifida, disc protrusion, and achondroplasia. In patients with a mildly narrowed
lumbar canal, any additional encroachment, such as by a small disc protrusion,
may result in the development of symptoms. Actions or postures that involve
extension of the lumbar spine usually precipitate symptoms, which are relieved
when the patient leans forward or squats. Hyperextension of the lumbar spine
displaces the cauda equina roots posteriorly and causes the roots to thicken
because their course is shortened, and this results in increased compression and
hence the production of symptoms. Only occasionally are symptoms precipitated by exercise of the extremities, presumably because of relative ischaemia
of active cauda equina roots during exercise (Blau and Logue 1961; Evans
1964). Experimental studies in the mouse by Blau and Rushworth (1958)
showed that after exercise of the hind limb, vessels of the regional spinal nerve
roots dilate widely. When symptoms of cauda equina claudication are precipitated specifically by exercise, it is probable that they relate not only to
compression of nerve roots but also to a limitation of the extent to which the
blood supply can increase with activity because of impaired blood flow through
radicular arteries at points of constriction (Blau and Logue 1961).

Clinical evaluation must distinguish between a neurogenic basis for intermittent claudication and peripheral vascular disease. In peripheral vascular
disease, intermittent claudication is characterized by pain in exercised muscles,

without spread such as typically occurs in neurogenic intermittent claudication. Other sensory disturbances are rare and, apart from some tightening of ischaemic muscles with activity, there is no motor deficit. Examination generally reveals cutaneous evidence of peripheral vascular disease, diminished or absent peripheral pulses, and a proximal arterial bruit; arteriography is diagnostic.

Intermittent Claudication of the Spinal Cord

This rare disorder may occur in patients with syphilitic arteritis, atherosclerosis (Henson and Parsons 1967), terminal aortic thrombosis (Ratinov and Jimenez-Pabon 1961), and pronounced lumbar spondylosis or lower thoracic disc protrusion (Bergmark 1950; Garcin et al. 1959), but the most common cause nowadays is probably a spinal AVM (Wyburn-Mason 1943; Aminoff 1976). When it occurs in coarctation of the aorta, the reduced blood supply to the cord below the narrowed aortic segment (Tyler and Clark 1958) or aortic steal from the anterior spinal artery (Kendall and Andrew 1972) may be responsible.

Initial symptoms may consist of a heaviness in one or both legs that comes on with activity and is relieved by rest, or of sensory symptoms, pain or sphincter disturbances that show a similar relationship to activity (Garcin et al. 1962; Aminoff 1976). Examination at rest is generally normal or reveals only minor abnormalities. After exercise, however, there is weakness of one or both legs, with hyperreflexia and extensor plantar responses; there may also be a sensory deficit, sometimes severe enough to cause gait ataxia. The syndrome is occasionally the prelude to infarction (Garcin et al. 1959; Garcin et al. 1962; Henson and Parsons 1967), but frequently there is no change or only gradual progression over a long period of time, with reduction in exercise tolerance until a lasting deficit is present.

The regional blood flow in the cord (and appropriate nerve roots) increases with leg exercise (Blau and Rushworth 1958), presumably to meet increased metabolic requirements. In patients with intermittent claudication of the cord, it seems likely that the underlying lesion prevents the increased circulatory requirements of activity from being met.

Haemorrhage

Haematomyelia and Spinal Subarachnoid Haemorrhage

Haematomyelia or spontaneous spinal subarachnoid haemorrhage occurs most commonly from AVMs (Wyburn-Mason 1943; Aminoff 1976), which are discussed on p. 291. It may also occur from other types of spinal hamartoma, such as telangiectases, and following trauma (Fig. 18.1). Subarachnoid haemorrhage may be associated with intradural spinal neoplasms located particularly about the conus or cauda equina, such as ependymomas, neurofibromas, meningiomas, and meningeal sarcomas. It may occur with coarctation of the aorta (Wyburn-Mason 1943; Blackwood 1958); with rupture of mycotic or other

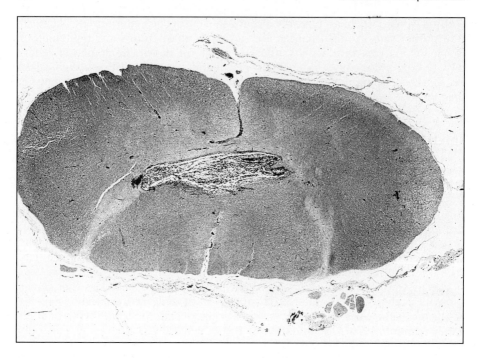

Fig. 18.1. Low power photomicrograph showing a traumatic haematomyelia of recent onset. (Courtesy of R.L. Davis, MD, Pathology Department, UCSF.)

spinal aneurysms; in certain connective tissue diseases, such as polyarteritis nodosa (Henson and Croft 1956), systemic lupus erythematosus (Fody et al. 1980) and Sjögren's syndrome (Alexander et al. 1982); in association with blood dyscrasias or anticoagulant drug therapy; in such toxic-infectious conditions as typhoid fever; and in relation to lumbar puncture (King and Glas 1960). In some cases, no specific cause can be recognized.

The onset of spinal subarachnoid haemorrhage is typically with sudden severe back pain overlying the site of bleeding, spreading rapidly to the rest of the back. Radicular pain, particularly bilateral sciatica, may occur as blood passes into the lumbar sac. With small and purely intramedullary haemorrhages, however, pain may not be conspicuous. When subarachnoid haemorrhage arises in the cervical region, distinction from intracranial haemorrhage may be impossible clinically. Symptoms of cerebral dysfunction may ultimately develop, and include vomiting, photophobia, a disturbance of consciousness, and seizures. Such symptoms tend to be milder and more short-lived than symptoms of cord dysfunction, which result from haematomyelia or compression of the cord or nerve roots by blood or blood clot. The cord dysfunction may lead to flaccid limb weakness, sensory disturbances, and impaired sphincter function.

Signs of meningeal irritation are usually conspicuous. Cranial nerve palsies, nystagmus, and a depressed level of consciousness reflect cerebral involvement, while motor, sensory or reflex abnormalities in the limbs usually relate to spinal cord or root disturbances. The presence of a cutaneous angioma or

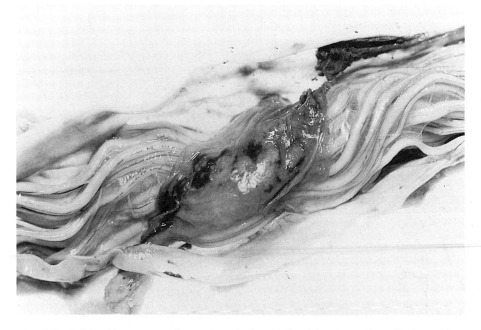

Fig. 18.2. Subdural haematoma of several weeks duration involving the cauda equina in a patient with systemic lupus erythematosus, who had undergone several lumbar punctures. (Courtesy of R.L. Davis, MD, Pathology Department, UCSF.)

spinal bruit suggests an underlying spinal vascular malformation, and careful inspection and auscultation of the spine is therefore important in patients with subarachnoid haemorrhage of uncertain cause.

The diagnosis of subarachnoid haemorrhage is confirmed by the presence of blood in the CSF or by the findings on CT scanning. Recognition of a spinal vascular malformation or neoplasm will generally depend upon the findings at myelography or with other imaging techniques such as MRI and CT scanning.

Prognosis depends on the severity of the haemorrhage and on its cause. Surgical treatment may be necessary if the spinal lesion is neoplastic, or there are signs of cord compression by blood or blood clot. If the myelogram suggests a spinal vascular malformation, angiographic delineation and operative treatment may be necessary, as discussed on p. 295. Collagenoses, blood dyscrasias, and anticoagulant-induced haemorrhage require appropriate medical management.

Spinal Subdural Haematoma

Spinal subdural haematomas are rare. They may occur spontaneously or after lumbar puncture (Fig. 18.2) in patients with blood dyscrasias that predispose to bleeding, such as haemophilia or thrombocytopenia, or in patients taking anticoagulant drugs. They may also occur spontaneously or after trauma of varying severity in patients without a bleeding diathesis, and are said to be an important cause of perinatal paraplegia (Towbin 1969).

Symptoms characteristically begin with sudden severe back pain, often accompanied by root pain. The clinical features of a spinal cord or cauda equina syndrome, due to compression by the haematoma, may then develop. When haemorrhage follows lumbar puncture, the clinical deficit usually develops within about 24 hours.

Myelography reveals a filling defect or a block at the site of the haematoma, or fixed displacement of the contrast material to one side. CT scan or MRI may also be helpful in visualizing the lesion and in suggesting its nature, but experience with it in this context is limited. Complete recovery may follow early evacuation of the haematoma, whereas any delay in surgical intervention often leads to an irreversible neurological deficit. Patients with blood dyscrasias require appropriate therapy; if anticoagulant drugs are being taken, they should be discontinued and their effect reversed.

In order to reduce the chances of haemorrhage, lumbar puncture must be undertaken with particular care in patients with a haematological disorder that predisposes to bleeding, being performed by a skilled physician and only when really necessary, using a small needle; consideration must also be given to correcting the haematological disorder by transfusion if feasible. In thrombocytopenic patients, spinal haematoma may be more likely to complicate lumbar puncture as the platelet count declines, and in patients with a rapidly dropping platelet count (Edelson et al. 1974); platelet transfusion just before lumbar puncture should be considered if the platelet count is below $20\,000/\text{mm}^3$ or dropping rapidly.

Spinal Epidural Haematoma

Spinal epidural heamatoma may occur at any age, but in children the haematoma is most often in the lower cervical region, whereas in adults the lower thoracic or thoracolumbar region is also a common site for haematomas.

Epidural haemorrhage may relate to trauma, particularly in neonates (Towbin 1969). In adults it may follow minor injuries without accompanying vertebral fracture or dislocation, symptoms of a progressive cord lesion commencing within a few hours or days of the trauma. It may also occur in patients with epidural vascular malformations (Cube 1962; Dawson 1963) or tumours, and in patients with blood dyscrasias or an iatrogenic predisposition to bleeding. Spinal epidural haemorrhage may occur spontaneously (Markham et al. 1967; Posnikoff 1968), occasionally in relation to pregnancy (Bidzinski 1966), and after lumbar puncture or epidural anaesthesia (Gingrich 1968), especially in anticoagulated patients (De Angelis 1972).

Clinical presentation is usually with a sudden, severe, constant back pain that may begin in relation to minor straining, overlies the site of haemorrhage, and is enhanced by percussion over the back, movements of the spine, or manoeuvres that increase the pressure in the vertebral venous plexus. Girdle pain, or radicular or diffuse pain in the extremities may also be present. After an interval of several hours (but, rarely, up to a few weeks), a cord or cauda equina syndrome develops. It may be impossible to distinguish epidural from subdural haematoma save by imaging studies or at operation.

Imaging studies demonstrate the site and nature of the lesion. MRI is particularly helpful for detecting a haematoma and defining its relationship to the cord and thecal sac, as well as for distinguishing it from other epidural lesions. Treatment is by urgent evacuation of the haematoma at laminectomy. Rebello and Dastur (1966) reported that 29 of 59 patients coming to operation recovered satisfactorily, 16 made a partial recovery and 14 failed to benefit, whereas only 1 of 11 treated conservatively recovered completely. Most of those who recovered were operated on within 72 hours of the onset of symptoms, emphasizing the importance of early diagnosis and prompt surgical treatment. The prognosis for functional recovery is generally worse in patients with a severe or rapidly progressive deficit. In patients on anticoagulant therapy, treatment should be stopped and vitamin K or fresh frozen plasma provided.

Spinal Aneurysms

Isolated arterial aneurysms of the spinal vasculature are rare. They usually lead to subarachnoid haemorrhage or a focal cord lesion (Henson and Croft 1956; Leech et al. 1976), but are rarely the cause of patients presenting in such a way. Marked aneurysmal distension of spinal arteries may occur in coarctation of the aorta (Wyburn-Mason 1943; Blackwood 1958), and in association with spinal AVMs (Herdt et al. 1971; Vogelsang and Dietz 1975; Caroscio et al. 1980). In the latter circumstance the aneurysm may be a more frequent source of haemorrhage than the AVM. Thus, in one series of 50 cases of spinal AVM, all patients with a history of spinal subarachnoid haemorrhage had a coexistent aneurysm intimately associated with their AVM (Herdt et al. 1971).

Dural and Intradural Spinal AVMs

AVMs, which are the most common kind of hamartoma related to the spinal cord, consist of an abnormal nidus of vessels between the arterial and venous systems, without intervening capillaries. In rare instances there may be a true fistula rather than a nidus of abnormal vessels between the main artery and vein involved in the malformation (Gueguen et al. 1987; Aminoff et al. 1988). Telangiectasias and cavernous angiomas uncommonly involve the spinal cord and are usually asymptomatic, although they occasionally bleed or lead to a focal neurological deficit.

Spinal AVMs may be associated with other vascular anomalies, including cutaneous, vertebral, paraspinal and epidural angiomas, cerebral or cerebellar angiomas, Osler-Weber-Rendu syndrome, and lymphatic anomalies (Aminoff 1976). The association with spinal aneurysms has already been discussed.

Most spinal AVMs are located below the T3 cord segment. These are usually wholly or partially extramedullary, lie behind the cord, and are fed by one or more arteries that either do not supply the cord at all or only supply the posterior spinal circulation. In many instances the site of the arteriovenous shunt is actually on the dura rather than intradural (Oldfield et al. 1983; Symon et al. 1984), but it is not possible to distinguish between these lesions either clinically or myelographically, and they will therefore be considered together. There is a marked male preponderance among reported cases, and patients may present at any age.

The 20% of AVMs located in the cervical or upper thoracic segments have an approximately equal sex incidence, and are usually diagnosed earlier than more caudal lesions because they are more likely to bleed. Most of these lesions are wholly or partially intramedullary, are anteriorly situated, and are supplied by vessels contributing also to the anterior spinal circulation. Multiple feeders are common, and the arteriovenous shunt is usually of large volume.

Clinical Features

Spinal AVMs may present with subarachnoid haemorrhage or with a myelo-radiculopathy. The most common cause of non-traumatic spinal subarachnoid haemorrhage is an AVM. About 10% of all spinal AVMs and over 40% of cervical AVMs will cause subarachnoid haemorrhage, at least once (Aminoff 1976). The features of such haemorrhage were described on p. 288. The overall mortality of the initial bleed is at least 15%, and approximately half of the survivors will have a second haemorrhage. Half of the subsequent survivors have further haemorrhages unless the underlying lesion is treated. The second bleed occurs within one year of the first in about 40% of cases with recurrent haemorrhage.

The myeloradiculopathy resulting from spinal AVMs may have an insidious onset and progression or, less commonly, follows a relapsing and remitting course, sometimes with long intervals between relapses. Aminoff and Logue (1974a) reported initial symptoms to consist of pain in 25 of 60 patients (42%), other sensory symptoms in 20 (33%), leg weakness in 19 (32%), disturbed sphincter or sexual function in 6 (10%), and subarachnoid haemorrhage in 3 (5%); most (two-thirds) had developed weakness, sensory symptoms, pain and a disturbance of bladder function by the time of diagnosis, and 6 (10%) had experienced a subarachnoid haemorrhage.

In 19 of the 60 patients there were symptoms suggestive of neurogenic claudication of the cord or cauda equina, and in 14 symptoms were precipitated or aggravated by certain postures. Exercise tolerance varied among these patients, but tended to diminish with time. Less common precipitants of symptoms include pregnancy, trauma, increased body temperature, non-specific infective illnesses, straining at stool, the menstrual cycle, and a heavy meal.

Although examination sometimes reveals no abnormalities, even after exercise, most patients with thoracolumbar AVMs have a mixed upper and lower motor neurone deficit in the legs, with an accompanying sensory disturbance, by the time of diagnosis. Occasionally a purely motor deficit is present, simulating motor neurone disease (except for the restricted distribution). With cervical AVMs, abnormal findings may be present in the arms as well as the legs. Although sensory deficits may have an upper level on the trunk, this sometimes correlates poorly with the angiographic level of the lesion. Occasional patients have coexisting cutaneous vascular lesions, which may relate segmentally to the spinal anomaly and which are more easy to recognize while patients perform the Valsalva manoeuvre. The presence of a spinal or paraspinal bruit is helpful in suggesting the underlying diagnosis, but its absence does not exclude an AVM.

The myeloradiculopathy is often rapidly progressive. Thus, within 6 months of the onset of any leg weakness or gait disturbance, 10 of the 60 patients reported by Aminoff and Logue (1974b) required two sticks or crutches to get about, or had become unable to walk at all, and 28 were so disabled within 3 years. Among the remaining patients, the disability was often sufficient to interfere with normal daily activities.

Pathophysiology

The myeloradiculopathy is not due to cord compression as judged by the radiological, operative or autopsy findings. Intravascular thrombosis may contribute to the clinical deficit, but this would not account for the marked fluctuations in symptoms that sometimes occur spontaneously or in relation to exercise, posture, or the other factors mentioned earlier. Moreover, thrombotic vascular occlusion is conspicuously absent in some autopsied cases. A common belief is that cord ischaemia results from diversion or "steal" of blood from the normal spinal circulation by the AVM. However, except in the cervical region, the supply to the AVM is usually distinct from that to the cord and does not even arise from the same segmental stem as a vessel supplying the anterior spinal artery, so that steal cannot normally occur by this route. Steal might occur via connections between the intramedullary circulation and the AVM, but such interconnections are usually inconspicuous at operation; further, if steal occurred by this route, ligation of the AVM's main feeders should enhance it (by reducing the pressure in the AVM) rather than producing clinical benefit.

The most likely explanation for the myeloradiculopathy is that the anomalous arteriovenous shunt increases the pressure in veins draining the cord, and intramedullary venous pressure therefore rises. This, in turn, reduces the intramedullary arteriovenous pressure gradient, diminishes intramedullary blood flow, and thus produces cord ischaemia beyond the territory of any individual spinal artery (Aminoff et al. 1974). This sequence of events would account for the cord syndrome described by Logue (1979) in a patient with an epidural AVM lying in the hollow of the sacrum; a large vein passed intradurally to ascend on the cord's surface, and division of this vessel reversed the patient's symptomatology.

An acute onset or exacerbation of symptoms probably relates to intramedullary haemorrhage or thrombotic occlusion of a major extramedullary vessel, whereas a steady progression of symptoms relates to increasing cord ischaemia resulting from the reduced intramedullary arteriovenous pressure gradient (Fig. 18.3). Transient spontaneous fluctuation of symptoms probably reflects minor variations in cord blood flow (for example, by posture) or requirements (which are increased by activity). Intramedullary malformations may also cause symptoms by displacement of adjacent structures. Radicular symptoms presumably relate to ischaemia of nerve roots or to compression of roots by enlarged vessels.

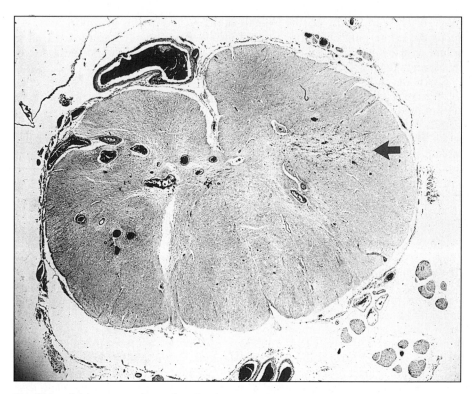

Fig. 18.3. Subacute necrotic myelopathy due to a spinal AVM. Low power photomicrograph shows large abnormal vascular channels in the subarachnoid space and spinal cord parenchyma. An incomplete infarct (arrow) is also seen. Original magnification ×5. (Courtesy of R.L. Davis, MD, Pathology Department, UCSF.)

Radiological Investigations

Plain radiographs of the spine are usually of little help. In most cases, the diagnosis is suggested by myelography, the length of the cord being visualized in both the prone and supine positions. The characteristic myelographic appearance is of localized or extensive vermiform defects due to vascular impressions in the column of contrast material (Fig. 18.4). In the thoracic region they are usually most conspicuous on the posterior aspect of the cord, and may not be seen except on supine films.

When the myelographic appearance suggests the presence of an AVM, selective spinal arteriography is undertaken to confirm its presence and to determine the level and extent of the vascular anomaly, its position in relation to the spinal cord, and the vessels feeding the AVM and the anterior spinal artery in the region of the malformation. Spinal angiography is usually unrewarding when a technically satisfactory myelogram, with both prone and supine views, fails to suggest an AVM.

The angiographic appearances of AVMs depend in considerable part upon their location. Cervical malformations usually lie in front of the cord and may

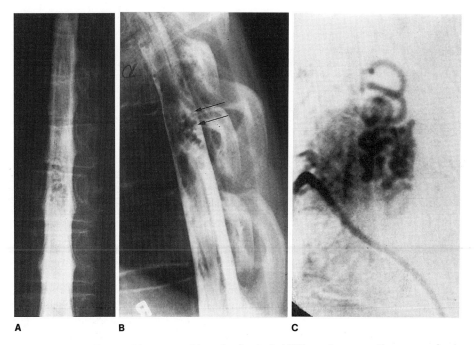

A   **B**   **C**

Fig. 18.4A–C. 65-year-old woman with a dural spinal AVM causing a spastic paraparesis. **A** Myelogram showing serpiginous defects in the column of contrast material in the lower thoracic region, suggestive of an AVM. **B** Myelogram, lateral view, showing serpiginous filling defects (arrows) mainly behind the cord, at about T9 level. **C** Arteriogram following injection of the right T9 intercostal artery, which is supplying an extramedullary spinal AVM. (Courtesy of Grant Hieshima, MD, Radiology Department, UCSF.)

be partly intramedullary. Such malformations are often fed by several different vessels, which may also supply the cord itself. More caudal AVMs usually lie more posteriorly and are supplied by only one or two vessels that generally do not contribute to the cord circulation (Fig. 18.4). Many of these caudal lesions are actually dural in location. The site of the fistula is usually projected lateral to the spinal cord, generally outside the plane of the dura and often encroaching into an intervertebral foramen (Kendall and Logue 1977). Surgical treatment of the latter malformations is thus simple in most instances.

Spinal AVMs can sometimes be visualized with contrast-enhanced CT scans and MRI, but a normal study does not exclude the possibility of an underlying AVM.

Indications for Treatment

Surgical excision of the AVM or the embolic occlusion of its feeding vessels may arrest a rapidly progressive myeloradiculopathy and may also prevent recurrence of bleeding in patients with subarachnoid haemorrhage. Whether patients with mild symptoms and no incapacity should undergo surgery can only be decided on an individual basis, with the general condition of the patient, the available angiographic and surgical facilities, and the risks of surgery in mind. The potential benefits of surgery are greater at this stage, but must be balanced against the operative risks.

An asymptomatic malformation discovered incidentally is best left undisturbed until it becomes clinically evident.

Feasibility of Treatment

Surgical treatment of dural or intradural extramedullary malformations situated posteriorly and fed by vessels not contributing to the cord circulation is usually uncomplicated. Feeders to the malformation can be ligated, and the fistulous portion ("nidus") of the AVM removed if desired. Alternatively, feeding vessels can be occluded by embolization. This is generally a simple and safe technique, although occasionally AVMs become revascularized by the enlargement of small feeders that were not recognized in the original angiographic studies because their contribution to the blood supply of the malformations was so insignificant.

It may not be possible to excise malformations in front of or within the cord and fed by the anterior spinal artery or vessels supplying it. Many such AVMs are cervical. However, accessible feeders can be ligated or embolized, and inaccessible ones sometimes occluded by embolization. Because the anterior spinal artery is fed by several vessels in the cervical region, a multistaged procedure, with occlusion of only one or two feeding vessels at any one time, is often well tolerated. The occasional thoracolumbar malformation supplied directly by the anterior spinal artery or one of its feeders is also difficult to treat. However, advances in radiological techniques have permitted better delineation of such lesions, and in some centres the operative treatment of intramedullary or mixed AVMs supplied by long sulcocommissural arteries is feasible (Riche et al. 1982). Inoperable AVMs supplied by short, sulcocommissural arteries feeding directly into them may sometimes be treated successfully by embolization (Riche et al. 1982).

In rare instances there is a direct arteriovenous fistula involving the anterior spinal artery and a draining vein, without an intervening nidus of abnormal vessels. Depending upon the angiographic appearance, a direct surgical approach is sometimes feasible, while in other instances embolization or treatment with detachable balloons may be possible (Riche et al. 1983; Gueguen et al. 1987; Aminoff et al. 1988).

Surgical Procedure

The optimal surgical approach to the treatment of most intradural AVMs is ligation of feeding vessels within the spinal canal, provided that all the feeding vessels are occluded. The procedure is best combined with excision of the fistulous portion of the malformation in case small feeding vessels are unrecognized at angiography or operation and are left intact. If the AVM is actually dural in location, the draining vessels on the surface of the cord can be left undisturbed, thereby reducing the risk of neurological complications.

References

Alexander EL, Craft C, Dorsch C, Moser RL, Provost TT, Alexander GE (1982) Necrotizing arteritis and spinal subarachnoid hemorrhage in Sjögren syndrome. Ann Neurol 11:632–635

Alexander GE, Provost TT, Stevens MB, Alexander EL (1981) Sjögren syndrome: central nervous system manifestations. Neurology 31:1391–1396

Aminoff MJ (1976) Spinal angiomas. Blackwell, Oxford

Aminoff MJ, Logue V (1974a) Clinical features of spinal vascular malformations. Brain 97: 197–210

Aminoff MJ, Logue V (1974b) The prognosis of patients with spinal vascular malformations. Brain 97:211–218

Aminoff MJ, Barnard RO, Logue V (1974) The pathophysiology of spinal vascular malformations. J Neurol Sci 23:255–263

Aminoff MJ, Gutin PH, Norman D (1988) Unusual type of spinal arteriovenous malformation. Neurosurgery 22:589–591

Andrianakos AA, Duffy J, Suzuki M, Sharp JT (1975) Transverse myelopathy in systemic lupus erythematosus. Report of three cases and review of the literature. Ann Intern Med 83:616–624

Beattie EJ, Nolan J, Howe JS (1953) Paralysis following surgical correction of coarctation of the aorta. Case report with autopsy findings. Surgery 33:754–760

Bergmark G (1950) Intermittent spinal claudication. Acta Med Scand Suppl 246:30–36

Bidzinski J (1966) Spontaneous spinal epidural hematoma during pregnancy. Case report. J Neurosurg 24:1017

Blackwood W (1958) Discussion on vascular disease of the spinal cord. Proc R Soc Med 51:543–547

Blau JN, Logue V (1961) Intermittent claudication of the cauda equina. An unusual syndrome resulting from central protrusion of a lumbar intervertebral disc. Lancet 1:1081–1086

Blau JN, Rushworth G (1958) Observations on the blood vessels of the spinal cord and their responses to motor activity. Brain 81:354–363

Bots GTAM, Wattendorff AR, Buruma OJS, Roos RAC, Endtz LJ (1981) Acute myelopathy caused by fibrocartilaginous emboli. Neurology 31:1250–1256

Boudin G, Pepin B, Cassan J-L, Vernant J-C, Gazengel J (1966) Le retentissement médullaire des thromboses ou stenoses de l'artère vertébrale. (A propos de 3 observations). Rev Neurol (Paris) 114:263–270

Brust AA, Howard JM, Bryant MR, Godwin JT (1959) Coarctation of the abdominal aorta with stenosis of the renal arteries and hypertension. Clinical and pathologic study of two cases and review of the literature. Am J Med 27:793–802

Caroscio JT, Brannan T, Budabin M, Huang YP, Yahr MD (1980) Subarachnoid hemorrhage secondary to spinal arteriovenous malformation and aneurysm. Arch Neurol 37:101–103

Cook AW (1959) Occlusion of the abdominal aorta and dysfunction of the spinal cord. A clinical syndrome. Bull NY Acad Med 35:477–489

Cube HM (1962) Spinal extradural hemorrhage. J Neurosurg 19:171–172

Dawson BH (1963) Paraplegia due to spinal epidural haematoma. J Neurol Neurosurg Psychiatry 26:171–173

De Angelis J (1972) Hazards of subdural and epidural anesthesia during anticoagulant therapy: a case report and review. Anesth Analg 51:676–679

DiChiro G, Wener L (1973) Angiography of the spinal cord: a review of contemporary techniques and applications. J Neurosurg 39:1–29

Dickson AP, Lum SK, Whyte AS (1984) Paraplegia following saddle embolism. Br J Surg 71:321

Edelson RN, Chernik NL, Posner JB (1974) Spinal subdural hematomas complicating lumbar puncture. Occurrence in thrombocytopenic patients. Arch Neurol 31:134–137

Evans JG (1964) Neurogenic intermittent claudication. Br Med J ii:985–987

Fody EP, Netsky MG, Mrak RE (1980) Subarachnoid spinal hemorrhage in a case of systemic lupus erythematosus. Arch Neurol 37:173–174

Garcin R, Godlewski S, Lapresle J, Fardeau M (1959) Syndromes vasculaires aigus probables de la partie inférieure de la moelle chez des sujets porteurs de lesions discarthrosiques du rachis dorso-lombaire. Rev Neurol (Paris) 100:212–229

Garcin R, Godlewski S, Rondot P (1962) Etude clinique des médullopathies d'origine vasculaire. Rev Neurol (Paris) 106:558–591

Garland H, Greenberg J, Harriman DGF (1966) Infarction of the spinal cord. Brain 89:645–662

Gelfan S, Tarlov IM (1955) Differential vulnerability of spinal cord structures to anoxia. J Neurophysiol 18:170–188

Gingrich TF (1968) Spinal epidural hematoma following continuous epidural anesthesia. Anesthesiology 29:162–163

Goodin DS (1989) Neurological sequelae of aortic disease and surgery. In: Aminoff MJ (ed) Neurology and general medicine. Churchill Livingstone, New York, pp 23–48

Gruner J, Lapresle J (1962) Etude anatomo-pathologique des médullopathies d'origine vasculaire. Rev Neurol (Paris) 106:592–631

Gueguen B, Merland JJ, Riche MC, Rey A (1987) Vascular malformations of the spinal cord: intrathecal perimedullary arteriovenous fistulas fed by medullary arteries. Neurology 37:969–979

Hayes MA, Creighton SR, Boysen BG, Holfeld N (1978) Acute necrotizing myelopathy from nucleus pulposus embolism in dogs with intervertebral disk degeneration. J Am Vet Med Assoc 173:289–295

Henson RA, Croft PB (1956) Spontaneous spinal subarachnoid haemorrhage. Q J Med 25:53–66

Henson RA, Parsons M (1967) Ischaemic lesions of the spinal cord: an illustrated review. Q J Med 36:205–222

Herdt JR, DiChiro G, Doppman JL (1971) Combined arterial and arteriovenous aneurysms of the spinal cord. Radiology 99:589–593

Herrick MK, Mills PE (1971) Infarction of spinal cord. Two cases of selective gray matter involvement secondary to asymptomatic aortic disease. Arch Neurol 24:228–241

Herron PW, Foltz EL, Plum F, Bruce RA, Merendino KA (1958) Partial Brown-Séquard syndrome associated with coarctation of the aorta: review of literature and report of a surgically treated case. Am Heart J 55:129–134

Hughes JT (1970) Thrombosis of the posterior spinal arteries. A complication of an intrathecal injection of phenol. Neurology 20:659–664

Jellinger K, Neumayer E (1962) Myelopathies progressives d'origine vasculaire. Rev Neurol (Paris) 106:666–669

Jurcovic I, Eiben E (1970) Fatal myelomalacia caused by massive fibrocartilaginous venous emboli from nucleus pulposus. Acta Neuropathol (Berl) 15:284–287

Kendall BE, Andrew J (1972) Neurogenic intermittent claudication associated with aortic steal from the anterior spinal artery complicating coarctation of the aorta. Case report. J Neurosurg 37:89–94

Kendall BE, Logue V (1977) Spinal epidural angiomatous malformations draining into intrathecal veins. Neuroradiology 13:181–189

Kepes JJ (1965) Selective necrosis of spinal cord gray matter. A complication of dissecting aneurysm of the aorta. Acta Neuropathol (Berl) 4:293–298

Killen DA, Foster JH (1960) Spinal cord injury as a complication of aortography. Ann Surg 152:211–230

King OJ, Glas WW (1960) Spinal subarachnoid hemorrhage following lumbar puncture. Arch Surg 80:574–577

Krause GS (1983) Brown-Séquard syndrome following heroin addiction. Ann Emerg Med 12:581–583

Leech PJ, Stokes BAR, ApSimon T, Harper C (1976) Unruptured aneurysm of the anterior spinal artery presenting as paraparesis. Case report. J Neurosurg 45:331–333

Logue V (1979) Angiomas of the spinal cord: review of the pathogenesis, clinical features, and results of surgery. J Neurol Neurosurg Psychiatry 42:1–11

Madow L, Alpers BJ (1949) Involvement of the spinal cord in occlusion of the coronary vessels. Arch Neurol Psychiatry 61:430–440

Markham JW, Lynge HN, Stahlman GEB (1967) The syndrome of spontaneous spinal epidural hematoma. Report of three cases. J Neurosurg 26:334–342

Matthews WB (1965) Sarcoidosis of the nervous system. J Neurol Neurosurg Psychiatry 28:23–29

Naiman JL, Donohue WL, Prichard JS (1961) Fatal nucleus pulposus embolism of spinal cord after trauma. Neurology 11:83–87

Oldfield EH, DiChiro G, Quindlen EA, Rieth KG, Doppman JL (1983) Successful treatment of a group of cord arteriovenous malformations by interruption of dural fistula. J Neurosurg 59:1019–1030

Posnikoff J (1968) Spontaneous spinal epidural hematoma of childhood. J Pediatr 73:178–183

Ratinov G, Jimenez-Pabon E (1961) Intermittent spinal ischemia. Neurology 11:546–549

Rebello MD, Dastur HM (1966) Spinal epidural hemorrhage. (A review and two case reports.) Neurol India 14:135–145

Riche MC, Modenesi-Freitas J, Djindjian M, Merland JJ (1982) Arteriovenous malformations of the spinal cord in children. A review of 38 cases. Neuroradiology 22:171–180

Riche MC, Scialfa G, Gueguen B, Merland JJ (1983) Giant extramedullary arteriovenous fistula supplied by the anterior spinal artery: treatment by detachable balloons. AJNR 4:391–394

Richter RW, Rosenberg RN (1968) Transverse myelitis associated with heroin addiction. JAMA 206:1255–1257

Roger H, Poursines Y, Roger J (1955) Les aspects neurologiques de la periarterite noueuse. Rev Neurol (Paris) 92:430–464

Ross RT (1985) Spinal cord infarction in disease and surgery of the aorta. Can J Neurol Sci 12:289–295

Shaw PJ (1986) Neurological complications of cardiovascular surgery. II. Procedures involving the heart and thoracic aorta. Int Anesthesiol Clin 24:159–200

Skillman JJ (1986) Neurological complications of cardiovascular surgery. I. Procedures involving the carotid arteries and abdominal aorta. Int Anesthesiol Clin 24:135–157

Skinhoj E (1954) Arteriosclerosis of the spinal cord. Three cases of pure "syndrome of the anterior spinal artery". Acta Psychiatr Neurol Scand 29:139–143

Spiller WG (1909) Thrombosis of the cervical anterior median spinal artery; syphilitic acute anterior poliomyelitis. J Nerv Ment Dis 36:601–613

Srigley JR, Lambert CD, Bilbao JM, Pritzker KPH (1981) Spinal cord infarction secondary to intervertebral disc embolism. Ann Neurol 9:296–301

Symon L, Kuyama H, Kendall B (1984) Dural arteriovenous malformations of the spine: clinical features and surgical results in 55 cases. J Neurosurg 60:238–247

Symonds CP, Meadows SP (1937) Compression of the spinal cord in the neighbourhood of the foramen magnum. Brain 60:52–84

Syrjanen J, Iivanainen M, Kallio M, Somer H, Valtonen VV (1986) Three different pathogenic mechanisms for paraparesis in association with bacterial infections. Ann Clin Res 18:191–194

Towbin A (1969) Latent spinal cord and brain stem injury in newborn infants. Dev Med Child Neurol 11:54–68

Tyler HR, Clark DB (1958) Neurologic complications in patients with coarctation of aorta. Neurology 8:712–718

Vogelsang H, Dietz H (1975) Cervical spinal angioma combined with arterial aneurysm. Neuroradiology 8:223–228

Watson P, Fekete J, Deck J (1977) Central nervous system vasculitis in rheumatoid arthritis. Can J Neurol Sci 4:269–272

Weenink HR, Smilde J (1964) Spinal cord lesions due to coarctatio aortae. Psychiatr Neurol Neurochir 67:259–269

Wells CEC (1966) Clinical aspects of spinovascular disease. Proc R Soc Med 59:790–796

Williamson RT (1894) Spinal thrombosis and haemorrhage due to syphilitic disease of the vessels. Lancet 2:14–16

Wilson CB (1969) Significance of the small lumbar spinal canal: cauda equina compression syndromes due to spondylosis. Part 3: intermittent claudication. J Neurosurg 31:499–506

Wolman L, Bradshaw P (1967) Spinal cord embolism. J Neurol Neurosurg Psychiatry 30:446–454

Wyburn-Mason R (1943) The vascular abnormalities and tumours of the spinal cord and its membranes. Kimpton, London

Zulch KJ (1962) Réflexions sur la physiopathologie des troubles vasculaires médullaires. Rev Neurol (Paris) 106:632–645

Chapter 19

Decompression Illnesses and the Spinal Cord

R.R. Pearson

Although diving as a purposeful activity has been going on since at least 5000 BC and almost certainly pre-dates any recorded history, the decompression illnesses which can result from diving are a comparatively recent phenomenon and were not even described in detail until well into the 19th century. The reason for this is that despite many attempts to produce a means of breathing underwater, most of which were dangerously impractical with little or no understanding of either the physics or physiology involved, breath-hold diving from the surface or from submerged diving bells was the only way of venturing underwater. However, the advent of an effective and relatively safe underwater breathing capability came with the 1819 introduction of Augustus Siebe's diving helmet, a device which allowed the diver to be provided with compressed air from a pump on the surface. Apart from the much greater freedom given to the diver by this equipment, divers were provided with a much easier means of achieving depth-time limits underwater which were capable of causing decompression sickness. Indeed, it is said that when Greek sponge divers began to use the 1839 version of Siebe's helmet, which by now was combined with a suit and heavy boots, 50% of them died within the first year! The very fact that it was now possible to breathe underwater also made divers vulnerable to decompression pulmonary barotrauma, the second decompression illness capable of damaging the central nervous system. Developments of Siebe's helmet, which remained remarkably close to the original design, were used almost exclusively by military and commercial divers up to World War II when, as is so often the case, accelerated technological development for military purposes led to the first effective self-contained underwater breathing apparatus (SCUBA) and with it, a further dramatic increase in underwater freedom and flexibility. The initial use of this equipment was by the so-called "frogmen" who used closed-circuit breathing apparatus with pure oxygen as a breathing mixture. Similar closed-circuit apparatus using oxygen or nitrogen/oxygen breathing mixtures is still much used by specialist military divers for a variety of offensive and defensive purposes. The advent of recreational diving as a popular pastime dates mainly from the 1946 invention of the "demand valve" by Cousteau and Gagnan. The demand valve is a self-regulating device which automatically provides the diver with a breathing mixture at the same pressure as the surrounding water. This simple and cheap device, combined with compressed air cylinders strapped to the diver, led to a dramatic change in routine commercial and military diving practice and, even more importantly, also provided the impetus for what was to become a veritable explosion in recreational or "sports" diving. It is in this population of recreational divers that the decompression illnesses and their sequelae are most commonly seen and, in the United Kingdom, approximately 50 000 active "sports" divers give rise to more than 150 decompression illnesses each year, the majority of which require recompression therapy. Table 19.1 shows that the cases requiring Royal Navy advice and/or treatment (approximately 70% of the total occurring in the United Kingdom) have risen dramatically over the last five years and that the incidence of central nervous system (CNS) involvement (Table 19.2) has also risen significantly. A similar rise in the incidence of CNS involvement has occurred in the United States where the Divers Accident Network (DAN), a central reporting agency, deals with 250–300 decompression illnesses each year from an estimated diver population of about 2 million. However, it is estimated that these accidents represent only about one-half of the decompression illnesses treated each year in the United States and the Caribbean.

Regrettably, the world over, there is an all-too-common failure in the timely diagnosis of decompression illnesses and, with it, inevitable delays in definitive treatment. These delays can result in permanent sequelae, many of them disabling neurological deficits, and there is nothing more true concerning the treatment of decompression illnesses than the simple fact that the sooner recompression is initiated, the better the prognosis is for full recovery.

Decompression Illnesses

The two decompression illnesses which may involve the CNS and, more specifically, cause spinal cord damage, are decompression sickness (DCS) and decompression pulmonary barotrauma (DPB). The various manifestations of DCS are due to the direct and indirect effects of bubbles of inert gas which can result from inadequate decompression after exposure to hyperbaric pressure whereas in DPB, alveolar gas may enter the pulmonary venous return and become arterialized via the left heart to give the condition known as arterial gas embolism (AGE).

Decompression Sickness

DCS may occur in divers or compressed air workers who are exposed to a hyperbaric environment in tunnelling and caisson work. It may also result from decompression to altitude from normal ambient pressure at ground level. The latter situation may arise in altitude chambers or unpressurized aircraft. In the case of individuals who breathe compressed air during their hyperbaric exposure and those who are decompressed to altitude, the inert gas responsible for DCS will be nitrogen but other inert gases such as helium and, more rarely, neon and hydrogen, are used in deep diving as carrier gases or diluents for the essential oxygen fraction of the breathing mixture. The use of these inert gases is exclusive to military and commercial diving and they avoid the problems of nitrogen narcosis and gas density which effectively limit air as a breathing

Table 19.1. Recreational diving accidents requiring Royal Navy advice and/or treatment

	1985	1986	1987	1988	1989
Uncomplicated pulmonary barotrauma	1	2	2	1	1
Cerebral arterial gas embolism	5	4	4	9	8
Type 1 (mild) DCS	19	15	14	13	37
Type 2 (serious) DCS	20	28	30	82	92

Table 19.2. Incidence of CNS involvement in cases of DCS requiring Royal Navy advice and/or treatment

Year	Type 2 (serious) DCS with CNS involvement (%)
1985	51
1986	65
1987	68
1988	86
1989	71

mixture. In the United Kingdom, legislation forbids diving on compressed air to depths in excess of 165 feet of sea water (fsw). The toxic effects on the CNS of oxygen breathed at increased pressure limit the use of pure oxygen as a breathing mixture to depths shallower than 26 fsw.

In general, the rate at which inert gases are taken up and released by body tissues during hyperbaric exposure and the subsequent decompression is controlled by both perfusion and diffusion, the former being the more important. For practical purposes, the process of uptake and elimination of inert gas may be regarded as exponential and, quite simply, well perfused tissues will take up inert gas more rapidly than relatively poorly perfused tissues. A further factor controlling the actual amount of inert gas taken up by any tissue is the solubility of inert gases in that particular type of tissue and, in this respect, it is unfortunate that nitrogen is much more soluble in fatty tissue than helium. Helium is expensive and generally reserved for breathing mixtures used in deep diving. It is generally accepted that this is the reason for the well-established fact that DCS involving the CNS in divers breathing helium/oxygen (heliox) mixtures is quite rare but when it does occur, it is largely similar to CNS involvement in DCS arising from compressed air diving. All further comment will, therefore, relate to DCS arising from breathing air and, therefore, the result of nitrogen bubbles. This is, in any case, the type of DCS seen in recreational divers who generally use compressed air. Also, apart from a lower incidence of cases with neurological involvement, DCS arising from work in compressed air or altitude exposure has no other major difference from that seen in divers and these groups will not be considered separately.

The decompression phase of any hyperbaric exposure is, at least in theory, capable of causing nucleation of inert gas and bubble formation as tissues and blood release gas taken up during compression and the time spent at pressure. However, decompression tables exist to allow divers to either limit their depth/

time exposure to enable a direct return to the surface or, if this limit is exceeded, to carry out a controlled decompression with stops at various depths during the ascent to allow an orderly and safe elimination of inert gas. Formal tables for air diving were first designed for the Royal Navy by Haldane in 1908 although the relatively simple concepts of the factors involved in elimination of inert gas during decompression which were used in the design of these tables have since been shown to be inappropriate for some of the more extreme exposures encountered in air diving. However, a reliable mathematical model of the complex processes involved in single or multiple dives to a wide range of depth/time exposures has yet to be developed despite numerous attempts. Apart from those which are evolved stochastically, many of these models are based on notional tissues which take up and release inert gas at different rates. These rates are expressed as "half-times", a term which refers to the time taken for the notional tissue to become half-saturated with inert gas. Saturation occurs when the partial pressure of the inert gas in solution in any given tissue is in equilibrium with the partial pressure of that gas in the breathing mixture. It is a process which may take as long as 24 hours or more to occur in very poorly perfused tissues but may occur extremely quickly in well perfused tissues such as the cerebral cortex. A largely empirical evolution of decompression tables and techniques for air diving has been going on for long enough to have evolved suitably safe decompression rules for air diving and the great majority of cases of DCS occur when these rules are ignored. Nevertheless, it is vitally important to recognize that severe DCS may occasionally arise from dives that are in full compliance with accepted diving tables.

Inert Gas Bubbles

Inert gas bubbles are generally categorized as being either extra- or intra-vascular and although good evidence does not, as yet, exist to suggest that they may also be intracellular, the smallest "bubble" is two molecules of gas and there is no theoretical reason why bubbles should not be intracellular. The effects of these bubbles may be direct and mechanical, or indirect, mainly as a result of activation of the acute inflammatory response with all its complexities.

Although it is essential to consider DCS as a particularly complex disease process with the potential to have a multi-organ and multi-system impact, the current, almost universally used classification (Golding et al. 1960) is based on

Table 19.3. Classification of decompression sickness (after Golding et al. 1960)

Type 1 (mild) – Joint pain ("niggles" to severe pain)
          – Cutaneous (pruritus, erythema, lividity)
          – Lymphoedema
          – Constitutional (fatigue, malaise)

Type 2 (serious) – CNS (spinal cord and/or brain)
             – Audiovestibular ("staggers")
             – Respiratory ("chokes")
             – Cardiovascular (hypovolaemia)

organ- or system-related symptoms and signs, particularly those associated with the presentation and progression of the illness. Most treatment regimes are based on this classification but it must be seen as limited and potentially dangerous in that it tends to disguise the potentially widespread impact of the condition. The classification referred to divides DCS into Type 1 (mild) and Type 2 (serious) and Table 19.3 details the various manifestations of these categories including the descriptive names that have, over the years, become associated with various presentations ("staggers", "chokes", etc). The term "bends" originated in the 19th century as a descriptive term for the musculo-skeletal manifestations of DCS but is now widely used to indicate any form of DCS.

Extravascular Inert Gas Bubbles

Before discussing the potential of DCS to damage the spinal cord, it is necessary to outline the respective role of extra- and intravascular inert gas bubbles. Without doubt, extravascular gas bubbles do occur and have been visualized both macro- and microscopically in a variety of tissues in man and experimental animals. It is fashionable to refer to such bubbles as "autochthonous" which literally means "formed in the region where found". If they arise in subcutaneous tissues, they can result in histamine and other vasoactive substance release and it is logical to attribute the cutaneous manifestations of itching, erythema and "marbling" or lividity to such substances. Inert gas bubbles may also block cutaneous lymphatic drainage channels and cause localized swelling and oedema. Expansion of autochthonous bubbles occurring in poorly perfused tissues such as cartilage and ligamentous tissues associated with joints is assumed to produce direct pressure on sensitive nerve endings (Nims 1951) and cause the varying degrees of pain in or adjacent to joints which are a characteristic feature of Type 1 DCS. Although no incontrovertible evidence exists to support this concept, and it has been suggested that such pain may be centrally mediated as a consequence of spinal cord or nerve root involvement, the great majority of such cases respond so rapidly to recompression and, where it can be applied, local pressure, that it is difficult to attribute the pain to anything other than some local phenomenon involving autochthonous bubbles. Further, no pathology attributable to DCS has ever been described in nerve roots or peripheral nerves. The role of autochthonous bubbles in the pathogenesis of CNS involvement is becoming increasingly recognized and will be discussed later.

Intravascular Bubbles

As with extravascular bubbles, intravascular inert gas bubbles have been seen and recorded by a variety of methods on numerous occasions commencing with Sir Robert Boyle (1670) whose 17th century experiments in subjecting a variety of animals to a vacuum resulted in visible intravascular bubbles which he described as "... choking up some passages and vitiating the figure of others ...". Paul Bert (1878), the famous French physiologist, also described intravascular bubbles in his famous treatise *La pression barometrique* and not only correctly attributed these bubbles to release of nitrogen during decompression but identified them as the cause of DCS.

It is generally accepted that, during decompression, the first intravascular gas emboli to occur are venous and pass to the microcirculation of the lungs which acts as a filter, allowing the inert gas to diffuse into the alveoli. The size of detectable decompression-induced venous gas emboli (VGE) probably ranges from 15 to 200 microns (Hills and Butler 1981) and ultrasonic doppler transducers can detect VGE as they transit the right heart (Spencer and Clarke 1972; Powell and Johanson 1978). It is evident from numerous studies of divers during decompression that a certain degree of bubbling is tolerable and equally numerous animal experiments show that surprising amounts of venous gas can be tolerated, particularly if they are given as an infusion of bubbles. VGE have been recorded on many occasions in asymptomatic divers but they can, in sufficient quantity, lead to rises in pulmonary artery and right ventricular pressures, both factors which assist the migration of VGE through the pulmonary microcirculation (Butler and Hills 1985) or a patent foramen ovale (Moon and Camporesi 1989; Wilmshurst et al. 1989) to give arterial gas emboli (AGE) which are a much less tolerable form of intravascular gas.

Notwithstanding the embolic potential of intravascular gas, it is also a particularly potent initiator of the acute inflammatory response. Powerful electrochemical forces at the blood–gas interface of bubbles can result in denaturation of proteins with formation of globules of free fats and fat emboli may result from release of fatty acids from cell membranes. Platelet and leucocytes also adhere to bubbles (Philp et al. 1972) and the net effect may be a cascade of events commencing with Hageman Factor activation which, in turn, leads to kinin, complement, clotting and fibrinolytic system activation. At worst, these reactions can add to the embolic action of bubbles by further occluding blood vessels and also have an adverse effect on vascular endothelial permeability. Further, the stability of bubbles may be enhanced by the formation of a very thin (20 nm) "shell" of precipitated protein on their surface and this shell may also fragment to form circulating microemboli. At worst, DCS may result in disseminated intravascular coagulation although this requires major decompression stress and is a rare event. A number of sources are available for a more comprehensive description of these events (Bove 1982; Francis et al. 1990). It is sufficient to add that intravascular gas may not only cause ischaemia but also that this ischaemia will further hinder the elimination of inert gas from tissues. The CNS may also be vulnerable to this complex chain of events.

Decompression Pulmonary Barotrauma (DPB)

If gas trapping occurs in the lungs or exhalation is inadequate during decompression, DPB, sometimes called the "pulmonary overinflation syndrome" may occur. The gas in the lungs must expand in accordance with Boyle's Law and overpressures necessary to cause alveolar rupture, be they localized or general, are surprisingly modest. Experiments with cadavers (Malhotra and Wright 1961) and animal models (Schaefer et al. 1958) suggest that as little as 100 mmHg overpressure can cause alveolar rupture. This degree of overpressure will be generated if gas trapping occurs during an ascent from depths as shallow as 4 fsw, a fact confirmed by a number of recorded cases of DPB occurring after ascents from such depths in swimming baths where SCUBA divers have not exhaled during the ascent. Once alveolar rupture has occurred, the gas may track to the lungs along the perivascular sheaths to give mediastinal emphysema or, much more frequently, it will go to the left heart via the pulmonary veins and become arterialized to give AGE. By far the most frequent destination of AGE is via the carotid arteries to give cerebral arterial gas embolism (CAGE), a dramatic event with potentially lethal consequences. The gas emboli usually end up in the areas of brain served by the anterior and middle cerebral arteries, particularly the "watershed" areas between the two circulations. Occasionally, the brain stem will be involved by gas emboli that have entered the vertebrobasilar arteries and it has been postulated that sudden death, a not uncommon outcome of CAGE, is due to cardiac arrest or arrhythmias following brain stem involvement (Greene 1978). Once in the cerebral circulation, AGE tend to arrest in the precapillary arteriolar circulation to give ischaemia and the exposure of the endothelium to gas leads to a very rapid loss of integrity of the blood–brain barrier. On restoration of the circulation, either spontaneously or as a result of recompression therapy, oedema of the "vasogenic" type may occur to produce secondary deterioration (Pearson 1984). It is difficult to believe that any AGE arresting in the microcirculation of the spinal cord will behave any differently.

Animal models have been used to show that the distribution of bubbles in the arterial circulation is influenced strongly by their buoyancy (Van Allen and Hrdina 1929). However, the bubbles used by Van Allen and Hrdina were relatively large and small bubbles (<100 microns) are much less buoyant which indicates that more widespread systemic arterial embolization is possible, particularly if the victim is not erect when the embolic gas reaches the aorta. Coronary artery embolization is also a possibility but remarkably few such cases are recorded of which only one fatal case had undeniable evidence of such an outcome (Harveyson et al. 1956). Evidence of other organ involvement by AGE is even more rare and only three cases of spinal cord involvement which were undeniably due to DPB are known to the author. Although it will be evident that the embolizing gas in DPB is whatever gas is being breathed, which contrasts with the inert gas emboli of DCS, the effect of AGE of a variety of gases is qualitatively virtually identical with the exception of carbon dioxide which is sufficiently soluble to effectively preclude it as a potentially embolic gas. Also, whereas DCS requires a sufficiently stressful depth/time profile and subsequent decompression to initiate a critical degree of bubbling, and this will be evident in most cases, DPB can occur after minimal time at equally minimal depths. That said, emergency ascents often occur after submerged times that would also give DCS and an accurate differential diagnosis may be almost impossible. Indeed, the two conditions frequently coexist. If the apparent frequency with which venous inert gas emboli become arterialized is also taken into account, the need to distinguish between the two decompression illnesses becomes almost academic, especially when the recommended recompression therapy for both is identical in a number of commonly used therapeutic regimes.

Presentation of the Decompression Illnesses

Decompression Sickness

Historically, the first descriptions of DCS appear to be by Triger, a French engineer, whose 1839 description of joint pain in caisson workers is cited both by Pol and Watelle (1854) and Bert (1878). The former described a variety of more serious manifestations in caisson workers during the use, also in 1839, of another caisson to sink a mine shaft. Pol and Watelle also must take the credit for recommending recompression as "the most certain way of easing" the symptoms of DCS. The building of a bridge across the Mississippi at St. Louis in 1867–74 involved much use of caissons and led to 19 deaths from DCS as well as 91 other cases, some severe and permanently disabling. These events were recorded in detail by Doctors Clark (1870–71) and Jaminet (1871), two physicians who treated these cases. Jaminet was successful in reducing both morbidity and mortality by empirically adjusting the length and frequency of the hyperbaric exposures. He also provided a graphic account of his own episode of DCS which involved transient quadriplegia and aphasia for which he was given Jamaica rum and beef tea. The value of alcohol in the treatment of DCS is a myth which, unfortunately, persists and it is all too frequently the first therapeutic choice of sports divers. Neither Jaminet nor Clark seems to have been aware of the use of recompression to treat DCS. Numerous accounts of DCS in compressed air workers then began to appear but some years elapsed before the problem was described as a specific hazard of diving (Khrabrostin 1888). Further accounts of DCS in divers then began to appear at regular intervals including one particularly graphic account of the short- and long-term sequelae of DCS (Blick 1909). Blick described over 200 cases of "divers' palsy" in Australian pearl divers. Many of these divers had long-standing bladder paralysis and a catheter was regarded as a standard "do-it-yourself" item of their equipment. Since then, a vast amount of literature has accumulated concerning DCS in individuals and groups of divers and compressed air workers.

Table 19.4. Distribution and percentage incidence of presenting symptoms and signs in 935 cases of DCS with CNS involvement

	Incidence (%)		Incidence (%)
Numbness/paraesthesia	21.2	Unconsciousness	2.7
Motor weakness	20.6	Personality change	1.6
Paralysis	6.1	Agitation/restlessness	1.3
Urinary disturbance	2.5	Convulsion	1.1
Muscular twitching	1.2	Equilibrium disturbance	0.7
Incoordination	0.9	Auditory disturbance	0.3
Dizziness/vertigo	8.5	Cranial nerve deficits	0.2
Nausea/vomiting	7.9	Aphasia	0.2
Visual disturbance	6.8	Dyspnoea	2.0
Headache	3.9	Fatigue	1.2

After Rivera 1963.

The symptoms and signs of DCS may appear singly or in combination and CNS involvement may be accompanied by any or all of the other categories listed in Table 19.3. However, CNS involvement is always regarded as a form of Type 2 DCS and qualifies inevitably for the designation of "serious". Evidence of CNS involvement tends to appear shortly after surfacing from the causative decompression, occasionally even occurring during decompression. Francis et al. (1988a) analysed the latency of 1070 cases of CNS DCS occurring in divers and compressed air workers. He showed that 66% presented within 10 minutes of surfacing and 84% within 1 hour. Of those cases exhibiting unequivocal evidence of cerebral involvement, either on its own or associated with spinal cord DCS, 76% had presented within 10 minutes and 96% within 1 hour. In contrast, the onset of joint pain and other less serious manifestations tended to be significantly more delayed. This study confirmed that 99% of all DCS occurs within 24 hours of the causative dive and that anything over 48 hours is extremely rare. It reinforces the belief that any unusual symptom or sign occurring within 48 hours of a dive should be treated as a decompression illness unless there is compelling evidence to the contrary.

The neurological manifestations of DCS range from minor, localized sensory disturbances and/or weakness in one or more limbs to profound quadriplegia, unconsciousness and convulsions. Virtually all severe cases where spinal cord involvement has occurred will demonstrate bilateral deficits but those in less serious cases may be unilateral and involve only a single modality. Loss of bladder and bowel sphincter control may occur and urinary retention is a frequent accompaniment of spinal cord DCS. From onset, symptoms and signs may progress and extend with extreme rapidity or remain relatively static. Spontaneous remission, sometimes complete, may occur in quite dramatic fashion and may be seen to some degree in as many as 30% of cases. However, a secondary relapse, with a return or extension of the original symptoms and signs, frequently follows spontaneous remission and is usually much less responsive to recompression therapy. Often, the symptoms and signs occur in seemingly bizarre combinations which are difficult to explain on a rational basis but must be seen as evidence of the very widespread involvement of the nervous system which may occur with DCS. Traditionally, it has been the custom to believe that, in the absence of clear evidence of cerebral involvement, virtually all neurological deficits in limbs and the trunk were indicative of spinal cord involvement, and no doubt many neurological examinations of divers have been carried out in the past with this assumption in mind. The most frequently encountered evidence of cerebral involvement in DCS is usually some combination of visual disturbance, headache and alteration in level of consciousness but a number of studies show that a much wider variety of indications of cerebral involvement occur, some of them very subtle and often ignored against a background of more florid symptoms. Table 19.4 lists the incidence of CNS symptoms and signs in the study by Rivera (1963) of 935 cases of DCS using his choice of categories.

Although the reported incidence of obvious cerebral involvement in DCS is about 20% (Pearson 1981; Francis et al. 1988a), a recent study which used radioisotopes to study cerebral perfusion deficits after decompression illnesses (Adkisson et al. 1989) suggested that some degree of cerebral involvement may be much more common, perhaps even universal, in DCS where there is any evidence whatsoever of CNS involvement. Although this study is continuing, there is no doubt that every case of DCS deserves the most detailed neurological examination that time will allow before treatment, and expert neurological assessment as soon as possible afterwards. As will be seen later, it is probable that quite different mechanisms are responsible for spinal cord and cerebral involvement.

One especially sinister, fortunately relatively rare, presentation of serious DCS is so-called "girdle pain" which is characteristic of severe spinal cord involvement. Such pain may be lower thoracic or upper abdominal and invariably comes on within 5 minutes of surfacing. It is a presentation requiring the most urgent recourse to recompression therapy and the response to therapy is often incomplete and disappointing.

If the spinal cord is involved in DPB, it can only be as a result of systemic AGE. In the three cases known to the author, sudden uncontrolled decompressions from shallow depths resulted in the very rapid onset of profound paraplegia with a sharply demarcated upper level for the motor and sensory losses involved. Although all these cases were treated promptly, the response was universally poor and significant residual disability ensued. In each case, it was presumed that a gas embolus had occluded a major nutrient artery to the cord resulting in an acute ischaemic/anoxic process which, despite the probable restoration of perfusion on recompression, was sufficient to cause a considerable degree of irreversible damage. The presentation of the cerebral AGE (CAGE) may be equally dramatic and almost always occurs within 10 minutes of surfacing, often immediately the surface is reached. Table 19.5 gives an analysis of the presentation of 188 cases of CAGE arising from submarine escape training and diving accidents.

Table 19.5 shows the presentation of CAGE generally is characterized by the high incidence of alterations of levels of consciousness, with or without convulsions, as well as a predominance of unilateral motor and sensory deficits. This is in contrast to DCS affecting the spinal cord where bilateral deficits are more common.

Pathogenesis and Pathology of Decompression Illnesses

Decompression Sickness

It is most surprising that the precise way in which inert gas bubbles give rise to spinal cord DCS still remains a matter of controversy and even what is known about the associated pathology is not too helpful in some respects. The arguments are largely concerned with the respective roles of embolic and autochthonous gas bubbles.

Gas Embolism. The possible contribution of VGE was first proposed by Haymaker and Johnston (1955) and demonstrated by Hallenbeck (1976) who, using a laminectomy to view the spinovertebral epidural venous plexus in decompressed dogs, recorded a dramatic accumulation of VGE in this system leading to stasis. It was argued that such a degree of stasis could lead to venous infarction and, in turn, the lesions in white matter of the cord (see below)

Table 19.5. Presentation of 188 cases of cerebral arterial gas embolism arising in submarine escape training and diving

Symptoms and signs	Incidence (%)
Coma with convulsions	14
Coma without convulsions	29
Stupor and confusion	21
Acute vertigo	12
Visual disturbances	8
Headache	2
Unilateral paresis	17
Unilateral sensory deficit	10
Unilateral motor and sensory deficits	4
Bilateral paresis	4
Bilateral sensory deficit	˙1

which have been described as the most prominent feature of spinal cord DCS by numerous authors over the past 100 years. Other studies in animals and humans (Kitano et al. 1977; Wolkiciwcz et al. 1979) have tended to support this theory but Hills and James (1982) argued that it has some fundamental limitations and the observed stasis may be the result rather than the cause of DCS. They also challenged the concept that stasis in the epidural venous plexus would affect the white matter preferentially. It is also difficult to explain the well-described vulnerability of certain levels and elements of the cord on such a basis. Dutka et al. (1990) have repeated Hallenbeck's experiment using somatosensory evoked potential (SEP) monitoring to correlate intravascular events with spinal cord function. They found that occlusion of the epidural venous plexus by a foam of bubbles did not, in itself, seem to cause any dramatic loss of SEP amplitude but that the appearance of AGE in the small arteries on the surface of the cord usually led to a rapid and profound loss of SEP amplitude and electrophysiological function. The source of the observed AGE could not be determined and AGE were seen to travel in different directions in the same vessel at different times which suggested that gas emboli might be arising from within the cord and moving in retrograde fashion. Another possibility is that the vessels studied were in a "watershed area" where alternating flow is normal.

Arterialization of VGE. This, or de novo origin of AGE within the lungs, has also been proposed as an important factor in the pathogenesis of spinal cord DCS (Gersh and Catchpole 1951; Behnke 1955; Hempleman 1972). One fundamental objection to this theory was voiced by Hallenbeck et al. (1976) who pointed out that the brain is almost universally involved in all other embolic conditions and that this did not seem to be the case in DCS, although this latter observation is now less tenable. Despite the AGE seen by Dutka, other experiments involving the injection of inert gas microemboli (50–200 microns) into the thoracic aorta of dogs (Francis et al. 1989; Pearson et al. 1990) produced profound loss of electrophysiological function in the cord but the associated pathology, namely acute anoxic-ischaemic damage, was confined

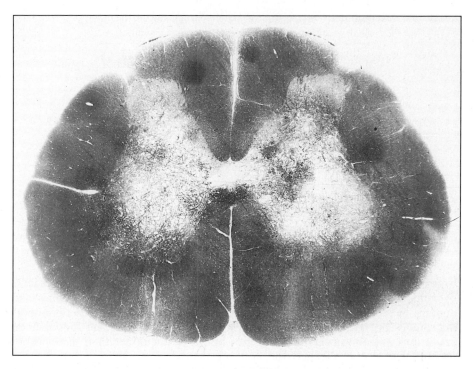

Fig. 19.1. Low power cross-section of cord (L1) following introduction of inert gas microemboli (50–200 μm) into thoracic aorta. Note severe disruption of grey matter with sparing of white matter.

to the grey matter with complete sparing of the white matter. Fig. 19.1 shows the severe degree of grey matter damage resulting from this experiment. There is no reason to believe that the process involved in the very few recorded cases in divers of spinal cord involvement secondary to DPB is any different to the lesions produced in this animal model and that acute ischaemic/anoxic damage will result, a process to which the grey matter will be most vulnerable.

Autochthonous Bubbles. Historically, the role of autochthonous bubbles of inert gas arising in the tissues of the cord and causing mechanical damage by expansion as decompression continues has long been popular. Paul Bert (1878) discussed such a possibility but Hills and James (1982) were perhaps the first to attempt to describe and model the process in a scientific manner. Certainly, bubbles of what was always assumed to be inert gas had been described on many occasions in autopsy reports following fatal decompression accidents. Many of these reports also described "lacerations" of the cord tissue in association with these bubbles. Sykes and Yaffee (1985) described decompression-induced myelin sheath abnormalities seen with electron microscopy in the cords of decompressed dogs and presumed these were evidence of gas bubbles. Francis et al. (1988b) used the same animal model, admittedly one producing DCS with an acute and very early onset, to demonstrate numerous non-staining space-occupying lesions in the white matter of the cord. The lesions were clearly extravascular and could be seen to be causing either displacement or disruption of axonal sheaths. These lesions were also transient and had largely disappeared within 6 hours to be replaced by discrete haemorrhagic areas with leucocyte infiltration and early organization. Francis et al. suggested that these bubbles had three possible injurious effects: mechanical disruption of conducting tissue, pressure on adjacent axons and pressure on the adjacent microcirculation to give ischaemia, the last having the added effect of hampering inert gas elimination. The transient nature of these bubbles no doubt explains why they have not been identified previously. It may be that the ''girdle pain'' referred to previously is the result of a degree of tissue disruption and laceration so severe that the resulting damage is irreversible and unresponsive to recompression and hyperbaric oxygen.

To sum up, convincing evidence now exists to implicate autochthonous bubbles in the pathogenesis of very acute, early onset DCS of the cord. The precise role of VGE and AGE remains less well understood and it may be that their ability to produce ischaemia is most important in the genesis of autochthonous bubbles. The delayed and less acute presentations of DCS may be also be due to ischaemia secondary to embolic phenomena.

Cerebral involvement in DCS, on the other hand, is rather easier to understand and almost certainly due to arterialized VGE. In unpublished work by the author and colleagues, a cranial window was used to study the effects of decompression, and the appearance of AGE in the pial arterial circulation can be positively correlated with loss of cortical evoked potentials. Further, it has been possible to identify positively, and for the first time, the pathology associated with cerebral DCS in an animal model and there is little doubt that the changes seen are entirely compatible with an embolic process. These changes are discrete infarcts mainly concentrated at the grey-white matter marginal areas supplied by the anterior and middle cerebral arteries. Small perivascular haemorrhages are also seen in the white matter but are a less prominent feature. These lesions are entirely compatible with the numerous descriptions of the pathology of CAGE secondary to DPB and a variety of iatrogenic accidents. Although the extent and severity of the lesions are dependent on the amount and, to some extent, size of embolic bubbles, the basic nature of the lesions is similar. It is this feature that leads to the previous comment that the distinction between cerebral manifestations of DCS and CAGE secondary to DPB is, to a large extent, academic. The luxurious nature of cerebral perfusion almost certainly precludes the formation of autochthonous bubbles of inert gas in all but the most extreme situations.

The distribution of the lesions of DCS in the cord in compressed air induced DCS seems to be a function of the amount of fatty tissue in different segments and this may be the explanation for the relative frequency with which the lower thoracic and upper lumbar cord are involved (Kidd and Elliott 1969; Desola and San Pedro 1984). Certainly, these sections of the cord would be more likely to produce autochthonous bubbles in view of the solubility of nitrogen in fatty tissue.

Pathological material relevant to the acute process of DCS in the spinal cord in humans is surprisingly scanty and not a lot of autopsy evidence is available. Fig. 19.2 shows the presence of autochthonous bubbles in the white matter of the cord of a diver who died from fulminating DCS within 2 hours of surfacing and there is remarkably little reaction to the bubbles at this stage.

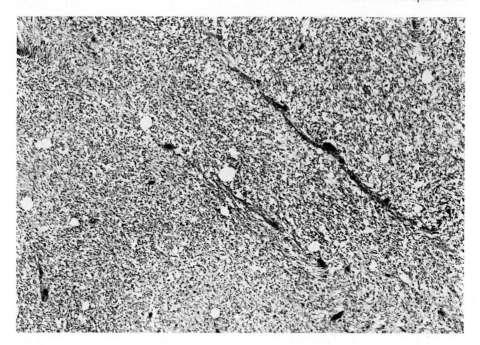

Fig. 19.2.   Acute DCS. Autochthonous bubbles in white matter (×125).

    The overall appearance of the white matter in Fig. 19.2 is remarkably similar
to that seen by Francis et al. (1988b) in an animal model of acute DCS. The
grey matter of the cord shown in Fig. 19.2 appeared to be essentially normal.
Later stages of the development of the white matter lesions begin to show
typical punctate haemorrhages (Calder 1986) and demyelination of axons both
distally and proximally.
    The chronic changes associated with DCS of the cord have been described
more often and reinforce the evidence for sparing of the grey matter in this
process as well as showing that the dorsal and lateral columns of the white
matter are most often involved (Palmer 1986). Cases have been described
where the degree of scarring in the white matter was extensive and seemingly
out of proportion to the degree of functional disability (Palmer et al. 1981). Of
some concern is the discovery of less specific degenerative changes in the cords
of a number of divers who died from non-diving related causes and who had no
history of overt DCS (Palmer et al. 1988). These changes were mainly in the
posterior, lateral and anterior columns of the white matter and, in the posterior
columns, suggested a degree of damage to the afferent fibres from the nerve
roots. Whatever the significance of these changes, they add to the growing
concern that diving may result in hitherto unrecognized chronic damage to the
CNS. The pathogenesis of these changes can only be speculative but it is
proposed that they result from chronic asymptomatic arterialization of VGE
although the relative sparing of the grey matter in this process remains difficult
to understand.

Treatment of Decompression Illnesses

The treatment of decompression illnesses is a specialist subject in itself but it is important to note that the earliest possible recompression remains the definitive treatment for any decompression illness affecting the CNS. A number of regimes exist for such therapy which, despite some significant differences in the amount of pressure used, aim to "crush" bubbles of inert gas to either alleviate their space-occupying effects or allow them to transit the blood vessels where they have become arrested. In the case of arterial bubbles, the aim is to allow them to pass through the capillary bed and return to the lungs where gas exchange into the alveoli can eliminate them. The breathing of pure oxygen at pressure is also commonly used to facilitate inert gas removal from bubbles and provide enhanced oxygenation of tissues at risk from anoxia/hypoxia. The majority of regimes use "treatment tables" which detail the pressures and breathing mixtures to be used. By far the most commonly used tables are those which involve recompression to a pressure equivalent to 60 fsw on pure oxygen for cases of DCS and to 165 fsw for CAGE. Those contained in the Diving Manuals of the United States and Royal Navies are typical of such an approach and used widely. However, some other regimes make no distinction between the two decompression illnesses and treat all cases at 60 fsw. As yet, there is insufficient evidence to recommend which of the approaches to CAGE gives the best results. A high cure rate for both DCS and CAGE is possible given timely recompression but success diminishes with delays.

A number of forms of first-aid and adjuvant therapy are frequently advocated although good scientific evidence for the benefit of most does not exist. There is no doubt that oxygen breathing prior to recompression therapy can be beneficial and should be started as soon as possible. There is also good reason to initiate intravenous fluid replacement therapy in all cases of serious DCS and crystalloid solutions are normally recommended. Similarly, a reasonable argument may be produced in favour of intravenous glucocorticoids such as dexamethasone which, in theory at least, protect against the effects of bubbles on vascular endothelium thereby reducing vasogenic oedema. Starting doses in the order of 16 mg are frequently recommended. A rational approach to the adjuvant therapy of DCS and CAGE is that recommended by Bove (1982). The arguments for diuretics, anticoagulants and even ethyl alcohol, all have their advocates but none are of proven value. Fortunately, expert advice on the therapy of decompression illnesses is always available from a number of centres in the United Kingdom and should always be consulted when a decompression illness is suspected.

Relapses may occur during or after recompression treatment, particularly where it has been delayed or the choice of initial treatment has been inadequate. Secondary deterioration is perhaps more common with CAGE and may be life-threatening (Pearson and Goad 1982). All promulgated treatment regimes give guidance on the management of such cases and usually recommend extension of time spent under pressure with addition of extra periods of oxygen breathing. However, such relapses are notoriously difficult to treat and an incomplete response frequently ensues. The most common approach to an incomplete response after a formal treatment is to carry on with shorter hyperbaric oxygen (HBO) sessions on a daily or twice daily basis

(Pearson and Leitch 1979). The risk of pulmonary oxygen toxicity (POT) must be borne in mind with all extensions to formal treatment tables, particularly when they are repeated over a period of days. In the absence of limiting POT, it is customary to carry on with HBO sessions until a plateau of response has occurred and no sustained objective improvement has occurred after two consecutive sessions.

With appropriate supportive and remedial therapy, the long-term prognosis for residual deficits following spinal cord DCS is much the same as for many other types of injury to the cord. A truly surprising degree of recovery may continue for as long as two years, or even more, after which no further improvement is seen. This slow, continued improvement is generally attributed to the processes of adaptation and the redundancy within the CNS. However, a number of the more serious cases treated by the author eventually begin to deteriorate again although the degree and amount of this further deterioration are variable. One interesting feature that has been observed is the emergence of severe limb pain where it had not previously featured in the symptomatology.

One of the most vexed questions that follows CNS DCS is whether a return to diving can be recommended. Resort may be made to a number of specialized investigations such as evoked potential testing, CAT scans and MRI, to attempt to establish whether any permanent damage has resulted. However, the use of these techniques in the study of DCS is evolving and they have not, as yet, been shown to be markedly superior to a detailed clinical examination. It seems prudent in such situations to advise against a return to diving where there is any evidence of permanent neurological sequelae, no matter how minor. This advice should be extended to all cases where a CNS deficit has not responded quickly and completely to recompression therapy.

References

Adkisson GH, Hodgson M, Smith F, et al. (1989) Cerebral perfusion deficits in dysbaric illnesses. Lancet 2:119–122

Behnke AR (1955) Decompression sickness. Milit Med 117:257–271

Bert P (1878) La pression barometrique. Recherches de physiologie experimentale. Masson, Paris. (Translated by MA and FA Hitchcock, 1943, Columbus, Ohio: College Book Co and reprinted Bethesda, MD: Undersea and Hyperbaric Med Soc 1978)

Blick G (1909) Notes on diver's paralysis. Br Med J ii:1796–1798

Bove AA (1982) The basis for drug therapy in decompression sickness. Undersea Biomed Res 9:91–111

Boyle R (1670) New pneumatical observations about respiration. Phil Trans R Soc 5:2011–2056

Butler BD, Hills BA (1985) Transpulmonary passage of venous air emboli. J Appl Physiol 59:543–547

Calder IM (1986) Dysbarism: a review. Forensic Sci Int 30:237–266

Clark EA (1870–1871) Effects of increased atmospheric pressure on the human body. A report of thirty five cases brought to the City Hospital from the St. Louis and Illinois Bridge. Med Arch St Louis 5:1–30

Desola AJ, San Pedro AG (1984) Epidemiological study of 146 dysbaric diving accidents. In: Desola AJ (ed) Diving and hyperbaric medicine. Proc IX Congress of Eur Undersea Biomed Soc, Barcelona

Dutka AJ, Knightly J, Collins J, Pearson RR, Mink RB, Hallenbeck JM (1990) The presence of bubbles in vessels surrounding the spinal cord correlates with changes in spinal somatosensory evoked potential (SSEP) amplitude. Undersea Biomed Res 17 (suppl):137

Francis TJR, Pearson RR, Robertson AG, Hodgson M, Dutka AJ, Flynn ET (1988a) Central nervous system decompression sickness: latency of 1070 human cases. Undersea Biomed Res 15:402–411

Francis TJR, Pezeshkpour GH, Dutka AJ, Hallenbeck JM, Flynn ET (1988b) Is there a role for the autochthonous bubble in the pathogenesis of spinal cord decompression sickness? J Neuropathol Exp Neurol 47:475–487

Francis TJR, Pezeshkpour GH, Dutka AJ (1989) Arterial gas embolism as a pathophysiologic cause for spinal cord decompression sickness. Undersea Biomed Res 16(6):439–451

Francis TJR, Dutka AJ, Hallenbeck JM (1990) Pathophysiology of decompression sickness. In: Bove AA, Davis JC (eds) Diving medicine. Saunders, Philadelphia, pp 170–187

Gersh I, Catchpole HR (1951) Decompression sickness: physical factors and pathologic consequences. In: Fulton JF (ed) Decompression sickness. Saunders, Philadelphia, pp 165–181

Golding FC, Griffiths P, Hempleman HV, et al. (1960) Decompression sickness during the construction of the Dartford Tunnel. Br J Ind Med 17:167–180

Greene KM (1978) Causes of death in submarine escape training casualties: analysis of cases and review of the literature. AMTE(E) report R78–402, Alverstoke, Hampshire

Hallenbeck JM (1976) Cinematography of dog spinal vessels during cord-damaging decompression sickness. Neurology 26:190–199

Hallenbeck JM, Bove AAS, Elliott DH (1976) Decompression sickness studies. In: Lambertsen CJ (ed) Underwater physiology V. FASEB, Bethesda, MD, pp 273–286

Harveyson KB, Hirschfield BEE, Tonge J (1956) Fatal air embolism from use of compressed air diving unit. Med J Aust 1:658–660

Haymaker W, Johnston AD (1955) Pathology of decompression sickness: a comparison of lesions in airmen with those in caisson workers and divers. Milit Med 117:285–306

Hempleman HV (1972) The site of origin of gaseous emboli produced by decompression from raised pressures of air and other gases. In: Fructus X (ed) Proc 3rd Int Conference on Hyperbaric Med Underwater Physiol, Doin, Paris, pp 160–162

Hills BA, Butler BD (1981) Size distribution of intravascular air emboli produced by decompression. Undersea Biomed Res 8:163–174

Hills BA, James PB (1982) Spinal decompression sickness: mechanical studies and a model. Undersea Biomed Res 9(3):185–201

Jaminet A (1871) Physical effects of compressed air. (Privately printed), St Louis, MO, pp 1–7

Khrabrostin MN (1888) Work under water and diseases of divers. Medits Pribavl 68:68–84

Kidd DJ, Elliott DH (1969) Clinical manifestations and treatment of decompression sickness in divers. In: Bennett PB, Elliott DH (eds) The physiology and medicine of diving and compressed air work, Ballière-Tindall and Cassell, London, pp 464–490

Kitano M, Hayashi K, Kawashima M (1977) Three autopsy cases of acute decompression sickness. Consideration of pathogenesis about spinal cord damage in acute decompression sickness. Jpn Orthop Traum 26:402–408

Malhotra MS, Wright HC (1961) The effects of a raised intrapulmonary pressure on the lungs of fresh unchilled cadavers. J Path Bact 82:198–202

Moon RE, Camporesi EM (1989) Patent foramen ovale and decompression sickness. Lancet 1:513–514

Nims LF (1951) Environmental factors affecting decompression sickness. In: Fulton JF (ed) Decompression sickness. Saunders, Philadelphia, pp 264–278

Palmer AC (1986) The neuropathology of decompression sickness. In: Cavanagh JB (ed) Recent advances in neuropathology, 3rd edn. Churchill Livingstone, New York, pp 141–162

Palmer AC, Calder IM, McCallum RI, Mastaglia FL (1981) Spinal cord degeneration in a case of "recovered" spinal decompression sickness. Br Med J 283:288

Palmer AC, Calder IM, Hughes JT (1988) Spinal cord damage in active divers. Undersea Biomed Res 15 (suppl):70

Pearson RR (1981) The aetiology, pathophysiology, presentation and therapy of pulmonary barotrauma and arterial gas embolism arising from submarine escape training and diving. MD Thesis, Durham University.

Pearson RR (1984) Diagnosis and treatment of gas embolism. In: Shilling CW, Carlston CB, Mathias RA (eds) The physicians guide to diving medicine. Plenum Press, London, pp 333–367

Pearson RR, Goad RF (1982) Delayed cerebral edema complicating cerebral arterial gas embolism: case histories. Undersea Biomed Res 9(4):283–296

Pearson RR, Leitch DR (1979) Treatment of air or oxygen/nitrogen mixture decompression illnesses in the Royal Navy. J R Nav Med Serv 65(2):53–62

Pearson RR, Francis TJR, Pezeshkpour GH, Dutka AJ (1990) Spinal cord dysfunction and pathology following arterial gas embolism. Undersea Biomed Res 17 (suppl):32–33

Philp RB, Ackles KN, Inwood MJ, et al. (1972) Changes in the hemostatic system and in blood and urine chemistry of human subjects following decompression from a hyperbaric environment. Aerospace Med 43:498–505

Pol B, Watelle T (1854) Mémoire sur les effets de la compression de l'air appliqué au creusement des puits à houille. Ann Hyg publ et med leg, Paris

Powell MR, Johanson DC (1978) Ultrasound monitoring and decompression sickness. In: Shilling CW, Beckett MW (eds) Underwater physiology IX. Undersea and Hyperbaric Med Soc, Bethesda, MD, pp 503–510

Rivera JC (1963) Decompression sickness amongst divers: an analysis of 935 cases. Milit Med 129:314–334

Schaefer KE, McNulty WP, Carey CR, Liebow AA (1958) Mechanisms in development of interstitial emphysema and air embolism in decompression from depth. J Appl Physiol 13:15–29

Spencer MP, Clarke HF (1972) Precordial monitoring of pulmonary gas embolism and decompression bubbles. Aerospace Med 43(7):762–767

Sykes JJW, Yaffee LJ (1985) Light and electron microscopic alterations in spinal cord myelin sheaths after decompression sickness. Undersea Biomed Res 12:251–258

Van Allen CM, Hrdina LS (1929) Air embolism from the pulmonary vein. Arch Surg 19:567–599

Wilmshurst PT, Byrne JC, Webb-Peploe MM (1989) Neurological decompression sickness. Lancet 1:731

Wolkiewiez J, Martin PJ, Lapoussiere JM, Kermarec J (1979) Spinal cord accidents. Med Aeronaut Spat Med Subaquat Hyp 18:313–317

Chapter 20

Hereditary and Nutritional Disorders of the Spinal Cord

B. Pentland

The existence of numerous uncommon but fascinating disorders contributes to the joy and the frustration of the study of neurology. Hereditary disorders affecting the spinal cord are uncommon, incompletely understood and many lack autopsy confirmation of lesions directly affecting the spinal cord. By their very nature nutritional disorders resulting from vitamin deficiency tend to have widespread effects on the nervous system and often features of peripheral nerve involvement overshadow those caused by central nervous system damage. The conditions described here are those in which spinal cord involvement is considered to be a major component of the disease process.

Hereditary Ataxias and Paraplegias

The term "hereditary ataxias" is given to a large group of inherited conditions, none of which are common and which exhibit a variety of clinical manifestations consequent upon degeneration of various parts of the nervous system including the spinal cord. This group name is far from satisfactory and, although no universally accepted classification of these conditions exists, two fairly comprehensive systems have been described (Barbeau et al. 1984; Harding 1984) which include some 70 or so diseases. Congenital ataxias and most of the ataxic disturbances associated with metabolic disorders of the urea cycle or disturbances of pyruvate and lactate metabolism have their main pathological effects on the cerebellum and result in death during early childhood (Harding 1984). Friedreich's ataxia and related syndromes, hereditary spastic paraplegias and abetalipoproteinaemia do result in significant spinal cord damage.

Friedreich's Ataxia

Nicolaus Friedreich (1825–1882), professor of medicine at Heidelberg, described the commonest of the hereditary ataxias in nine patients from three families in a series of papers between 1863 and 1877. He noted the characteristic onset before adulthood, the predominance of ataxia as a symptom, the hereditary nature of the disorder and many of the typical pathological changes.

Epidemiology and Aetiology

The prevalence of Friedreich's ataxia is of the order of 1 in 50000 of the population (Harding and Zilkha 1981; Romeo et al. 1983). The sex incidence is equal (Bell and Carmichael 1939). It is an autosomal recessive condition although controversy exists as to whether dominant inheritance of the classical disorder or sporadic mutations occur (Harding 1984). The site of the defective gene has been localized to the centromeric region of the short arm of chromosome 9 (Chamberlain et al. 1988). This recent finding makes the prenatal diagnosis of Friedreich's ataxia possible.

Pathology

Friedreich's original detailed account of the pathology has been expanded by many subsequent authors and there is general agreement concerning the principal pathological changes (Mackay 1898; Greenfield 1954; Kinnier Wilson 1954).

Macroscopically the spinal cord is smaller that usual. Degeneration and reactive gliosis are most marked in the posterior columns, particularly the fasciculus gracilis which correlates with the usual finding that atrophy is most marked in the lumbosacral area. The lateral columns are also affected with involvement of the corticospinal and spinocerebellar tracts. Changes are more severe in the posterior than the anterior spinocerebellar tracts. The cells of the dorsal nucleus are also usually affected by the degenerative process. The anterior corticospinal tracts and anterior horn cells may also be involved in some cases.

The cell bodies of the dorsal root ganglia undergo degenerative change and there is selective degeneration of the large myelinated axons from these cell bodies but there is relative sparing of the fine unmyelinated fibres (Hughes et al. 1968).

Other parts of the CNS may show pathological changes but on a less consistent basis. Examples are a patchy loss of Purkinje cells in the cerebellum, gliosis of the dentate nucleus and degeneration of the superior cerebellar peduncle (Oppenheimer 1979).

Clinical Features

The onset of symptoms is generally apparent during the patient's school years, several large series reporting a mean age of onset around the age of 10 years (Geoffroy et al. 1976; Harding 1984). Although the diagnosis may be made in the under five-year-old child, especially if there is an affected sibling, most children achieve their normal motor milestones in infancy and the impairment of motor performance is noted later. The great majority of cases present before the age of 20 years but occasional exceptions with first symptoms occurring in slightly older adults have been reported.

The presenting symptom is usually ataxia of gait but individuals may initially come to medical attention because of spinal and foot deformities, cardiac symptoms, dysarthria or other characteristic manifestations of the established disease.

Ataxia

Unsteadiness of gait is often noted first during school gymnastics or sports or on attempting to learn to cycle. The gait tends to be broad based with clumsiness on pivotal, turning movements. Truncal ataxia is present in addition to lower limb incoordination with resultant swaying particularly on rising from a sitting position and on changing direction. Falls are a frequent accompaniment of progression of the disease. The lurching, wide-based walking pattern in the adolescent sufferer not uncommonly is wrongly attributed to drunkenness by casual adult observers.

It is often impossible to isolate the particular pathology most responsible for the disturbance of stance and gait. Indeed in the established case the combination of cerebellar, pyramidal and proprioceptive tract damage is responsible for the characteristic pattern of disability and one cannot reliably quantify their relative contributions.

Upper limb incoordination tends to become evident at a later date with deterioration in writing, doing and undoing buttons or laces and other fine manual tasks. Clumsiness in hand function is variable in degree and rate of progression. Many individuals have severe impairment of walking but have well-preserved upper limb function for some years. The finger nose test may reveal only slight intention tremor for instance in a patient who is wheelchairbound because of truncal and lower limb ataxia.

Muscle Tone and Weakness

Fatiguability is a common complaint, again predominantly in the legs. Thus the patient who may cope with a 100 yard walk fairly well after a period of rest but be unable to repeat the performance is in functional terms severely compromised by fatigue.

Muscle weakness is usually apparent on formal testing of power in the legs at an early stage and muscle tone tends to be flaccid reflecting the posterior column and dorsal root damage. In some cases because of lateral column involvement of the corticospinal tracts spasticity may be detectable.

Reflexes

In most patients the pattern is of progressive diminution and loss of tendon reflexes with ankle jerks lost first followed by knee and upper limb responses. In some cases corticospinal tract damage leads to pathologically brisk arm or knee jerks in combination with absent ankle jerks but loss of lower limb reflexes is characteristic of established disease. The pyramidal tract involvement usually results in extensor plantar responses and impairment or loss of superficial reflexes.

Sensory Changes

Sensory symptoms are fairly common and, while they are often not volunteered, the patient usually admits to aches and cramps on enquiry. Some suffer from shooting pains or uncomfortable paraesthesiae.

Posterior column sensation is impaired or lost distally in the lower limbs in most cases. There may be diminished vibration and joint position sense in the upper limbs also but this is less reliably found. Anterolateral pathway damage with impaired pain and temperature sensibility may also be found particularly in the legs in advanced cases.

Nystagmus

Some form of nystagmus is present in the majority of cases. The commonest variety is a horizontal nystagmus on lateral gaze but fixation nystagmus and vertical or rotatory nystagmus may be found.

Dysarthria

Dysarthria of cerebellar type is a cardinal feature of established Friedreich's ataxia. The severity of the disturbance tends to increase progressively over time so that it may be absent or mild in the earliest stages but can lead to unintelligible speech in some very advanced cases.

Optic Atrophy

Modern accounts agree that about one-quarter of patients have optic atrophy although only the minority of those with this sign have reduced visual acuity.

Deafness

A minority of patients suffer from a sensorineural deafness. This was rated as severe in only three of Harding's series of 115 cases (Harding 1981a).

Involuntary Movements

Head nodding or titubation and irregular movements of the limbs, which are often inaccurately described as choreiform, occur in a proportion of cases and are probably an expression of the ataxia itself rather than an independent feature of the disease (Tyrer 1975).

Pes Cavus

Deformities of the feet are found in most, some would claim all, patients with Friedreich's ataxia and indeed were noted by Friedreich himself. Tyrer and

Sutherland (1961) described four features of the deformity: pes equinus/pes equinovarus; pes cavus; claw toes and small muscle wasting of the sole of the foot. Salisachs (1974) added pes planus to the repertoire. Claw hand, manus cava, may also occur but is a relatively infrequent finding. Although small muscle wasting in the hands can be severe in advanced cases resulting in a claw hand this is not analagous to pes cavus as there is no abnormality of the "midcarpal" joint (Tyrer 1975).

Scoliosis

Scoliosis or kyphoscoliosis is another almost invariable accompaniment of the disease. Controversy persists about whether the spinal deformity is secondary to the neurological disturbances or is the direct result of a genetic factor (Tyrer 1975). The scoliosis of Friedreich's ataxia does not follow the pattern of a neuromuscular conditon but behaves more like an idiopathic scoliosis in the age of onset, course, nature of the curve and the absence of a relationship to muscle weakness (Labelle et al. 1986).

Cardiomyopathy

It is increasingly recognized that cardiomyopathy is probably a universal finding. Even in studies of individuals with no cardiac symptoms, abnormalities are detectable in cardiological investigations such as electrocardiography and echocardiography (Pentland and Fox 1983; Child et al. 1986). Only 46 of 115 cases had cardiac symptoms in one series (Harding 1981a) but in a detailed retrospective study of 82 fatal cases Hewer (1968) described evidence of cardiac dysfunction during life in 60 and death from cardiac failure in 46 cases. Exertional dyspnoea, palpitations and ankle swelling are among the commoner symptoms and clearly one cannot always reliably attribute these directly to cardiac involvement. Both concentric and asymmetric hypertrophic cardiomyopathies occur (Child et al. 1986) and, in addition to cardiac muscle abnormalities, a so-called cardioneuropathy has been described in that extensive degeneration of the myelinated and unmyelinated nerves of the heart and of the cardiac ganglia has been demonstrated pathologically (James et al. 1987).

Diabetes Mellitus

There is an increased incidence of diabetes in association with Friedreich's ataxia probably affecting about one in 10 patients. Those without overt diabetes do show insulin resistance which correlates with the duration of neurological symptoms and the degree of immobility (Khan et al. 1986).

Establishing the Diagnosis

It is useful for clinical, counselling and research purposes to establish firmly whether an individual patient has Friedreich's ataxia, the commonest hereditary

Table 20.1.   Friedreich's ataxia: major symptoms and signs

Most (> 2/3) cases:
Progressive ataxia of limbs and gait
Absent knee and ankle jerks
Extensor plantar responses
Dysarthria
Weakness of lower limbs
Distal posterior column sensory impairment in lower limbs
Scoliosis
Foot deformity

---

ataxia, or one of the other varieties. The diagnosis of Friedreich's ataxia is a clinical one. However, well-established diagnostic criteria schedules exist (Geoffroy et al. 1976; Harding 1984) which differ only slightly in detail. Table 20.1 lists the major features from these schedules and is not an attempt to create a hybrid. Clinicians should hopefully find it adequate but researchers would be advised to consult the original descriptions.

Harding (1984) includes in her list of essential criteria motor nerve conduction velocity greater than 40 metres per second in the upper limbs with small or absent sensory action potentials. This pattern of abnormalities has also been described as characteristic by other authors (Peyronnard et al. 1976; Ouvrier et al. 1982).

Somatosensory evoked potentials (Jones et al. 1980), visual evoked potentials (Carrol et al. 1980; Livingston et al. 1981b) and brain stem auditory evoked potentials (Satya-Murti et al. 1980; Ell et al. 1984) all commonly show reduced amplitude or flat responses in this condition. Minor non-specific electroencephalogram findings have been reported in one-third of cases (Remillard et al. 1976) but are of little diagnostic help.

Glucose tolerance testing and non-invasive cardiological screening with electro-, vector- and echocardiography should be considered as routine in these patients.

Treatment

There is no specific medical treatment which can be recommended for routine use in Friedreich's ataxia. Minor improvements in ataxia have been claimed for the anticholinesterase, physostigmine (Kark et al. 1977, 1981). Although in a controlled trial some improvement in ataxia was reported with choline chloride (Livingstone et al. 1981a) similar trials with lecithin, which should more effectively raise plasma choline levels, failed to show a beneficial effect (Pentland et al. 1981; Melancon et al. 1982). Other reports have suggested improvement in ataxia scores using 5-hydroxytryptophan and benserazide (Trouillas et al. 1982) and amantadine (Peterson et al. 1988) in small open trials but these can not be recommended for routine use at present.

Symptomatic treatment of associated diabetes and cardiomyopathy is obviously important. There is also a place for orthopaedic surgical treatment of the bony deformities associated with Friedreich's disease. Posterior spinal fusion using either Harrington or Luque instrumentation for scoliosis when the curve is greater than 40 degrees is recommended rather than the use of bracing which has been shown to be ineffective (Cady 1983; Daher et al. 1985). While good results from surgical correction of the foot deformities was reported in 30 of 34 cases described by Makin (1953), others suggest that surgical treatment of pes cavus is generally inadvisable because of the poor long-term prognosis and the presence of neuromuscular problems (Fitton 1988). As in most progressive neurological disorders the value of remedial therapy input cannot be under-estimated even if scientific proof of its efficacy is lacking. The guidance of a physiotherapist in a rest-exercise programme and education about gait can help the individual maintain optimal motor function. The occupational therapist can advise on activities of daily living, vocational and leisure activities and, with the social worker, can guide the individual about benefits, housing matters and voluntary and statutory support agencies. The patient's needs in terms of orthoses, walking aids and wheelchair provision may be the responsibility of therapists or physicians but, in either event, review to determine changing needs with progression of the disability is usually necessary. Although the degree of dysarthria is variable, speech therapists can help maximize the individuals's communication skills.

Although D'Ambrosio et al. (1987) reported that most patients described low dependency and a satisfactory quality of life on a postal questionnaire, it is important that patients have ready access to expert advice regarding their condition in view of the progressive nature of the disorder.

Death commonly results from cardiac failure or intercurrent infection and Hewer (1968) and Harding (1981a) reported very similar mean ages of death in their series of 36.6 and 37.5 years respectively. A significant proportion of patients do survive into late middle age or older.

Syndromes Similar to Friedreich's Ataxia

Friedreich's ataxia is the commonest early onset hereditary ataxia and the value of describing the many conditions reported over the last hundred years as variants of the disease, often in only a single family, is dubious. Harding (1984) and Barbeau et al. (1984) have provided extensive reviews on this subject and suffice it to say that among the associated features in this group of early onset ataxias are: deafness, myoclonus, retinal pigmentary changes, optic atrophy, cataract, mental retardation and extrapyramidal features. One hopes that the geneticists will eventually provide definitive guidance to the clinician faced with such diagnostic dilemmas.

Hereditary Spastic Paraplegia

Within the myriad of uncommon hereditary conditions which include para-plegia in their descriptions it does appear that a "pure" form exists which can be designated as hereditary spastic paraplegia (HSP) (Holmes and Shaywitz

1977; Harding 1981b). Matters are, however, still not simple as at least two different types are recognized within this category.

Aetiology

Holmes and Shaywitz (1977) in a review of 104 families noted a dominant form of inheritance in 73 and recessive form in 31. Within 22 families seen in her personal survey Harding (1981b) found 19 followed an autosomal dominant and 3 recessive inheritance. The condition is thus described as genetically heterogeneous.

Pathology

Degeneration is most marked in the corticospinal tracts from the medullary pyramids downwards. Changes are also found in the posterior columns without loss of posterior root fibres (Holmes and Shaywitz 1977).

Clinical Features

Harding (1981b) describes two forms of dominant HSP: type I with age of onset below 35 and type II with onset after 35.

In type I delay in age of walking in childhood was not uncommon and the major feature was spasticity rather than weakness in the legs. Progress of disability tended to be slow and severity very variable with 23% asymptomatic and 53.5% symptomatic but able to walk reasonably well and work. Sensory impairment was uncommon in this group and urinary difficulties were noted in slightly more than a third.

Those developing the condition over 35 years of age showed a more rapid progression of symptoms; weakness and sensory impairment were more prominent and twice as many had urinary difficulties, particularly urgency, in addition to their spastic paraplegia. None of the type II cases was classed as asymptomatic and 56% required a walking aid or were chairbound.

The recessive forms appeared similar to the dominant form in clinical features in Harding's cases. Combining her cases with those reported and reviewed from the literature by Holmes and Shaywitz (1977), 27 out of 37 (73%) had onset of symptoms in the first decade.

Management

Where spasticity is marked, the use of agents such as baclofen and dantrolene sodium can be beneficial and other approaches to the management of spasticity such as phenol injections may have a place. The advice and intermittent review by a physiotherapist are also very useful to help maintain optimal motor function and to recommend appropriate walking aids. As with other cases of spasticity there is sometimes symptomatic benefit from such techniques as relaxation therapy and hydrotherapy.

Other Hereditary Spastic Paraplegias

In addition to the pure form of HSP a complex array of variants exist much as with Friedreich's ataxia. Thus syndromes associated with optic atrophy or other eye pathology; with mental retardation; and with cerebellar or extrapyramidal signs have been described and faced with an individual case the clinician must consider first checking other family members, documenting accurately the constellation of features present and searching for a diagnostic label.

Abetalipoproteinaemia

Abetalipoproteinaemia is a rare inborn error of lipoprotein metabolism of autosomal recessive inheritance. Originally described by Bassen and Kornzweig in 1950 and 1957, the major neurological features are polyneuropathy and progressive ataxia but the effects are more widespread with haematological and gastrointestinal features also prominent.

Pathology

Few pathological studies have been reported and the emphasis has tended to be on the patchy demyelination and axonal loss in peripheral nerves (Miller et al. 1980; Wichman et al. 1985). The spinal cord is also affected with demyelination of the spinocerebellar tracts and posterior columns and loss of anterior horn cells in some cases (Sobrevilla et al. 1964).

Clinical Features

Presentation is usually in childhood with failure to thrive, and neurologically with progressive ataxia and learning difficulties. The original case did not walk until the age of 2 years, at which time she developed persistent diarrhoea, and visual problems were noted when she was 6 but unsteadiness of gait was described for the 2 years prior to presentation aged 18 (Bassen and Kornzweig 1950). Neurological findings included diminished abdominal reflexes, abnormal plantars and distal impairment of position, vibration and touch sensation as well as cerebellar signs. Her 9-year-old brother had no neurological complaints when first seen but developed ataxia, muscle weakness and signs of a myeloneuropathy in the following 2 years (Kornzweig and Bassen 1957). Subsequent reports have confirmed the common features of progressive ataxia, loss of tendon reflexes, impaired joint position and vibration sense and retinitis pigmentosa (Miller et al. 1980). Diarrhoea or steatorrhoea are major complaints in addition to the eye and neurological problems.

Investigations

The primary abnormality in abetalipoproteinaemia is the absence of apoprotein B, an essential component of low density lipoproteins; consequently cholesterol, phospholipid, triglyceride and free fatty acid levels are all reduced in the blood and chylomicrons are absent. Fat-soluble vitamin absorption is reduced and vitamin E levels are undetectable (Muller et al. 1983), Red blood cells become thorn-like or acanthrocytic in the majority but not all cases.

Treatment is essentially "dietary" with reduction in the intake of long-chain fatty acids for which medium-chain triglycerides are substituted and fat-soluble vitamin A, K and E supplementation. High dose vitamin E intake can prevent the development of neurological and retinal complications (Sokol 1988) but there is still controversy as to whether fat-soluble vitamin supplementation can stabilize neurological and retinal dysfunction once it is established in adults (MacGilchrist et al. 1988).

Ataxia Telangiectasia

This uncommon autosomal recessive condition is classified with the phacomatoses rather than the hereditary ataxias. Progressive early onset cerebellar ataxia is accompanied by conjunctival and skin telangiectases and an immune deficiency which leads to susceptibility to infection (McFarlin et al. 1972). A DNA repair defect has been identified in this condition (Bridges and Harnden 1981).

The brunt of the neuropathological damage is on the cerebellum with loss of Purkinje cells especially in the vermis but there is neuronal loss in the granular layer and the dentate and inferior olivary nuclei (McFarlin et al. 1972). It has also been shown that, as the disease advances, demyelination of the posterior columns and spinocerebellar tracts is common (Sedgewick and Boder 1972).

Progressive cerebellar ataxia begins in infancy, becoming evident when the child first walks. Both truncal and limb incoordination occur and some degree of dysarthria is universal. Eye movements are disturbed by oculomotor dyspraxia and choreoathetoid and other involuntary movements are common. Deep reflexes are usually diminished or absent. Most patients who survive beyond adolescence develop spinal cord signs such as impaired vibration and joint position sense (Sedgewick and Boder 1972). Telangiectasia usually appears in early childhood slightly later than ataxia, being noted first in the bulbar conjunctivae and later in the skin. Recurrent sinus and chest infections are common relating to the immune deficiency, particularly of immunoglobulin A.

The course and prognosis are variable but the majority of patients are wheelchair-bound by the age of 10 years and most die in adolescence from infection or, less frequently, from lymphoreticular malignancy. A small proportion do however survive even to the fifth decade. There is no specific treatment but antibiotic therapy for infective episodes is important (Harding 1984).

Vitamin B12 Deficiency: Subacute Combined Degeneration of the Spinal Cord

Vitamin B12, or cobalamin, deficiency can result in degenerative changes of the white matter of the spinal cord but also results in lesions in the brain and peripheral nerves. There is consequently a number of rather incomplete and unsatisfactory terms for the neurological syndromes which occur. The spinal cord damage has long been described as "subacute combined degeneration" as originally coined by Leichtenstein in 1884. Alternatives of posterolateral sclerosis and combined system disease have sometimes been in favour. The effects of deficiency on the brain have been described as vitamin B12 dementia, "megaloblastic madness" (Smith 1960) or by extension of the original title to subacute combined degeneration of the spinal cord and brain (Walton 1987), a rather cumbersome name. Peripheral neuropathy is perhaps the commonest neurological accompaniment of cobalamin deficiency and the term vitamin B12 neuropathy, possibly due to its relative brevity, has largely superseded others as the general title for the neurological features of the deficiency. It is, however, important to note that the syndrome can be a combination of brain, spinal cord and peripheral nerve signs and might be better described as cobalamin deficiency encephalomyeloneuropathy. Rather than advocate such a clumsy neologism, the term vitamin B12 neuropathy will be espoused here.

Epidemiology

By far the commonest cause is Addisonian pernicious anaemia and it is estimated that about 16% of untreated patients may have neurological signs (Shorvon et al. 1980). Pernicious anaemia has a prevalence rate in the UK of 127/100 000 (Scott 1960). The condition is uncommon before the age of 40 years and is slightly more common in females.

Aetiology

Addisonian pernicious anaemia is an autoimmune disorder characterized by severe atrophic gastritis with failure of intrinsic factor production. Antibodies to intrinsic factor are found in about 60% of cases and antiparietal cell antibodies in 90%. The lack of intrinsic factor leads to reduced vitamin B12 absorption in the lower ileum. Although most cases of vitamin B12 neuropathy are associated with pernicious anaemia, any cause of severe vitamin B12 deficiency can be responsible.

Lack of intrinsic factor can result from total gastrectomy and less commonly from partial gastrectomy. In the rare Zollinger-Ellison syndrome, a gastrin-secreting tumour, usually of the pancreas, causes intense gastric hyperacidity which lowers intestinal pH and impairs cobalamin absorption.

Any disease or surgery to the lower ileum can result in defective absorption of the intrinsic factor/vitamin B12 complexes. Thus idiopathic steatorrhoea, tropical sprue, Crohn's disease, ileal diverticulae or fistulae and small bowel resections can all be responsible. One could add the legendary fish tapeworm, Diphyllobothrium latum, infestation to this group of causes.

Dietary deficiency is an unusual cause of vitamin B12 deficiency. It is, however, important to consider the possibility in vegans. Chanarin et al. (1985) describe paraesthesiae as occurring in 10% of a population of 138 vegetarian Hindus with megaloblastic haemopoeisis, including a case of subacute combined degeneration. There can be diagnostic difficulties in Indians with the thalassaemia trait which results in a microcytosis which can mask the macrocytic tendency of vitamin B12 deficiency.

The oral hypoglycaemic biguanide, metformin and the antimitotic agent, methotrexate can also cause significant impairment of vitamin B12 absorption (James et al. 1987).

Pathology

Macroscopically the cord and brain may show pale greyish areas in their white matter. The characteristic histological changes are of scattered demyelination throughout the cord, particularly in the posterior and lateral columns. The areas of demyelination are often accompanied by accumulations of lipid-filled macrophages and gliosis. The areas of damage may coalesce resulting in holes in a glial network where myelin sheaths and axis cylinders have disappeared (Pant et al. 1968). In the peripheral nerves there is usually atrophy of the larger myelinated sensory fibres.

Pathogenesis of Neurological Lesions

The presentation with neurological symptoms and signs in the absence of megaloblastic anaemia has been recognized for many years and has provided an intriguing riddle as to the metabolic basis of the neuropathy (Victor and Lear 1956; Beck 1988). Fashionable hypotheses include the possibilities that the neuropathy results from a defect in one of two major cobalamin-dependent enzymes: methionine synthase or methylmalonyl CoA mutase which depend on methylcobalamin and adenosylcobalamin respectively. Methionine synthase is indirectly involved in DNA synthesis. Methylmalonyl CoA mutase is relevant to fatty acid synthesis and consequently to myelin synthesis (Beck 1988).

Clinical Features

In the majority of patients the neurological symptoms and signs occur on a background of features of the anaemia. The patient may, therefore, complain of tiredness and fatigue, exertional dyspnoea and ankle swelling; and may exhibit the classical lemon-tinted or biscuit-like complexion, a glossitic tongue, haemic murmurs and splenomegaly. Gastrointestinal complaints such an anorexia and diarrhoea or more florid features of malabsorption may occur depending upon the cause of the vitamin B12 deficiency.

As one might suspect, the onset of neurological symptoms is usually insidious and reflects the damage to spinal cord, peripheral nerve and brain. Occasionally an acute, fulminating course may be seen.

Usually the initial neurological symptoms are paraesthesiae or dysaesthesia of the feet. These may take the form of pins and needles, tingling, coldness or numbness but a wide variety of descriptions may be reported including the feeling of walking on pebbles or tight, constricting sensations. The hands are usually similarly affected and occasionally are troubled first. As the condition progresses these sensory features spread to the trunk. Posterior column damage leads to what the patient usually describes as clumsiness, either with a tendency to trip or stagger or to drop things when the upper limbs are affected. By this stage the picture is often complicated by motor features, with muscle weakness aggravating the tendency to fall or stagger when walking.

Examination reveals loss of vibration sense in the toes followed by more widespread loss, impairment of joint position sense and a "glove and stocking" loss of pain and temperature pathway senses. The gait is ataxic and Romberg's sign may be present. Either flaccidity or spasticity may be found depending upon the relative dominance of posterior column and corticospinal tract damage. Correspondingly, reflexes may be diminished or exaggerated and the plantars can be normal or extensor. Advanced cases will often show the classical combination of absent ankle jerks and extensor plantars beloved by postgraduate examiners.

The mental effects of vitamin B12 deficiency are protean (Lindenbaum et al. 1988). Memory loss, disorientation and even frank confusional psychosis can occur. Personality change or affective disturbances are also described, particularly depression.

Other associated problems of a neurological nature are optic atrophy and sphincter disturbance usually in the form of urgency of micturition.

Investigation

While a full blood count and film are the obvious initial investigations, megaloblastic features may not be present and the essential test is estimation of serum B12. Supplementary studies include a bone marrow sample; a B12 absorption test such as the Schilling urinary excretion test with cobalt-57 B12; and assays for autoantibodies.

Treatment

Intramuscular hydroxocobalamin is given initially in high doses such as 1000 μg daily for one to two weeks, followed by 250 μg at one to two month intervals. Response is often rapid in terms of resolution of the symptoms of polyneuropathy but spasticity and sensory ataxia from spinal cord damage is less likely to improve. The main aim of treatment is prevention of further lesions.

Folic Acid Deficiency

Deficiency of folic acid, like that of vitamin B12, can result in megaloblastic anaemia with associated neurological features of polyneuropathy, myelopathy and encephalopathy (Reynolds 1981; Lever et al. 1986).

Subacute combined degeneration is a rare complication of folate deficiency and Lever et al. (1986) review previous literature and indicate 28 reported cases including their own patient. The combination of reduced tendon reflexes, extensor plantar responses and reduced sensation is similar to that occurring in vitamin B12 deficiency. In seven cases described in detail in the report of Lever et al. alcohol was described as the aetiological factor in five.

Treatment with methyl folate, the reduced form of folate, is recommended for neurological syndromes associated with folate deficiency.

Vitamin E Deficiency

In addition to its importance in the pathogenesis of the neurological lesions in abetalipoproteinaemia, deficiency of vitamin E can be responsible for similar problems in other patients (Sokol 1988). Prolonged steatorrhoea over 10–20 years, e.g. after lengthy surgical resections for Crohn's disease, can lead to such a syndrome in adults. Isolated vitamin E deficiency inherited as an autosomal recessive condition has been described. There is debate as to whether the defect involved is in the absorption of vitamin E or in its hepatic metabolism. Sokol suggests that it is necessary to examine vitamin E status in all patients with unexplained neuropathy.

References

Barbeau A, Sadibelouiz M, Sadibelouiz A, Roy M (1984) A clinical classification of hereditary ataxias. Can J Neurol Sci 11:501–505

Bassen FA, Kornzweig AL (1950) Malformation of the erythrocytes in a case of atypical retinitis pigmentosa. Blood 5:381–387

Beck WS (1988) Cobalamin and the nervous system. N Engl J Med 318:1752–1754

Bell J, Carmichael EA (1939) On hereditary ataxia and spastic paraplegia. In: Fisher RA (ed) Treasury of human inheritance vol IV part III. Nervous diseases and muscular dystrophies. Cambridge University Press, pp 141–196 and p 281

Bridges BA, Harnden DG (1981) Untangling ataxia-telangiectasia. Nature 289:222–223

Cady RB (1983) Natural history and treatment of scoliosis and Friedreich's ataxia. Orthop Trans 7:430

Carroll WM, Kriss A, Baraitser M, Barrett G, Halliday AM (1980) The incidence and nature of visual pathway involvement in Friedreich's ataxia. Brain 103:423–434

Chamberlain S, Shaw J, Rowland A, et al. (1988) Mapping of mutation causing Friedreich's ataxia to human chromosome 9. Nature 334:248–250

Chanarin I, Malkowska V, O'Hea AM, Rinsler MG, Price AB (1985) Megaloblastic anaemia in a vegetarian Hindu community. Lancet 2:1168–1172

Child JS, Perioff JK, Bach PM, Wolfe AD, Perlman S, Kark RAP (1986) Cardiac involvement in Friedreich's ataxia: a clinical study of 75 patients. J Am Coll Cardiol 7:1370–1378

Daher YH, Lonstein JE, Winter RB, Bardford DS (1985) Spinal deformities in patients with Friedreich's ataxia: a review of 19 patients. J Pediatr Orthop 5:553–557

D'Ambrosio R, Leone M, Rosso MG, Mittino D, Brignolio F (1987) Disability and quality of life in hereditary ataxias: a self-administered postal questionnaire. Int Dis Studies 9:10–14

Ell J, Prasher D, Rudge P (1984) Neuro-otological abnormalities in Friedreich's ataxia. J Neurol Neurosurg Psychiatry 47:26–32

Fitton J (1988) Other neurological disorders. In: Helal B, Wilson D (eds) The foot, vol 1. Churchill Livingstone, Edinburgh pp 353–377

Geoffroy G, Barbeau A, Breton A, et al. (1976) Clinical description and roentologic evaluation of patients with Friedreich's ataxia. Can J Neurol Sci 3:279–286

Greenfield JG (1954) The spino-cerebellar degenerations. Blackwell, Oxford

Harding AE (1981a) Friedreich's ataxia: a clinical and genetic study of 90 families with an analysis of early diagnostic criteria and intrafamilial clustering of clinical features. Brain 104:589–620

Harding AE (1981b) Hereditary "pure" spastic paraplegia: a clinical and genetic study of 22 families. J Neurol Neurosurg Psychiatry 44:871–883

Harding AE (1984) The hereditary ataxias and related disorders. Churchill Livingstone, Edinburgh

Harding AE, Zilkha KJ (1981) "Pseudo-dominant" inheritance in Friedreich's ataxia. J Med Genet 18:285–287

Hewer RL (1968) Study of fatal cases of Friedreich's ataxia. Br Med J 3:649–652

Holmes GL, Shaywitz BA (1977) Strumpell's pure familial spastic paraplegia: case study and review of the literature. J Neurol Neurosurg Psychiatry 40:1003–1008

Hughes JT, Brownell B, Hewer RL (1968) The peripheral sensory pathway in Friedreich's ataxia. Brain 91:803–818

James WPT, Broom J, Ralph A (1987) Nutrition. In: Girdwood RH, Petrie JC (eds) Textbook of medical treatment, 15th edn. Churchill Livingstone, Edinburgh, pp 151–163

Jones SJ, Baraitser M, Halliday AM (1980) Peripheral and central somatosensory nerve conduction defects in Friedreich's ataxia. J Neurol Neurosurg Psychiatry 43:495–503

Kark RAP, Blass JP, Spence MA (1977) Physostigmine in familial ataxias. Neurology 27:70–72

Kark RAP, Rodriguez-Budelli MM, Wachsner R (1981) Double-blind, triple-crossover trial of low doses of oral physostigmine in inherited ataxias. Neurology 31:288–362

Khan RJ, Andermann E, Fantus IG (1986) Glucose intolerance in Friedreich's ataxia: association with insulin resistance and decreased insulin binding. Metabolism 35:1017–1023

Kinnier-Wilson SA (1954) Neurology vol 2, 2nd edn. Bruce AN (ed) Butterworth, London, pp 1078–1098

Kornzweig AL, Bassen FA (1957) Retinitis pigmentosa, acanthocytosis and heredodegenerative neuromuscular disease. Archiv Ophthalmol 58:183–187

Labelle H, Tohme S, Duhaime M, Allard P (1986) Natural history of scoliosis in Friedreich's ataxia. J Bone Joint Surg 68A:564–572

Lever EG, Elwes RDC, Williams A, Reynolds EH (1986) Subacute combined degeneration of the cord due to folate deficiency. response to methyl folate treatment. J Neurol Neurosurg Psychiatry 49:1203–1207

Lindenbaum J, Healton EB, Savage DG, et al. (1988) Neuropsychiatric disorders caused by cobalamin deficiency in the absence of anemia or macrocytosis. N Engl J Med 318:1720–1728

Livingstone IR, Mastaglia FL, Pennington RJT, Skilbeck C (1981a) Choline chloride in the treatment of cerebellar and spinocerebellar ataxia. J Neurol Sci 50:161–174

Livingstone IR, Mastaglia FL, Edis R, Howe JW (1981b) Pattern of visual evoked responses in hereditary spastic paraplegia. J Neurol Neurosurg Psychiatry 44:176–178

MacGilchrist AJ, Mills PR, Noble M, Foulds WS, Simpson JA, Watkinson G (1988) Abetalipoproteinaemia in adults: role of vitamin therapy. J Inher Metab Dis 11:184–190

Mackay H (1898) Pathology of a case of Friedreich's disease. Brain 21:435–474

Makin M (1953) The surgical management of Friedreich's ataxia. J Bone Joint Surg 35A:425–436

McFarlin DE, Strober W, Waldmann TA (1972) Ataxia-telangiectasia. Medicine 51:281–314

Melancon SB, Vanasse M, Geoffroy G, et al. (1982) Oral lecithin and linoleic acid in Friedreich's ataxia. II Clinical results. Can J Neurol Sci 9:155–164

Miller RG, Davis CJF, Illingworth DR, Bradley W (1980) The neuropathy of abetalipoproteinemia. Neurology 30:1286–1291

Muller DPR, Lloyd JK, Wolff OH (1983) Vitamin E and neurological function. Lancet 1:225–228

Oppenheimer DR (1979) Brain lesions in Friedreich's ataxia. Can J Neurol Sci 6:173–176

Ouvrier RA, McLeod JG, Conchin TE (1982) Friedreich's ataxia – early detection and progression of peripheral nerve abnormalities. J Neurol Sci 55:137–145

Pant SS, Asbury AK, Richardson EP (1968) The myelopathy of pernicious anaemia: a neuropathologic reappraisal. Acta Neurol Scand 44 (suppl 35):7

Pentland B, Fox KAA (1983) The heart in Friedreich's ataxia. J Neurol Neurosurg Psychiatry 46:1138–1142

Pentland B, Martyn CN, Steer CR, Christie JE (1981) Lecithin treatment in Friedreich's ataxia. Br Med J 282:1197–1198

Peterson PL, Saad J, Nigro MA (1988) The treatment of Friedreich's ataxia with amantadine hydrochloride. Neurology 38:1478–1480

Peyronnard JM, Lapointe L, Bouchard JP, Lamontage A, Lemieux B, Barbeau A (1976) Nerve conduction studies and electromyography in Friedreich's ataxia. Can J Neurol Sci 3:313–317

Remillard G, Andermann F, Blitzer L, Andermann E (1976) Electroencephalographic findings in Friedreich's ataxia. Can J Neurol Sci 3:309–312

Reynolds EH (1981) Pathogenesis of subacute combined degeneration. Lancet 2:1109

Romeo G, Menozzi P, Ferlini A, et al. (1983) Incidence of Friedreich's ataxia in Italy estimated from consanguinous marriages. Am J Hum Genet 35:523–529

Salisachs P (1974) La historia natural de la enfermedad de Friedreich. A proposito de 13 casos. Med Clin 63:1–10

Satya-Murti S, Cacace A, Hanson P (1980) Auditory dysfunction in Friedreich ataxia: result of spinal ganglion degeneration. Neurology 30:1047–1053

Scott E (1960) The prevalence of pernicious anaemia in Great Britain. J Coll Gen Pract Research Newsletter 3:80–84

Sedgewick RP, Boder E (1972) Ataxia-telangiectasia. In: Vinken PJ, Bruyn GW (eds) Handbook of clinical neurology vol 14. North-Holland, Amsterdam, pp 267–339

Shorvon SD, Carney MWP, Chanarin I, Reynolds EH (1980) The neuropsychiatry of megaloblastic anaemia. Br Med J 281:1036–1039

Smith ADM (1960) Megaloblastic madness. Br Med J 2:1840–1845

Sobrevilla LA, Goodman ML, Kane CA (1964) Demyelinating central nervous system disease, macular atrophy and acanthocytosis (Bassen-Kornzweig syndrome). Am J Med 37:821–828

Sokol RJ (1988) Vitamin E deficiency and neurologic disease. Ann Rev Nutr 8:351–373

Trouillas P, Garde A, Robert JM, et al. (1982) Regression du syndrome cerebellaux sous administration à long terme 5-HTP ou de l'association 5-HTP-benserazide. Rev Neurol (Paris) 138:415–435

Tyrer JH (1975) Friedreich's ataxia. In: Vinken PJ, Bruyn GW (eds) Handbook of clinical neurology vol 21. North-Holland, Amsterdam, pp 319–364

Tyrer JH, Sutherland JM (1961) The primary spinocerebellar atrophies and their associated defects, with a study of the foot deformity. Brain 84:289–300

Victor M, Lear AA (1956) Subacute combined degeneration of the spinal cord. Am J Med 20:896–918

Walton JN (1987) Brain's diseases of the nervous system 9th edn. Oxford University Press, Oxford

Wichman A, Buchthal F, Pezershkpour GH, Gregg RE (1985) Peripheral neuropathy in abetalipoproteinaemia. Neurology 35:1279–1289

Chapter 21

Vertebral Body Collapse

J.P.R. Dick

Vertebral collapse is not an uncommon finding post mortem, present in 20%–30% of autopsies when sought (Fornasier and Czitrom 1978; Sartoris et al. 1986) and may be due to many aetiologies. In general, collapse of the anterior structures of the vertebral body is due either to infection or neoplasm, usually metastatic, or to a more generalized process causing osteopenia, e.g. metabolic, neoplastic or inflammatory disorders. In these conditions minor trauma may finally precipitate vertebral fracture. Involvement of the posterior vertebral structures by infection (Roberts 1988) or neoplasia is uncommon as metastatic disease usually involves the vascular tufts just deep to the end plate (Waldvogel et al. 1970). Inflammatory involvement of the facet joints is not uncommon, particularly in rheumatoid disease, but rarely causes vertebral collapse.

Pathology

In a study of 659 consecutive autopsies from a general hospital and a hospital specializing in the treatment of cancer, Fornasier and Czitrom (1978) found 133 spines with vertebral collapse: an incidence of 17.3% from the general hospital and 24% from the cancer hospital. Using radiographic and histologic techniques they studied from T3 downwards and found 372 collapsed vertebrae; the thoracic spine was involved twice as often as the lumbar spine and the most commonly involved vertebrae were T12 and T6, the least frequently T3 and T4. Of the 133 involved spines, 75 cases had cancer and 58 cases did not; malignant disease is over-represented as 70% of cases of vertebral collapse were due to benign disease in the series of Sartoris et al. (1986). In half of the 58 cases of non-malignant disease collapse was considered to be due primarily to osteoporosis and in two there was histologic evidence of osteomalacia. In the remainder, collapse was due to serious degenerative disc disease with end plate erosion and collapse; this tended to be in the lumbar spine. End plate erosion is more common in rheumatological conditions such as rheumatoid arthritis (RA) than in purely degenerative conditions such as osteoarthritis (Heywood and Meyers 1986) but as the latter is so common it tends to account for a high proportion of cases.

Rheumatic diseases (RA, Still's disease, ankylosing spondylitis), developmental conditions (Scheuermann's disease, spondylolisthesis) and traumatic vertebral body collapse are dealt with elsewhere in this book. Here we shall deal with collapse due to osteopenia, neoplasia and vertebral osteomyelitis.

Radiological Features

Typically, benign osteopenic conditions show a generalized decrease in bone density with a tendency for vertebral collapse in the low thoracic spine; collapse associated with severe disc disease tends to occur in the lumbar spine. Apart from erosion of a single pedicle, which has a high degree of specificity for neoplasia, the radiological features of malignant collapse are non-specific. In most cases there are multiple osseous deposits which are lytic with or without sclerotic margins, though certain tumours provoke a sclerotic response. As sclerosis around end plate deformities can occur in healing fractures the presence of excess osteoblastic or even excess osteoclastic activity, as seen in osteitis fibrosa cystica, is non-specific.

To establish criteria which might reliably differentiate benign from malignant collapse Sartoris et al. (1986) studied 300 nearly consecutive routine autopsies. They found vertebral collapse in 99 spines, 30 due to neoplastic disease and 69 due to benign metabolic bone disease (osteoporosis, osteomalacia, osteitis fibrosa cystica). They found that neither disc space narrowing nor diffuse involvement of the end plate region reliably differentiated between benign and malignant groups whereas the presence of angled end plates which occurred in 64% of malignant cases but in less than 25% of benign cases ($P < 0.001$) was useful in differentiating these aetiologies. A benign collapse was predicted by anterior wedging of the vertebral bodies at T6–7 or by vertebral collapse with an even concavity of both superior and inferior end plates in a low thoracic vertebra (cod fish vertebra). This is likely to occur in osteopenic spines that have normal intervertebral discs as the major mechanical forces of body weight are transmitted through the axis of the vertebral body (apex of the concavity) where the end plate tends to be more porous due to the presence of the nucleus pulposus (Schmorl and Junghanns 1971). In some cases of benign disease more angulated end plates were explicable by recent local trauma.

Metabolic Bone Disease

Osteoporosis is the commonest metabolic disorder associated with vertebral collapse though its coexistence with osteomalacia or hyperparathyroidism should be considered (Fornasier and Czitrom 1978). Radiological features of osteitis fibrosa cystica are seen better in the hands than in the spine but over the last 50 years the pattern of bone disease in primary hyperparathyroidism has changed. The more commonly encountered picture is of diffuse osteopenia similar to osteoporosis though less homogeneous; this disorder is associated with vertebral collapse (Fairney 1983). Rarely, Paget's disease of bone (osteitis deformans) may cause compression of the spinal cord or nerve roots though involvement of the skull is more usual (Fairney 1983)

Osteoporosis may be defined as a decrease in bone mass and strength leading to an increase in fractures, particularly of vertebral bodies, proximal femur and distal radius (Raisz 1988). This propensity to fracture requires trauma for its full expression and the wide variety of hormonal influences that are thought to be involved with the pathogenesis of osteoporosis may well also influence a patient's strength and stability (Raisz 1988). It is rare to develop myelopathic features consequent to osteoporotic collapse.

Osteoporosis is commoner in women than men, in white or asians than blacks and becomes more prevalent with age in both sexes, being particularly related to the female menopause. It may be reversed by the administration of oestrogens in women and is probably related to insufficient levels of androgen and testosterone in men as it is more prevalent in hypogonadal males. It has been associated with a wide range of endocrine disorders (hyperthyroidism, hypercortisolism, acromegaly, hyperprolactinaemia) as well as with disordered homeostasis of calcium and vitamin D. Surprisingly, osteoporosis is not directly correlated with abnormal parathormone (PTH) activity or vitamin D status (1,25 dihydroxyvitamin D). Serum concentrations of bioactive PTH increase with age but the levels are not correlated with decreased bone mass (Raisz 1988) and although a primary excess of PTH is associated with an increase of long bone fractures (Raisz 1988) it is not associated with an increased incidence of vertebral fractures (Raisz 1988). Serum levels of 1,25 dihydroxyvitamin D decrease with age and patients with vertebral crush fractures have lower mean levels than age-matched normals; however, the values are not particularly low and are within the normal range. In addition, although older patients have decreased intestinal absorption of calcium, and the administration of 1,25 dihydroxyvitamin D can reverse this abnormality, it does not reverse osteoporosis.

Osteomalacia typically presents with bone pain, often in the back and may be associated with a cod fish spine on X-ray. The differential diagnosis from osteoporosis may be difficult, if routine testing of calcium homeostasis is not abnormal, and may require bone biopsy. A wide variety of conditions predispose to osteomalacia (e.g. dietary deficiency, malabsorption, anticonvulsant medication, chronic renal diseases and chronic liver disease especially following transplantation); often osteoporosis and osteomalacia coexist (Fairney 1983).

Cancer

Primary

Of the three common primary malignant tumours of bone (myeloma, osteosarcoma and Ewing's sarcoma), only myeloma typically affects the spine. Osteosarcoma and Ewing's sarcoma affect the metaphyseal areas of long bones (Schajowicz and Araujo 1983). Myeloma has a particular propensity to affect the spine where it may cause diffuse osteopenia and vertebral collapse or cause epidural compression due to florid focal activity.

Secondary

Pathology

The skeleton, and in particular the vertebral column, is the third commonest site for distant metastases after lung and liver (Boland et al. 1982). This conclusion is based on autopsy data which may underestimate the real incidence of bony metastases (BMs) as it is rare to examine all vertebrae (Fornasier and Czitrom 1978). Jaffe's study (1958) showed that of all patients with cancer, 70% had BMs, 30% had clinically evident BMs, 10% had resulting pathological fractures and 5% had developed a compressive myelopathy. The commonest site for BMs was the thoracic spine and the body of each vertebra was more often affected than were the arches or spines (Boland et al. 1982). Radiological assessment tends also to underestimate the true incidence of BMs as 50% of trabecular bone must be destroyed before loss is discernible by conventional radiographic techniques (Edelestyn et al. 1967). Management of spinal cord compression due to malignant disease poses a significant problem as a one-year survival rate of 30% is not unusual (Gilbert et al. 1978) and preventing the inevitable myelopathy which occurs if left untreated has been difficult.

The commonest tumour types encountered have been breast, bronchus and lymphoma (Gilbert et al. 1978; Boland et al. 1982) though other tumours have a predilection for the spine (e.g. myeloma and prostatic carcinoma). Tumours of the gastrointestinal (GI) tract are seen more frequently than expected as they are common tumours. Gilbert et al. (1978) analysed 235 patients with surgically managed spinal cord compression due to malignant disease. They had been seen at the Memorial Sloan Kettering Cancer Center, New York over a nine-year period. Primary intraspinal tumours (sarcomata) accounted for 9% of cases and metastatic disease for the rest (breast 20%, lung 13%, lymphoma 11%, prostate 9%, kidney 7%, myeloma 4%, melanoma 3%, GI 4%, female reproductive tumour 2%, embryonal cell carcinoma 2%, neuroblastoma 2%). Sixty-eight per cent of tumours were in the thoracic spine though this figure was skewed by the high incidence of breast metastases. In none of their cases did they report intramedullary deposits; these are 20 times less common than epidural deposits (Edelson et al. 1972).

Tumours of breast and bronchus metastasize preferentially to the spine (Gilbert et al. 1978) and this may be related to the system of valveless vertebral veins which communicate with intercostal and lumbar veins (Batson 1940). This anatomical feature is well recognized in the pelvis and accounts for the high incidence of vertebral metastases from prostatic carcinoma but also accounts for the high incidence of thoracic vertebral metastases from breast carcinoma (Fornasier and Czitrom 1978). It has been suggested that marantic emboli enter the vertebral venous system, particularly during periods of raised intra-abdominal pressure, such as coughing. This has been demonstrated experimentally by the injection of rat femoral veins with malignant cells where normally 100% of metastases are pulmonary; with 15–60 seconds light abdominal pressure vertebral metastases become frequent (Coman and Delong 1951).

Clinical Presentation

Osteoporotic collapse in the thoracic spine may be asymptomatic but pathological fractures typically present with severe local pain. This was seen in 92% of patients in one series (Gilbert et al. 1978). It was constant, exacerbated by coughing or sneezing and was noticed particularly when rolling over in bed at night. Metastases in the cervical (72%) or lumbar spine (90%) were more commonly associated with a radiculopathy than those in the thoracic spine (55%) and the site of the pain usually localized the tumour accurately (Gilbert et al. 1978). Radiculopathy in the thoracic spine tended to be bilateral. Occasionally, pain was more diffuse (32%) but passive neck manipulation (cervical tumours), local percussion (thoracic tumours) and straight leg raising (lumbosacral tumours) helped localize the site of the lesion clinically.

Myelopathy developed after the onset of pain in all but two of this series; however, only 77% complained of weakness at presentation. Sensory and autonomic features developed subsequently, being present at the initial examination in 51% and 57% respectively. Gait ataxia, an unusual clinical manifestation, was seen in 9% of cases and was the main presenting complaint, in the absence of sensory or motor features, in two patients (Gilbert et al. 1978).

Plain radiographs of the spine may be normal at a time when a bone scan is abnormal but usually they show an absent pedicle and a mixture of lytic and sclerotic lesions; myeloma, lymphoma or highly anaplastic tissue may be predominantly lytic while Hodgkin's disease, prostatic carcinoma and carcinoid may be predominantly sclerotic. A bone scan shows multiple deposits in 90% of cases. In the presence of a myelopathy further investigation either by myelography and CT or by MRI is essential. The latter is non-invasive, shows the entire length of the vertebral canal clearly and demonstrates mild epidural disease (Smoker et al. 1987); when compared with myelography/CT it provided additional information in 13 of 22 patients.

Treatment

Management of these patients has been disappointing and several treatment regimes have been tried. The most important criterion defining outcome has been the extent of neurological deficit at presentation and the speed of appropriate referral (Findlay 1984). In the series of Gilbert et al. (1978), 15% of cases were paraplegic at the time of diagnosis, half of whom had a precipitate course. In none of these was a haemorrhagic tumour found at operation, none improved after surgery and it was assumed that cord infarction had occurred. It is therefore important to initiate therapy as early as possible (Greenberg et al. 1980).

Establishing that vertebral collapse is due to a malignant condition and not due to a metabolic bone disease or infective osteomyelitis may require biopsy. This can be done via a percutaneous route in the absence of cord compromise. However, if vertebral collapse is associated with a myelopathy, then a more aggressive approach is indicated. There was a vogue for decompressive laminectomy but the results of this approach proved singularly disappointing (Findlay 1984). Brice and McKissock (1965) noted that no patient with a severe neurological deficit and vertebral collapse improved after laminectomy and Findlay (1987) analysing 37 patients with a myelopathy due to malignant vertebral collapse found that laminectomy was associated with a significant neurological deterioration in 18 and an improvement in one. Laminectomy has therefore fallen into disfavour and other treatment regimes have evolved. Based on experimental work in the rodent, Posner's group in New York initiated treatment with radiotherapy alone (Ushio et al. 1977). After an initial phase of pulsed, high-dose dexamethasone therapy which substantially ameliorated pain, they gave an initially intense burst of local radiotherapy followed a few days later by a maintenance course. Their results were slightly better than those from surgery and radiotherapy and as a result radiotherapy alone became the standard treatment for metastatic disease of the spine. However, occasionally surgical therapy is still necessary for tissue diagnosis or in the face of clinical deterioration despite radiotherapy. As spinal instability had occurred following posterior surgical approaches and recalling experience from the management of chronic osteomyelitis, anterior decompression with or without stabilization was investigated (Siegal and Seigal 1985; Moore and Uttley 1989). Although there was a 30% postoperative mortality from the chest complications of thoracotomy (pneumonia and pulmonary emboli) the ability to walk returned in one series for 10 of 16 patients who could not walk preoperatively. This improvement was maintained till death an average of 7 months later (Moore and Uttley 1989).

Infection

Pyogenic Osteomyelitis

Osteomyelitis develops following septicaemia and tends to involve two adjacent vertebrae. This is due to the embryological origin of the arterial supply; a single segmental artery supplies the lower half of one vertebra and the upper half of the next vertebra. As a result, disc space narrowing is common and disc involvement not unusual. This radiographic finding is important in differentiating osteomyelitis from malignant collapse.

It is commoner in children than adults (Waldvogel et al. 1970); however, bacterial seeding in this group is to the actively growing ends of long bones. In one study there was involvement of the femur or humerus in 63%, the tibia in 19% and the vertebrae in 19% (Waldvogel et al. 1970). A bimodal age distribution was observed in this study, the first peak in childhood and a second peak in the sixth decade; patients in the second peak had vertebral osteomyelitis. Seeding in these cases seems to be to the richly vascularized bone of the vertebral end plates (Waldvogel and Vasey 1980).

Patients complain of constant spinal pain, exacerbated by mechanical manoeuvres, that has been present for weeks or months. Although they may be afebrile with a normal peripheral white blood cell count, the ESR is usually markedly elevated, particularly in pyogenic infections (Harris 1983). Plain radiographs of the spine may be unhelpful as several weeks are necessary before bone changes are seen in vertebral osteomyelitis though radionuclide bone scanning is more effective in the early detection of bony lesions (Boland et al. 1982).

An unequivocal source of infection is found in 40% of cases with pyogenic and mycobacterial infection. This is slightly less than in acute spinal epidural abscess, and has a different topography (Ross and Fleming 1976). This is, in order of frequency, the genitourinary tract, the skin and the respiratory tract. *Staphylococcus aureus* is again the commonest organism accounting for 60% of identified cases but Enterobacteriaceae are more prominent than in acute spinal epidural abscess (Sapico and Montgomerie 1979; Waldvogel and Vasey 1980) and in the vertebral osteomyelitis of drug abusers gram-negative aerobic bacilli account for 92% of infections (Sapico and Montgomerie 1980). *Pseudomonas* species have been observed most commonly in heroin addicts (Kaufman et al. 1980; Waldvogel and Vasey 1980). Occasionally unusual organisms are encountered. For example, *Brucella abortus* is a well-recognized cause of subacute, pyogenic vertebral osteomyelitis in the Middle East and 12% of cases develop signs of cord compression (Harris 1983), and fungal species may affect patients with diabetes, impaired immunity or those who abuse intravenous drugs. Fungal osteomyelitis occurs in less than 1% of patients with candidaemia and has a predilection for the spine (Harmon 1984).

Untreated, the osteitis leads to vertebral collapse and angulation; infection may spread to involve the intervertebral disc, rare in neoplastic vertebral collapse and, if partially treated, may lead to chronic osteomyelitis which is associated with anaemia, secondary amyloidosis and progressive deformity.

Confirmation that vertebral collapse is due to infection requires tissue and in the absence of neurological phenomena this may be undertaken by needle biopsy of the infected vertebra. Bed rest and antibiotics while monitoring spinal pain and the ESR are the mainstays of therapy for acute vertebral osteomyelitis and, as cortical bone is thin, sequestrum formation is uncommon in pyogenic osteomyelitis (Harris 1983). As a result surgical management is rarely necessary. If chronic osteomyelitis develops or it becomes necessary surgically to debride necrotic tissue, which may serve as a persistent source of infection, an anterior approach is used though fixation by bone graft is usually unnecessary (Harris 1983).

Vertebral Osteomyelitis Due to Tuberculosis

The spine is involved in about 50% of patients with bone and joint tuberculosis and is complicated by kyphoscoliosis which may lead to respiratory difficulties, and by paraplegia (Harris 1983). It is commoner in young adults and in the third world. Paraplegia occurs in about 20% of patients with spinal tuberculosis (Tuli 1975). It is associated with a greater tendency to local spread, e.g. psoas abscess, sinus formation and epidural abscess (Kaufman et al. 1980). Paraplegia may be either early when it is related to an expanding mass of infective tissue, or late when either the infection has been rekindled or chronic deformity has caused slowly progressive damage due to mechanical factors. Paraplegia due to the latter cause tends to respond poorly to surgical intervention though some improvement even after two years of paraplegia may occur. The best results are seen with anterior decompression and fixation by bone grafts or mechanical prostheses (MRC 1982).

References

Batson OV (1940) The function of the vertebral veins and their role in the spread of metastases. Ann Surg 112:138

Boland PJ, Lane JM, Sunderesan N (1982) Metastatic disease of the spine. Clin Orthop 169:95–102

Brice J, McKissock W (1965) Surgical treatment of malignant extradural spinal tumours. Br Med J i:1341–1344

Coman DR, Delong RP (1951) The role of the vertebral venous system in metastasis of cancer to the spinal column: experiments with tumour cell suspensions in rats and rabbits. Cancer 4: 610–618

Edelestyn GA, Gillespie PJ, Grebbell FS (1967) The radiological demonstration of osseous metastases: experimental observations. Clin Radiol 18:158–162

Edelson RN, Deck MDF, Posner JB (1972) Intramedullary spinal cord metastases: clinical and radiographic findings in 9 cases. Neurology 22:1222–1231

Fairney A (1983) Metabolic bone disease. In: Harris NH (ed) Postgraduate textbook of clinical orthopaedics. Wright and sons, Bristol, pp 307–338

Findlay GFG (1984) Adverse effects of the management of malignant spinal cord compression. J Neurol Neurosurg Psychiatry 47:761–768

Findlay GFG (1987) The role of vertebral body collapse in the management of malignant spinal cord compression. J Neurol Neurosurg Psychiatry 50:151–154

Fornasier VL, Czitrom AA (1978) Collapsed vertebrae a review of 659 autopsies. Clin Orthop 131:261–265

Gilbert RN, Kim JH, Posner JB (1978) Epidural spinal cord compression from metastatic tumour: diagnosis and treatment. Ann Neurol 3:40–51

Greenberg HS, Kim JH, Posner JB (1980) Epidural spinal cord compression from metastatic tumour: results with a new treatment protocol. Ann Neurol 8:361–366

Harmon DC (1984) Case records of the Massachussets General Hospital. N Engl J Med 311:455–462

Harris NH (1983) Bone and joint infections In: Harris NH (ed) Postgraduate textbook of clinical orthopaedics. Wright and sons, Bristol, pp 339–396

Heywood AWB, Meyers OL (1986) Rheumatoid arthritis of the thoracic and lumbar spine. J Bone Joint Surg 68B:362–368

Jaffe WL (1958) Tumors and tumorous conditions of bones and joints. Lea and Febiger, Philadelphia

Kaufman DM, Kaplan JG, Litman N (1980) Infectious agents in spinal epidural abscesses. Neurology 30:844–850

Medical Research Council working party on tuberculosis of the spine (1982) A 10 year assessment of a controlled trial comparing debridement and anterior spinal fusion in the management of tuberculosis of the spine in patients on standard chemotherapy in Hong Kong. J Bone Joint Surg 64B:393–401

Moore AJ, Uttley D (1989) Anterior decompression and stabilization of the spine in malignant disease. Neurosurgery 24:713–717

Raisz LG (1988) Local and systemic factors in the pathogenesis of osteoporosis. N Engl J Med 318:818–828

Roberts WA (1988) Pyogenic vertebral osteomyelitis of a lumbar facet joint with associated epidural abscess: a case report with a review of the literature. Spine 13:948–952

Ross PM, Fleming J (1976) Vertebral body osteomyelitis: spectrum and natural history, a retrospective study of 37 cases. Clin Orthop 118:190–198

Sapico FL, Montgomerie JZ (1979) Pyogenic vertebral osteomyelitis: report of nine cases and a review of the literature. Rev Infect Dis 1:754–776

Sapico FL, Montgomerie JZ (1980) Vertebral osteomyelitis in intravenous drug abusers: report of three cases and review of the literature. Rev Infect Dis 2:196–206

Sartoris DJ, Clopton P, Nemcek A, Dowd C, Resnick D (1986) Vertebral collapse in focal and diffuse disease: patterns of pathologic processes. Radiology 160:479–483

Schajowicz F, Araujo EH (1983) Cysts and tumours of the musculoskeletal system. In: Harris NH (ed) Postgraduate textbook of clinical orthopaedics. Wright and sons, Bristol, pp 605–639

Schmorl G, Junghanns H (1971) The human spine in health and disease, 2nd edn. EF Bersemann trans. Grune and Stratton, New York

Siegal T, Seigal T (1985) Surgical decompression of anterior and posterior malignant epidural tumours compressing the spinal cord. Neurosurgery 17:424–432

Smoker WR, Godersky JC, Knutzon R, Keyes WD, Norman D, Bergman W (1987) The role of MR imaging in evaluating metastatic spinal disease. AJR 149:1241

Tuli SM (1975) Results of treatment of spinal tuberculosis by "middle path" regime. Br J Surg 169:29

Ushio Y, Posner R, Kim JH, Shapiro WR, Posner JB (1977) Treatment of experimental spinal cord compression by extradural neoplasms. J Neurosurg 47:380–390

Waldvogel FA, Vasey H (1980) Osteomyelitis: the past decade. N Engl J Med 303:360–370

Waldvogel FA, Medoff G, Swartz MN (1970) Osteomyelitis: a review of clinical features, therapeutic considerations and unusual aspects. N Engl J Med 282:198–206 and 316–322

Chapter 22

Spinal Epidural Abscess

J.P.R. Dick

In an editorial describing his clinical experience of spinal epidural abscess, Heusner (1948) reminds us that "... the decisive factor in the outcome of most cases is the celerity with which the first physician suspects the probable nature of the ailment and summons expert aid". On pathological grounds he recognized three presentations: (1) an acute metastatic presentation which evolves over hours to days and where the epidural abscess cavity contains frankly purulent material; (2) a subacute presentation evolving over days to weeks where the epidural abscess cavity comprises granulation tissue without significant quantities of necrotic material; (3) a chronic presentation, most often associated with osteomyelitis. The last accounted for only 10% of his series and involved a broader differential diagnosis.

Anatomy

Infection is usually confined to the adipose tissue of the dorsal epidural space between the ligamenta flava where there is a rich venous plexus (Batson 1940). Thoracic and lumbar sites are equally represented in most series, cervical sites being less frequent but may be seen in those who abuse intravenous drugs. Infection usually extends vertically over 4–5 vertebral segments and may become circumferential, reaching the anterior epidural compartment in the lumbar region. Early reports commented on the rarity of extension to the anterior epidural space but Danner and Hartman (1987) have observed several patients with anterior epidural collections following low back surgery; they attributed this to the increased space available at this level. The dura mater limits the further spread of sepsis and subdural abscesses are unusual (Fraser et al. 1973; D'Angelo and Whisler 1978). Autopsy studies fail to show substantial compression of the cord and histological examination shows pan-necrosis with little or no inflammatory response suggesting infarction rather than infection (Hassin 1928); this mechanism probably accounts for the precipitate course of the myelopathy. Epidural infection will spread to the paravertebral muscles or subcutaneous tissues if left untreated (Dandy 1926).

Clinical Presentation

Acute Metastatic Epidural Abscess

This is the commonest syndrome in most series (Heusner 1948; Hancock 1973; Baker et al. 1975; Danner and Hartman 1987) and requires the greatest speed of clinical response. Several authors describe a typical clinical progression though errors of initial diagnosis are not infrequent (Baker et al. 1975; Heusner 1948; Hancock 1973; Danner and Hartman 1987). The patient presents with exquisite localized back pain associated with tenderness to percussion; in 2 of 39 cases reported by Baker et al. (1975) its severity was great enough to be associated with a florid behavioural syndrome leading, erroneously, to a psychiatric diagnosis. Epidural abscesses in the lumbar region are not infrequently associated with severe local and radicular pain but little neurological symptomatology (Adams and Victor 1989) and can be confused with musculoskeletal pain or disc prolapse. However, the presence of headache with neck stiffness and the systemic signs of sepsis, such as an elevated temperature, ESR and peripheral white blood cell count should help differentiate these conditions. Other alternative diagnoses have been recorded, particularly intraabdominal sepsis and transverse myelitis (Findlay 1987). The latter usually prompts urgent radiological investigation and is not often as painful as an epidural collection of pus nor is it associated with such striking local tenderness. Although severe abdominal pain and the systemic features of sepsis may simulate an intra-abdominal abscess, abdominal examination usually differentiates an epidural from an intra-abdominal abscess. By the second or third day of the illness, a recognizable clinical syndrome will have evolved with radicular pain in the absence of a vesicular rash and root signs. It is at this stage that investigation (radiological and bacteriological) should be undertaken urgently.

Plain radiographs of the spine are usually normal though disc space narrowing may be seen, helping to differentiate malignant epidural disease, and urgent myelography should be undertaken. Since infection is usually confined to the dorsal epidural space, spinal puncture may be hazardous and is best undertaken by the radiologist. This will usually be done via a lateral cervical route so as to avoid spinal coning and the introduction of bacteria into the subdural compartment; however, one can puncture the abscess directly as a therapeutic measure. There is usually a complete block to the flow of dye at the upper border of the abscess and in order to delineate the lower limit of the abscess, a second spinal puncture may be necessary. However, in view of the risks and the difficulty of such a puncture in a patient with rigid paraspinal muscles, contrast enhanced CT and MR imaging are currently the preferred methods of investigation (Angutaco et al. 1987). CSF is abnormal and this will help differentiate an epidural abscess from osteomyelitis. Typically there is an elevated protein concentration with a modest lymphocytic pleocytosis and a normal sugar. If the sugar is depressed an associated meningitis should be suspected.

Once the diagnosis has been made, neurosurgical intervention should be undertaken for bacteriological confirmation and to avoid clinical progression. This may occur after a few days when the patient suddenly will develop an ascending paralysis with double incontinence. The interval between presentation and the onset of myelopathy in Hancock's series (1973) of 49 patients ranged from 1–23 days. This change may be precipitous and once spinal cord damage has occurred it tends to be irreversible. Even with the most recent management criteria (Danner and Hartman 1987), only 6 of 20 patients with limb weakness at presentation made a complete recovery.

Although the mainstay of therapy is an adequate course of antibiotics, cure of an epidural abscess can rarely be achieved without surgical drainage (Findlay 1987). As the main collection of infected tissue is likely to be posterior, laminectomy is usually performed with antiseptic irrigation of the adjacent segments by soft catheter. There is debate as to whether the wound should be closed with or without drainage. For pan-spinal abscesses it may be necessary to perform two small laminectomies, one in the cervical and one in the lumbar areas (Findlay 1987).

The acute presentation is most frequently associated with haematogenous spread of infection from a distant focus, such as a furuncle, wound infection or decubitus ulcer, though in 40% of cases no source can be identified (Danner and Hartman 1987). Characteristically, the causative organism is *Staphylococcus aureus* which can be grown from blood cultures. In 40% of cases blood cultures are negative and culture from the abscess cavity is required for bacteriological confirmation.

Danner and Hartman (1987) point out that the incidence of spinal epidural abscesses in New York City has increased from 0.18/100000 during the period 1971–1973 to 2.8/100000 for the calendar year 1982. They suggest that this is not only due to the greater prevalence of intravenous drug abuse but also to the greater frequency of invasive medical procedures. A wide variety of organisms causing spinal epidural abscess have been recorded (*Staphylococcus aureus* 103/166, aerobic streptococci 14/166, aerobic gram-negative rods 30/166, anaerobic organisms 3/166, *Staphylococcus epidermidis* 4/166) (Danner and Hartman 1987). These infections are seen more usually in the immunosuppressed population and often present subacutely. In addition, *Staphylococcus aureus* is no longer the sole infecting organism as was the case in Heusner's series (1948) and they suggest that it would be prudent, pending further bacteriological data, to give antibiotic cover for gram-negative organisms and *Staphylococcus epidermidis* (Danner and Hartman 1987).

Subacute Osteomyelitic Epidural Abscess

This syndrome is more variable than the acute syndrome, is seen in the immunocompromised, in the diabetic and in the partially treated. The course may be protracted and merge with the chronic syndrome or may progress over two weeks merging with the acute syndrome. Baker et al. (1975) make no distinction between acute and subacute presentations. They defined as chronic all those with abscesses whose centres were non-purulent. These patients all had symptoms in excess of two weeks.

Although such patients usually present with spinal and radicular pain, and with signs suggestive of radicular and cord disease (Phillips and Jefferson 1979), diagnostic difficulties are frequent. In their series Danner and Hartman (1987) note that, due to a toxic confusional state, several patients failed to give any history of back pain while in others spinal tenderness was minimal (see also Hancock 1973); thus 64% of patients had no neurologic deficit on admission and in 15 of 35 cases the initial diagnosis was unrelated to the spine. In the series reported by Baker et al. (1975) 10 of 39 patients had an initial diagnosis unrelated to the back though 34 of 39 had root signs. One can anticipate difficulty in confused patients in whom there are no clinical or radiographic findings and in drug abusers, whose only symptom may be pain, whose only sign a mild pyrexia, and from whom a history may be unreliable. Koppel et al. (1988) describe their experience with this group of patients: they tend to have prolonged histories (1–2 months), prominent pain and little fever. As is seen in other series (Kaufman et al. 1980) there is a slight excess of patients with recent back trauma which may confound the issue. Whether the increase in incidence of epidural sepsis is due to impaired host immunity or due to the introduction of infection by frequent needling is not clear; the former is likely as there is an undue prevalence of cervical osteomyelitis in heroin abusers (Sapico and Montgomerie 1980). In Koppel's series only 2 of 18 were HIV positive whereas 13 of 18 were due to *Staphylococcus aureus* (Koppel et al. 1988). The bacteriology is similar to that seen in individuals with normal immunity (Heusner 1948) though different from that seen in the vertebral osteomyelitis of drug abusers (Sapico and Montgomerie 1980) where gram-negative aerobic bacilli account for 92% of infections.

Plain radiographs are more helpful in this group and may show disc space narrowing or end plate erosion though the latter is best appreciated on tomography. Radionuclide scanning can be helpful in locating the site of the abscess and its extra axial extent (Koppel et al. 1988) but urgent myelography with CT scanning and MR imaging remain the investigations of choice (Berns et al. 1989). Once epidural infection has been demonstrated surgical decompression is necessary.

Chronic Epidural Abscess

This syndrome usually complicates pyogenic vertebral osteomyelitis (Findlay 1987) or tuberculous epidural cord compression (Kaufman et al. 1980). However, only 17% of patients with osteomyelitis develop neurological phenomena. This figure is similar for pyogenic osteomyelitis (Sapico and Montgomerie 1979), infection due to *Mycobacterium tuberculosis* (Waldvogel and Vasey 1980) and vertebral osteomyelitis in drug abusers (Sapico and Montgomerie 1980). By contrast, of patients with acute or subacute presentation, less than 35% had radiographic features suggestive of vertebral osteomyelitis (Baker et al. 1975; Danner and Hartman 1987).

The duration of history is usually more than 6 weeks (Heusner 1948; Kaufman et al. 1980) and patients may be relatively asymptomatic; however, once neurological complications have started they may proceed rapidly (Kaufman et al. 1980). Autopsy studies suggest thrombotic infarction of the cord occurs in these circumstances. If vertebral osteomyelitis is left untreated, osteitis may spread to involve the intervertebral disc, or the patient may develop vertebral collapse and kyphotic angulation. Waldvogel and Vasey (1980) suggest that neurological involvement in patients with tuberculous spondylitis is due to mechanical problems rather than epidural infection.

Confirmation of diagnosis requires tissue and in the absence of neurological phenomena this may be undertaken by needle biopsy of the infected vertebra; however, if epidural disease is evident, surgical intervention is usually necessary. Bed rest and antibiotics while monitoring spinal pain and the ESR are the mainstays of therapy for vertebral osteomyelitis. With neurological involvement, usually consequent to anterior epidural disease, anterior decompression with debridement is current practice; fixation is rarely necessary (Harris 1983) unless associated with tuberculous spondylitis (MRC 1982).

References

Adams RD, Victor M (1989) Principles of neurology, 4th edn. McGraw-Hill, New York, pp 168 and 728

Angutaco EJC, McConnell JR, Chadduck WM, Flanigan S (1987) MR imaging of spinal epidural sepsis. AJR 149:1249–1253

Baker AS, Ojemann RG, Swartz MN, Richardson EP (1975) Spinal epidural abscess. N Engl J Med 293:463–468

Batson OV (1940) The function of the vertebral veins and their role in the spread of metastases. Ann Surg 112:138

Berns DH, Blaser SJ, Modic MT (1989) Magnetic resonance imaging of the spine. Clin Orthop 244:78–100

Dandy WE (1926) Abscesses and inflammatory tumours in the spinal epidural space (so-called pachymeningitis externa). Arch Surg 13:477–494

D'Angelo CM, Whisler WW (1978) Bacterial infection of the spinal cord and its coverings. In: Vinken PJ, Bruyn GW, Klawans HL (eds) Handbook of clinical neurology 33:187–194

Danner RL, Hartman BJ (1987) Update of epidural spinal abscess: 35 cases and a review of the literature. Rev Infect Dis 9:265–274

Findlay GFG (1987) Compression and vascular disorders of the spinal cord. In: Miller JD (ed) Northfields surgery of the central nervous system. Blackwell Scientific, Oxford, pp 745–748

Fraser RAR, Ratzan K, Wolpert SM, Weinstein L (1973) Spinal subdural empyema. Arch Neurol 28:235–238

Hancock DO (1973) A study of 49 patients with acute spinal epidural abscess. Paraplegia 10:285–288

Harris NH (1983) Bone and joint infections. In: Harris NH (ed) Postgraduate textbook of clinical orthopaedics. Wright and sons, Bristol, pp 339–396

Hassin GB (1928) Circumscribed suppurative (non-tuberculous) peripachymeningitis. Arch Neurol Psychiatry 20:110–127

Heusner AP (1948) Non tuberculous spinal epidural infections. N Engl J Med 239:845–854

Kaufman DM, Kaplan JG, Litman N (1980) Infectious agents in spinal epidural abscesses. Neurology 30:844–850

Koppel BS, Tuchman AJ, Mangiardi JR, Daras M, Weitzner I (1988) Epidural spinal infection in drug abusers. Arch Neurol 45:1331–1337

Medical Research Council working party on tuberculosis of the spine (1982) A 10 year assessment of a controlled trial comparing debridement and anterior spinal fusion in the management of tuberculosis of the spine in patients on standard chemotherapy in Hong Kong. J Bone Joint Surg 64B:393–401

Phillips GE, Jefferson A (1979) Acute spinal epidural abscess. Observations from 14 cases. Postgrad Med J 55:712–715

Sapico FL, Montgomerie JZ (1979) Pyogenic vertebral osteomyelitis: report of nine cases and a review of the literature. Rev Infect Dis 1:754–776

Sapico FL, Montgomerie JZ (1980) Vertebral osteomyelitis in intravenous drug abusers: report of three cases and review of the literature. Rev Infect Dis 2:196–206

Waldvogel FA, Vasey H (1980) Osteomyelitis: the past decade. N Engl J Med 303:360–370

Chapter 23

Spinal Cord Compression and Spinal Cord Tumours

N.T. Gurusinghe

Surgical Anatomy

The spinal canal extends from the foramen magnum to the coccyx. The spinal intradural and subarachnoid compartments containing the neural elements end at the level of S2. The cord lies within these meningeal sleeves and in a normal adult, the conus medullaris tapers to an end at the L1/L2 intervertebral disc level. Below this the subarachnoid space is occupied by the filum terminale and the lumbosacral roots forming the cauda equina. (Fig. 23.1). At birth the cord terminates at L3 level, but due to differential growth rates of the cord and spinal column, the cord ascends to the adult position.

The cord measures 42–45 cm in men and is slightly shorter in women. It is divided into 31 functional units, but the segmentation is not externally recognizable except by the pairs of spinal roots emerging from each segment. There are 8 cervical, 12 thoracic, 5 lumbar, 5 sacral and 1 coccygeal segments. The diameter of the cord increases between C4 to T1 and L2 to S3 segments forming the cervical and lumbar enlargements supplying the innervation to the upper and lower extremities respectively.

As the spinal cord is shorter than the extent of the spinal canal, the cord segments are not situated opposite the corresponding vertebrae (Fig. 23.2). The spinous processes slope downwards especially in the dorsal region and their tips, as palpated by the surgeon externally, do not coincide with the plane of the corresponding vertebral body. The clinical examination will identify the level of the tumour according to the spinal segment(s) involved. The radiologist will identify the level of the lesion according to the vertebral body opposite the tumour. The discrepancy between the spinal segment, the vertebral body and the level of the spinous process is most significant in the dorsal region and must be considered carefully by the neurosurgeon attempting spinal tumour excision. It is sound practice to identify the spinous process of the vertebral level affected immediately preoperatively under radiological control and insert a needle percutaneously into this spinous process before moving the patient into the operating theatre.

A spinal nerve is formed by the union of an anterior (motor) and posterior (sensory) root within each intervertebral foramen. The roots are attached to the cord by a series of rootlets. The ganglion of the sensory root lies within the intervertebral foramen. The spinal nerves of C1 to C7 leave the vertebral canal

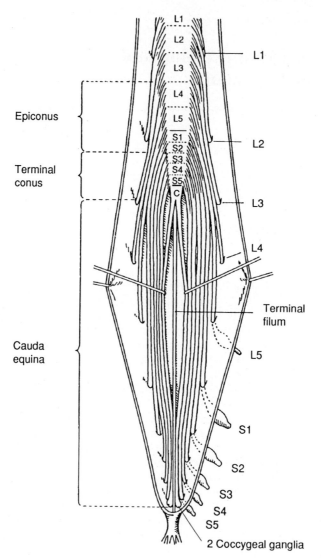

Fig. 23.1. Anatomy of epiconus, conus and cauda equina. (Reproduced with permission from Duus P, *Topical diagnosis in neurology*. Translation by R. Lindenberg, drawings by G. Spitzer. Georg Thieme Verlag 1989.)

rostral to the corresponding vertebrae, but all nerves from D1 downwards exist on the caudal side of the vertebral unit (Fig. 23.2). The recognition of spinal root dysfunction is of immense value in localization of a spinal lesion. Intradural tumours can arise from, or are related to spinal roots and malignant extradural lesions often irritate spinal nerves causing pain of radicular distribution.

The spinal canal is lined with a layer of extradural fat. Tumours occupying the canal can cause pressure necrosis and atrophy of the fat layers in that

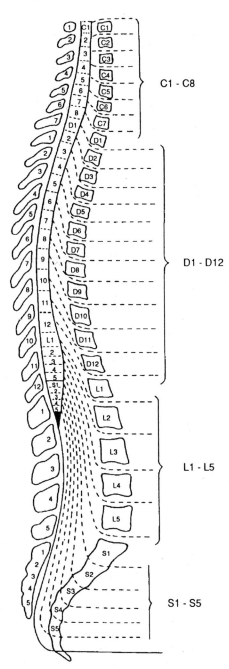

Fig. 23.2. Relationship of spinal root segments to vertebral bodies. (Reproduced with permission from Duus P, *Topical diagnosis in neurology*. Translation by R. Lindenberg, drawings by G. Spitzer. Georg Thieme Verlag 1989.)

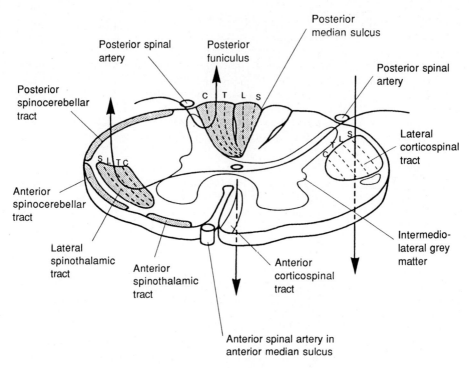

Fig. 23.3. Cross-section of spinal cord showing main ascending (shaded) and descending tracts and the somatopic arrangements in each tract.

region. This is a useful sign to the surgeon approaching a spinal tumour. Longitudinal, valveless venous channels lie in the extradural fat forming the internal vertebral plexus. They are in communication with the basivertebral plexus within the vertebral bodies and the pelvic veins as well as the superior vena cava. The internal vertebral plexus veins therefore communicate directly with the venous channels of the breast, thyroid and prostate gland. This fact may be significant in the dissemination of secondary cancer deposits to the vertebrae.

The spinal cord derives blood from the single anterior spinal artery and the pair of posterior spinal arteries (Fig. 23.3). Their rostral origin is from the vertebral arteries, and the three vessels have several communications with each other via circumferential branches around the cord and at their termination near the conus medullaris. The arterial input to these vessels is boosted at several points along their course by radicular arteries which arise from the vertebral artery, thyrocervical trunk as well as intercostal and lumbar arteries. These vessels will enter the spinal canal via the intervertebral foraminae. Of the 31 such pairs of arteries only 7 or 8 participate significantly in supplying blood to the cord. The other vessels supply only the roots and meninges. The radicular arteries reaching the cord along the ventral roots are larger (radiculomedullary arteries). The largest of these vessels usually entering the canal from the left between T12 and L2 is called the arteria radicula magna or artery of Adamkiewicz. This is an important vessel which boosts the blood supply even up to the upper dorsal region. The vascular dynamics of this arrangement creates watershed areas of relatively precarious blood supply. The most important of these is at D4 level which falls between the rostral subclavian supply and the caudal aortic contribution.

Radicular arteries must not be sacrificed at operation even when the root is divided. A tumour in the lower dorsal region may displace and occlude the arteria radicula magna causing a cord lesion as high as D4. The three main spinal arteries give off deep medullary branches which supply the grey and white matter of the cord. The anterior spinal arteries supply the anterior two-thirds of the cord while the posterior vessels provide blood to the posterior columns and the posterior horn of grey matter. An anteriorly placed spinal tumour may endanger the blood supply of the cord by compressing the anterior spinal artery. The wasting of the hand muscles seen in tumours of the foramen magnum may be due to ischaemia from a disturbance of the anterior spinal artery or a major radicular contributor thereof.

The pia mater envelops the cord closely and blends with the epineurium of nerve roots. At the conus it extends downwards as the filum terminale. A continuous lateral pial extension stretches between the cord and the dura at each spinal level. The intermittent dural attachment of this membrane on either side produces a scalloped edge and the tooth-like points of adhesion explain the term "ligamentum denticulatum". The anterior and posterior spinal roots pass on either side of the ligament to reach their intervertebral foramina. Since most neurinomas arise from the posterior spinal roots, these tumours are usually situated posterior to the dentate ligament. The ligament can be safely divided at its attachment to the dura during surgery and used as a means of gentle manipulation of the cord to gain access to the anterior spinal canal. The last dentate ligament is at the L1 level. The roots, dentate ligaments and filum suspend the spinal cord in the subarachnoid space, but allow a degree of movement of the cord within the canal during spinal flexion and extension.

The spinal subarachnoid space extends from C1 to S2 and communicates with the cranial subarachnoid compartment. The space is narrow at the cervical and lumbar enlargements of the cord, but is capacious in the region of the cauda equina. In this region, intradural tumours can enlarge as elongated sausages and grow to a large size before becoming symptomatic. In the cervical and dorsal regions however, a tumour, especially if situated intradurally, will "block" the subarachnoid space preventing the flow of CSF. The CSF below the block contains a high concentration of protein with no significant cellular reaction i.e., Froin's CSF loculation syndrome. The block will also result in a negative Quekenstedt's test in which jugular venous compression or abdominal pressure fails to cause a rise of lumbar CSF pressure. A "dry tap" may result when a lumbar puncture is attempted to perform a myelogram because CSF is scanty below the tumour. Alternatively, a tumour at the cauda equina may be traumatized by the unsuspecting radiologist who attempts the examination. Severe back pain or sciatic pain when CSF is withdrawn or contrast is injected, is almost pathognomonic of an intradural tumour occupying the lumbar spinal compartment.

Pathophysiology

The spinal canal is a closed compartment of finite volume akin to the cranial cavity. It contains neural tissue, meninges, fat, blood and CSF, the last two maintaining a dynamic but stable volumetric equilibrium. A spinal tumour expanding within the canal will displace CSF and blood initially to gain accommodation without impinging on neural tissue. Slow-growing tumours cause pressure atrophy of the extradural fat to achieve some territorial advantage. Eventually however, continued growth of a tumour will cause displacement and distortion of the neural elements. Similar effects on blood vessels would lead to partial or complete occlusion and cause ischaemia or venous congestion. These pressure effects will inevitably result in the neurological symptoms and signs of spinal cord compression.

The sequence of compensatory events is not identical in all cases. A tumour arising outside the cord (i.e., extramedullary) will typically go through the stages of attempted compensation and then decompensation causing neurological signs to appear. A tumour arising within the cord (i.e., intramedullary) may however produce neurological signs much earlier because the neoplastic process affects cord function before causing cord expansion. An intradural tumour within the large CSF sac of the cauda equina will grow to a large size before compromising neural structures. An extradural metastasis involving the vertebral body and pedicle will irritate the spinal nerve root causing radicular pain before the tumour encroaches into the spinal canal.

The mechanisms by which an expanding tumour causes neurological disturbances are complex and therefore the modes of clinical presentation variable. The deleterious effects to neural function are probably caused by the following mechanisms operating singly or in combination:

1. Mechanical compression
2. Arterial occlusion leading to neural ischaemia
3. Venous occlusion leading to congestion and infarction

Mechanical compression is by far the most important factor. The size and rate of growth of the tumour are important in determining the extent of the force inflicted on the cord. A rapidly expanding lesion will not allow sufficient time for the natural compensatory mechanisms to operate. On the other hand, a slow growing tumour, although causing significant cord displacement, will preserve neurological function because of the time allowed for neural and vascular adaptation. The surgeon is often impressed by the neurological state on initial presentation when visualizing a cord grossly displaced and flattened by a tumour at operation.

Large diameter nerve fibres such as those contained in the corticospinal tract are more vulnerable to the effects of mechanical forces. This may explain the early and inevitable occurrence of a spastic limb weakness in extramedullary spinal compression. Also, grey matter is less vulnerable to compression than white matter, probably explaining the rarity of lower motor neurone weakness in extramedullary lesions unless motor nerve roots are involved.

The concept that ischaemia due to arterial occlusion plays a role in producing the neurological disturbance of cord compression is well recognized. The occlusion of vessels from displacement caused by a tumour can operate on large vessels around the cord, the deep penetrating branches, or at the level of the microcirculation. The rapid deterioration of neurological function often seen in extradural lesions lends support to the vascular compression theory of cord decompensation. Since the venous drainage of the cord operates mainly via the extradural space it is possible that venous occlusion also plays an important part in this phenomenon. The microscopic changes observed in compressed spinal cord tissue are compatible with nutritional deficiency either from arterial ischaemia or venous congestion. Unlike compression, anoxia is more harmful to grey than white matter, the former being richer in vascularity but more vulnerable probably due to a greater demand for nutrients by the cell body.

The tumour may cause mechanical compression of the spinal cord nerve roots and blood vessels. The neurological disturbance is due to a combination of pressure and vascular inadequacy. The term *spinal neural compromise* which embraces these pathophysiological and anatomical concepts is suggested as an alternative to *spinal cord compression*.

Clinical Features

The term spinal cord compression is widely used in ordinary practice to indicate the pathological and clinical entity produced by any expanding lesion within the spinal canal. Strictly, cord compression can only occur with a lesion situated between C1 and L1/2. Below this level neural compromise can only involve the roots of the cauda equina. A lesion at the conus medullaris will invariably disturb the cord and the associated nerve roots. Similarly, a tumour compressing the cord in the cervical or dorsal region can also disturb nerve roots either within the dural sac or in the intervertebral foramen. Therefore a lesion between C1 and L1/2 will cause predominantly an upper motor neurone (spastic) paralysis associated with lower motor neurone features only if root involvement has also occurred. The exception is the early and significant lower motor neurone paralysis of an intramedullary tumour involving the cervical or lumbar enlargements of the cord or the flaccid paralysis due to spinal shock of acute extramedullary cord compression. Cauda equina compression by a spinal tumour produces a typical lower motor neurone paralysis.

Traditionally, three clinical stages of cord compression are recognized (Oppenheim 1923). The first or neuralgic stage is characterized by pain from root irritation often associated with mild motor and sensory signs due to segmental cord disturbance. Due to the paucity and subtle nature of the physical signs the diagnosis can be easily missed at this stage (Fig. 23.4). The second stage of incomplete cord transection is the commonest encountered in clinical practice. The neurological picture can vary from a typical Brown-Séquard syndrome to any possible combination of motor and sensory disturbance. The final stage of complete transection needs no description. Despite the wide availability of medical facilities and sophisticated diagnostic methods a small number of patients are in this unfortunate state when first referred to the neurosurgeon for attention. *A high index of clinical suspicion is the key to early diagnosis of a spinal tumour.*

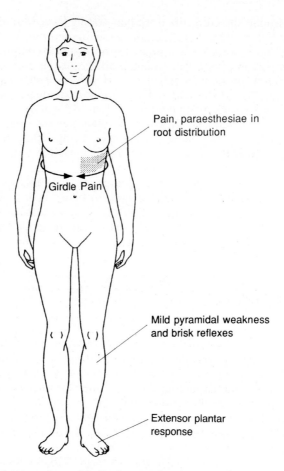

Pain, paraesthesiae in
root distribution

Girdle Pain

Mild pyramidal weakness
and brisk reflexes

Extensor plantar
response

Fig. 23.4. Clinical features of neuralgic (first) stage of cord compression.

Although a variety of clinical syndromes are possible, a spinal tumour usually produces a well recognized neurological picture. The symptoms and signs can be grouped into four broad categories:

1. Pain
2. Motor disturbances (paralysis)
3. Sensory disturbances (paraesthesiae)
4. Disturbances of sphincter and sexual function

A careful history and examination will reveal the anatomical site of the tumour. This deduction requires a basic knowledge of the arrangements of tracts and fibres within the spinal cord (Fig. 23.3). The clinical syndromes produced by a spinal tumour are determined by the function of the neurones affected by the lesion. In general, the symptoms and signs are dominated by motor pathway disease, spastic paraparesis being the commonest feature. The onset of sensory and sphincter symptoms signifies decompensation and a rapid clinical course can be expected thereafter.

For descriptive purposes it is customary to subdivide the neuronal disturbances into two categories: (1) segmental dysfunction i.e., roots and grey matter; (2) ascending and descending tract dysfunction. The neurological presentation is a product of these effects occurring singly or in combination.

Segmental Dysfunction

One or more segments of the cord are affected depending on the size of the tumour. Pain and flaccid weakness are the common symptoms of segmental origin. The former arises from involvement of the posterior nerve root, dura, vertebral body or the cord itself. The most important is pain arising from the posterior nerve root and the associated cord entry zone.

Radicular pain in a dermatomal or myotomal distribution is the classical symptom of such involvement. The nerve can be compressed within or outside the dural sac. Root involvement is commonly due to metastatic disease of the vertebra causing pedicle erosion or a neurofibroma. The radiation of pain can be along a limb or around the trunk and bilateral symptoms can occur. Numbness, paraesthesiae (pins and needles), hyperaesthesia and unpleasant dysaesthesia can be experienced in the same distribution. This pain is usually aggravated by coughing, sneezing and movement. The anatomical distribution of the radicular symptom accurately localises the lesion. Whilst radiculopathy from disc disease is the commonest cause of brachialgia and sciatica, atypical limb radicular pain is inevitably due to an intradural tumour. Superficial sensation may be diminished over the cutaneous innervation of the spinal root. Autonomic compression may result in pallor, redness or coldness of the affected peripheries.

Midline spinal pain can be experienced localized to the area of the tumour and probably arises from pain sensitive structures in the dura and extradural tissues. This symptom is commoner and more severe in extradural lesions and in metastatic disease is invariably due to collapse of a vertebral body. The pain of malignant extradural disease of the spine can be extremely severe. A dull aching or burning pain more widespread than radicular or segmental spinal pain can occur in cord compression. It involves a limb or the trunk below the lesion and probably arises from several spinal segments. The aetiology of this *central pain* remains obscure. *Radicular pain and midline spinal pain are of immense value in anatomical localization of a tumour.*

The segmental motor components are the anterior horn cells and the ventral root. Their involvement produces a flaccid weakness in the corresponding muscles with wasting, fasciculation and reduced tendon reflexes. Muscles are usually supplied by more than one root but disease affecting the dominant root or spinal segment will cause a profound weakness. The identification of the affected myotomes will signify the longitudinal extent of an intramedullary tumour situated in the cervical or lumbar enlargement of the cord. A similar lesion of the dorsal cord will cause paralysis of the intercostal and paraspinal muscles. This is more difficult to identify clinically and progressive scoliosis can be one manifestation.

Ascending and Descending Tract Dysfunction

The main ascending tracts subserve sensation. The ascending impulses of the spinocerebellar tracts do not reach consciousness and their integrity cannot be tested by clinical examination. The main sensory pathways which can be tested are:

1. Posterior columns
2. Lateral spinothalamic tracts
3. Anterior spinothalamic tracts

The *posterior columns* (fasciculus cuneatus and gracilis) convey joint position sense, vibration sense, stereognosis (i.e., the ability to recognize the shape of objects), light touch and two point discrimination. They ascend in the ipsilateral cord and cross at the brain stem level before reaching the cortex. The sacral fibres are situated medially and the cervical fibres laterally according to their order of entry into the cord. The clinical effects produced by loss of function are easily detectable by the standard methods of bedside examination. Loss of position sense causes gait ataxia especially in the dark. The patient cannot perceive the position of the feet in space whilst walking. The gait may thus acquire a "high-stepping" quality particularly accentuated by the concomitant presence of a foot drop. Standing posture is unstable with the eyes closed (positive Romberg's sign). Fine tingling paraesthesiae can be experienced below the level of the lesion. Occasionally, tight band-like sensations are felt around the trunk or limbs. These occur over a more widespread area than a single spinal segment and are akin to the central pain described above.

The *lateral spinothalamic tracts* convey pain and temperature sensation from the opposite side of the body. The fibres enter the cord and cross to the opposite side in the anterior commissure over two to three segments. In the tract the sacral fibres are outermost and the cervical fibres innermost according to their order of entry into the cord. The symptoms arising from dysfunction of this tract are usually more dramatic. Deep, poorly localized, unpleasant aching pain can occur in a limb or the trunk. The patient will be unable to recognize temperature sensation (e.g., of the bath water) with the affected area and accidental burns or injuries may go unrecognized because they are painless. Tingling hyperaesthesia, hypersensitivity or numbness may occur. Often patients mistakenly use the term numbness to mean the heaviness of a weak limb. A lesion of the lateral spinothalamic tract will cause impairment of pain and temperature sensation over the contralateral limb or trunk below the lesion. This classical feature of a sensory level is best demonstrated with a pin. The impairment of temperature sensation may not correspond exactly to the pain diminution.

The *anterior spinothalamic tract* is not clinically important and contains fibres conveying light touch and pressure sensation. The fibres have entered the cord on the opposite side and crossed in the same manner as the pain and temperature fibres. Light touch impulses are also conveyed in the posterior columns and the dual pathway system ensures that light touch is not totally abolished unless the cord is transected.

The main descending motor pathway is the *lateral corticospinal or crossed pyramidal tract*. The uncrossed or anterior corticospinal tract fibres cross at spinal segmental level to innervate their respective anterior horn cells. The uncrossed tract is unimportant for ordinary clinical purposes. The somatotopic arrangement of fibres places the cervical fibres innermost and the sacral fibres outermost in the order in which they will leave the tract to reach the anterior horn cells. A lesion of the crossed tract will cause a spastic (upper motor neurone type) paralysis of the ipsilateral limb(s) below the lesion. A bilateral lesion produces paralysis of both lower limbs (paraparesis) or all four limbs (quadriparesis). The earliest complaint is usually a heaviness or stiffness in the legs and an inability to run or hurry. Difficulty in managing stairs and tripping over the carpets and kerbs occurs due to weakness of hip flexion and ankle dorsiflexion. This pyramidal weakness has a particular distribution due to differential involvement of muscle groups. In the upper limbs, the extensor muscles (i.e., shoulder abductors, elbow extensors, wrist and finger extensors and finger abductors) are more affected by the paralysis than their corresponding antagonistic groups. In the lower limbs, the hip flexors, knee flexors and ankle and toe dorsiflexors are more affected than the extensor groups. The stronger muscles have increased tone due to involvement of the extrapyramidal fibres and this produces the classical limb posture of the chronic quadriplegic patient with elbow flexion and knee extension. In addition to the hyperreflexia which is typical, a lesion of the pyramidal tract above D9 cord level abolishes the ipsilateral abdominal, cremasteric and plantar reflexes. The last is replaced by the pathological Babinski (extension of the big toe) response.

Disturbance of Sphincter and Sexual Function

Disorders of sphincter (bladder and bowel) control and sexual function are common accompaniments of spinal compression by tumour. Their onset signifies decompensation and impending rapid deterioration of cord function. The symptoms are a result of disruption of spinal autonomic reflex pathways and/or their connections with the higher centres situated in the brain stem, frontal lobes and hypothalamus. These systems are complex and their normal anatomy and physiology are not well understood. As a result the suggested pathophysiology in disease conditions is often tentative. Only bilateral lesions cause significant disturbance of these autonomic functions.

Control of the bladder is predominantly subserved by the parasympathetic component which on stimulation induces contraction of the detrusor and relaxation of the internal sphincter. These impulses originate in the sacral segments (S2,3,4) on receiving afferent input indicating that the bladder is full. The cell bodies reside in the intermediolateral grey matter of the cord. The fibres subserving higher control are closely associated with the pyramidal tracts. The sympathetic innervation of the bladder originates in the intermediolateral grey matter of D12, L1 and L2. The precise function of this system is unknown and damage to the sympathetic pathway alone does not disturb bladder control significantly.

Traditionally, a variety of terms (i.e., automatic, autonomous, uninhibited, spinal bladder, etc.) have been applied to the different types of neurological disturbances of the bladder. These terms are confusing and do not really assist either in diagnosis or management. If the roots of the cauda equina or the S2,3,4 segments of the cord are disturbed, the spinal reflex is abolished resulting in acute retention or dribbling (overflow) incontinence. A lesion of the cord above 'S2,3,4 will obliterate the action of the higher centres causing hesitancy or urgency, the latter resulting in incontinence because of reflex bladder contraction. In practice, the symptoms of bladder dysfunction resulting from a spinal tumour are hesitancy, dribbling, incontinence, urgency with incontinence or acute retention.

Nevertheless, none of these symptoms are of value in localizing the anatomical site of the bladder disturbance and such a deduction may not be possible even after detailed urodynamic assessment. It is important to remember that patients, through embarrassment, can be reluctant to divulge symptoms such as incontinence and dribbling. The impairment of walking ability caused by the tumour often enhances the predicament of the sufferer. The control of bowel emptying is very similar to the bladder mechanism and mediated by the parasympathetic innervation of the rectum and internal sphincter originating in the S2,3,4 spinal segments. Fortunately, most patients with spinal compression tend to become constipated rather than incontinent of faeces. The former is far easier to treat and less distressing to the individual concerned. Faecal impaction causes mucosal irritation with the formation of liquid faeces which leads to incontinence especially with concomitant loss of the anal reflex due to the tumour.

Sexual function is also mediated by complex autonomic pathways. Parasympathetic impulses originating from the S2,3,4 segments of the cord produce erection and sympathetic messages originating from the L1,2 segments achieve ejaculation. These spinal centres are connected to higher function control by pathways in the central grey matter of the cord. Disorders of potency affect males only. However, lesions affecting the S2 roots will cause diminished genital sensation and thus impair sexual enjoyment in either sex. Cord lesions above L1 can lead to impotence or reflex priapism and lesions involving S2,3,4 may produce loss of erection and ejaculation ability. Lesions of the cauda equina can have similar effects but may also cause priapism or spontaneous ejaculation. Careful inquiry into these aspects of bodily function is required in establishing the nature of sexual inability. It must be remembered that psychiatric and endocrine diseases are the commonest cause of male impotence.

Recognized Clinical Syndromes

The neurological features caused by an intradural tumour sited posterolaterally on the left at D6, provides an ideal model to describe Oppenheim's three stages of compression.

Neuralgic Stage

The initial stage of compression (Fig. 23.4) will involve the left D6 posterior root with mild effects on the left hemicord. The clinical features can be summarized as:

1. Pain and paraesthesiae around trunk in the left inframammary region. This dermatomal area may be hypersensitive to touch and pin stimulus

2. Tight band-like sensations around the whole trunk affecting the lower costal area (girdle pain)
3. Subtle exaggeration of lower limb reflexes (more on the left), a left Babinski response and weakness of left hip flexion
4. Usually no sensory loss can be demonstrated
5. Urinary hesitancy or urgency

This is the stage when diagnosis is difficult because the physical signs are not obvious without a careful examination.

Hemicord Syndromes

With further expansion of tumour the cord becomes more compromised. Although the left hemicord will be particularly affected the signs are usually bilateral. The clinical picture will be a typical or atypical Brown-Séquard syndrome with the following neurological findings:

1. Pain and temperature lost over left D6 dermatome
2. Pain and temperature loss over right lower limb and trunk up to D8
3. Posterior column function impaired in left lower limb
4. Spasticity, weakness, brisk reflexes and Babinski response in left lower limb. The right lower limb is affected to a lesser extent
5. Sphincter disturbance i.e., urgency, incontinence or hesitancy

Similar to the hemisection syndrome of the cord as described by Brown-Séquard, in spinal compression due to a tumour the cord disturbance is usually asymmetrical at this stage.

Transection Syndromes

The transition from the first to the final stage can be slow or rapid. Gradually, both sides of the cord become equally affected. Eventually, all motor and sensory function is lost below the level of the lesion.

1. Bilateral sensory level at D6 below which all modalities are either impaired or absent. A zone of hyperaesthesia may be present at the upper part of the area of sensory loss. The upper margin of this represents the true sensory level and the level of the tumour. In extradural cord compression, sensation is often preserved over the lower sacral segments (sacral sparing)
2. Severe or complete paralysis affecting both lower limbs or all four limbs. Usually, it is an upper motor neurone disturbance but flaccidity and areflexia are seen in the stage of spinal shock
3. Acute retention of urine

Central Cord Syndrome (Intramedullary Tumour)

The intrinsic cord tumours have a unique clinical presentation virtually un-known in extramedullary spinal compression. They originate in the central grey matter and the anterior commissure. Therefore, the decussating fibres of the spinothalamic system are disturbed very early. Initially, the zone of pain and temperature loss which is usually bilateral, is confined to the dermatomes of the spinal segments occupied by the tumour and two or three segments caudal to the lesion because the fibres cross over gradually. As the tumour expands longitudinally within the cord more segments are affected and the sensory loss becomes more widespread, still adhering to the dermatomal pattern. The distribution of the sensory loss is an index of the longitudinal extent of the tumour. No other sensory modality is affected in the early stages whilst the tumour is confined to the central cord. This "dissociated" sensory loss is typical of the early central cord syndrome. An intrinsic tumour of the cervical cord will eventually produce a cape-like pattern of dissociated sensory loss over the face, arms and upper trunk.

The anterior horn cells are also disturbed at an early stage causing wasting and weakness in the myotomes corresponding to the cord segments involved by the tumour. As the tumour expands longitudinally the lower motor paralysis will extend similarly to the sensory loss.

Transverse growth of tumour affects the reflex arc and the reflexes disappear in the wasted muscles. Further expansion in the transverse plane disturbs the crossed pyramidal tracts producing a bilateral, probably asymmetric spastic paralysis below the level of the lesion. Similarly, the lateral spinothalamic tracts will be affected and the sensory loss will spread caudally following the somatotopic representation of fibres in the cord. Eventually all except perhaps the lower sacral segments will be involved and a sensory level with sacral sparing is detected. Even the sacral areas can be anaesthetic in the final stages. By this time the posterior columns are also affected by the transverse expansion and all modalities of sensation are involved so that the sensory loss is no longer "dissociated".

Cervical Intramedullary Tumour

The cervical enlargement from C5 to D1 is a common site of intramedullary tumours. The clinical features can be summarized:

1. Deep aching or burning pain in the shoulder girdle and/or arms
2. Painless burns or injuries in the hands
3. Wasting and weakness of upper limb muscles with loss of reflexes
4. Spastic paralysis of the lower limbs with brisk reflexes and Babinski responses
5. Cape distribution of dissociated sensory loss
6. Sensory level (with sacral sparing) for pain and temperature at first but all modalities affected eventually
7. Unilateral or bilateral Horner's syndrome
8. Urgency or incontinence of urine/faeces

Cervical Extramedullary Tumour

Cord compression between C5 to D1 (cervical enlargement) produces a clinical picture which is different to that due to a lesion in the high cervical or foramen magnum area. Therefore, the features of the latter will be considered separately. The neurological picture in the former is characterized by the differing types of motor involvement in the upper and lower limbs.

1. The radicular pain is situated along the radial (C5,6), medial (C8, D1) or posterior (C6,7) border of an upper limb. Root pain from C6 and C7 can be felt in the ipsilateral medial scapular border. The muscles supplied by each root affected may be painful and even tender in addition to being weak and wasted. The corresponding tendon reflex is depressed or absent. The root area may be anaesthetic or hyperaesthetic. Radicular syndromes can be recognized combining the above effects.

C5 root – wasting and weakness of deltoid and biceps. Reduced biceps reflex.
C6 root – wasting and weakness of brachioradialis. Reduced biceps and/or supinator jerk.
C7 root – wasting and weakness of triceps. Reduced triceps jerk.
C8,D1 roots – wasting and weakness of small hand muscles.
These effects are at the level of the tumour and usually ipsilateral to the tumour. The typical syndromes are much commoner with intradural tumours.

2. Below the level of the tumour a spastic paralysis results. The usual picture is of a quadriparesis/plegia with lower motor features in some upper limb muscles (from the root involvement) and upper motor paralysis in the remaining upper limb and all the lower limb muscle groups. The reflexes are brisk below the level of the lesion. With compression at C5,6 the supinator jerk may be inverted. Hyperreflexia in the upper limbs is manifested by finger jerks, positive Hoffman reflexes and even Wartenberg's sign.

3. The sensory level is often in the upper limbs and affects the trunk below D2. A suspended dorsal sensory level without sacral sparing is possible in cervical lesions due to lateral spinothalamic tract compression because the sacral fibres are sited outermost.

4. A Horner's syndrome can be observed in lesions between C8 and D2 due to interruption of the cervical sympathetic pathway within the cord or from extraspinal involvement of the stellate ganglion.

Foramen Magnum and High Cervical Compression

The tumours in this region are usually extramedullary but intrinsic cord lesions can occur. The clinical picture is well recognized but easily overlooked if one is careless. The region of the foramen magnum is difficult to visualize by routine radiological methods. Therefore, once clinical suspicion has been alerted the process of investigations must be pursued diligently to conclude or exclude the diagnosis. It is possible to be deceived by an incidental mid-cervical disc prolapse seen on X-rays and, accepting this as the diagnosis, missing the tumour entirely with disastrous consequences to the patient. MRI is extremely useful in investigating this region.

The clinical picture is as expected by the anatomical structures being compressed. Foramen magnum lesions may involve the lower brain stem and cranial nerves (IX,X,XI,XII), in addition to the upper part of the spinal cord. A lesion above C5, rostral to the upper limb outflow inevitably causes a spastic quadriparesis and all the tendon reflexes are pathologically brisk in the four limbs. Although lower motor type weakness is not expected, wasting of the small hand muscles is well described, probably occurring due to remote ischaemia caused by compression of the anterior spinal arteries. Any combination of the following list of clinical features is possible:

1. Pain in the occipitocervical region often radiating towards the vertex, commonly associated with neck stiffness due to spasm of paraspinal muscles
2. Wasting of suboccipital and paraspinal neck muscles noticeable especially if it occurs unilaterally. Also wasting and weakness of the sternomastoid and trapezius muscles often causing a head tilt (torticollis). These features are due to involvement of the motor roots of C2,3,4 and the accessory nerves
3. Wasting and paralysis of the tongue (uni- or bilateral)
4. Spastic quadriparesis with brisk reflexes and Babinski responses
5. Wasting and weakness of the small hand muscles
6. Downbeat nystagmus on horizontal gaze
7. Acroparaesthesiae in limb extremities with loss of position sense and/or stereognosis, initially in the hands (demonstrated by pseudo-tremor of the outstretched hands), the lower limbs being affected late
8. Spinothalamic sensory level anywhere between C1 to C5 but since the trigeminal sensory nucleus occupies the upper cervical cord, facial sensation can also be disturbed. Accurate knowledge of the dermatomal map and careful testing are essential to detect sensory levels over the neck and scalp
9. Lhermitte's sign

Dorsal Compression Syndrome

The following clinical features are possible:

1. Radicular pain is of intercostal nerve distribution. Unilateral pain can be mistaken for being of visceral origin. Bilateral pain is felt like a tight belt or girdle
2. Spastic paraparesis with brisk reflexes and Babinski responses. If spinal shock supervenes in rapidly progressive compression flaccid paralysis occurs. The relevant abdominal reflexes are lost in cord lesions above D9 or if the D8 to D12 roots are involved with tumour
3. Sensory level over the trunk at the level of the lesion, or a suspended level below groin (D12) level. Physiological sensory levels exist because the supraclavicular (C4) inframammary (D5,6) and groin (D12) regions are more sensitive to pain in most individuals. The patterns of involvement of posterior columns and spinothalamic tracts have already been described
4. Scoliosis due to wasting and weakness of paraspinal and intercostal muscles occurs especially with intramedullary tumours
5. Paralytic ileus especially in rapid compression due to involvement of splanchnic nerves
6. Bladder, bowel and sexual function disturbances (as discussed)

Lumbar and Sacral Compression Syndromes

The D12 cord segment lies behind the D10/D11 intervertebral disc. Therefore, a lesion at or below D11 vertebral level can cause compression of the lumbosacral cord and the corresponding roots. Certain root syndromes arising from this area can be identified by the distribution of the pain and the associated motor and sensory deficits.

L1,2 roots – pain in hip/groin; weakness of iliopsoas (hip flexion)

L2,3 roots – pain in medial aspect of thigh; weakness of hip adduction

L3,4 roots – anterior thigh pain; weakness and wasting of quadriceps with reduced knee (patellar) reflex

L5 root – lateral thigh and leg and dorsum of foot; weakness and wasting of glutei, hamstrings, extensor hallucis, tibialis anterior

S1 root – posterior thigh and leg and lateral foot; weakness and wasting of calf with reduced ankle reflex; weakness of peroneii (eversion of foot)

Paraesthesiae or hypalgesia can occur in the appropriate root distribution. The radicular pain of root compression due to tumour is often atypical and different from the sciatica of disc disease and yet increases with coughing, sneezing and certain postures. The midline spinal pain in contrast is worse when lying flat and often wakes the patient at night who then finds relief by walking about. Sensory impairment can occur over the appropriate areas and pain is more reduced than any other modality. Autonomic functions such as sweating and piloerection are absent and the skin may be blotchy and cold. Pain from the lower sacral segments localizes to the perineum, rectum and genitalia.

The anatomy of this region is seemingly complex (Fig. 23.1) and the motor and sensory features of compression are dependent on the extent and pattern of cord and nerve root disturbance. Nevertheless, several well-recognized syndromes occur.

The terminal part of the spinal cord is surrounded by a sheath of nerve roots. Pure intramedullary tumours usually do not disturb nerve roots but an ependymoma involving the lower sacral cord often sprouts through and intermingles with the corresponding roots. Extramedullary tumours between D11 and L1/2 invariably compress roots and the cord. Tumours sited below L1/2 cannot compress the cord and produce a pure cauda equina lesion. The possible clinical syndromes are:

1. Pure cord lesions (intramedullary)
   a) Cord between L1–L4.
   b) Epiconus (L4–S2)
   c) Conus (S3–S5)
   Examples: ependymoma, astrocytoma, dermoid/epidermoid cysts, lipoma
2. Mixed cord and root lesions (mostly extramedullary)
   a) High – involving cord or epiconus (Fig. 23.5)
   b) Low – involving conus
   c) Midline – intrinsic conus lesion involving lower sacral roots
   Examples: neurofibroma, metastases, lymphoma, ependymoma
3. Pure cauda equina lesion
   Examples: same as in 2 above

Epiconus Syndrome

Although the cord segments are L4 to S2, the roots of L2 to S2 are draped around this part. An intramedullary tumour can cause lower motor type weakness in all the muscles of the lower limbs except hip flexion (iliopsoas L1,2). True weakness of this muscle is often difficult to assess because of inhibition of movement due to pain but, when present, it is an important clue that the lesion is sited high in the lumbar spine. The knee (L3,4) and ankle (S1) reflexes are affected dependent on the extent of the tumour. Both are never preserved but often the former is intact while the latter is reduced. The spinothalamic loss can spread from L4–S2 segments but sacral sparing is not invariable because the lesion may extend into the conus eventually or transverse growth can disturb the ascending fibres. Bladder and rectal sphincter disturbance is inevitable and impotence common. Extramedullary compression is described under Mixed Cord and Root Compression Syndromes below.

Conus Syndrome

The cord segments affected are S3,4 and 5 but the roots from L3 to S5 are around the conus. The main features of a pure (intramedullary) conus syndrome centre around the innervation of the bladder and rectum by S2,3,4 and the sensory supply to the "saddle" area. These are:

1. Saddle anaesthesia
2. Acute urinary retention, incontinence or overflow with retention
3. Faecal incontinence
4. Impotence
5. Absent anal reflexes

It is important to note that there is no paralysis of the lower limbs and the ankle reflexes are preserved if the lesion remains confined to the conus.

Mixed Cord and Root Compression Syndromes

The clinical features of this variety of compression are best described by illustrating an intradural neurofibroma arising from the root of L4 on the left side (Fig. 23.5). The root syndrome will comprise the following:

1. Root pain over the left anterior thigh
2. Wasting of the left quadriceps muscle
3. Weakness of left knee extension and ankle inversion (L4 root)
4. Reduced left knee reflex

If cord compression occurs, additional physical signs will appear. These will vary in severity depending on the degree of compression. In the extreme situation complete motor and sensory loss will occur below L5 (cord level) associated with loss of autonomic function. In the early stages however the signs are:

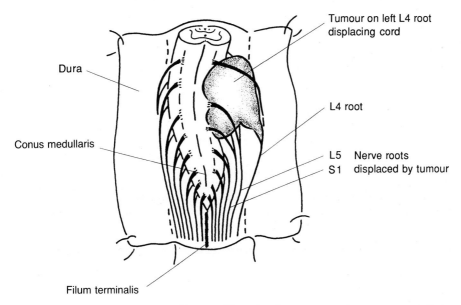

Dura

Conus medullaris

Tumour on left L4 root
displacing cord

L4 root

L5   Nerve roots
S1   displaced by tumour

Filum terminalis

Fig. 23.5.   Intradural tumour: neurofibroma with cord and root compression – conus medullaris.

5. Brisk ankle reflexes with clonus
6. Extensor plantar responses

An intrinsic tumour of the conus can extend into the extramedullary space and then compress sacral nerve roots. Usually, the root involvement will be bilateral and in descending order of root value. In addition to the features of a conus tumour described above the following can be noted in the clinical picture:

1. Rectal, genital or perineal pain
2. Loss of ankle reflexes
3. Weakness of muscles supplied by L5 and S1 roots
4. The sensory loss may extend beyond the "saddle" area

Cauda Equina Syndrome

A tumour sited below the L1/2 disc level can only cause a disturbance of the spinal roots. The L1 and L2 roots exit from the canal above L2 and are never affected. The L3 root has only a short course within the canal below L2 and is rarely disturbed. The L5 and all the sacral roots follow a long course within the canal and therefore can be affected by a tumour sited anywhere in that territory. The capacious subarachnoid space of the canal in this region will accommodate growth of a tumour. The nerve roots become draped around its outer surface. They are capable of accepting some displacement before neurological disturbance occurs. Vascular channels accompanying the roots and the filum terminale may also become compromised and cause further neurological dysfunction. The usual clinical features of a cauda equina tumour are:

1. Radicular pain in the anterior (L4), lateral (L5) or posterior (S1) thigh with paraesthesiae in the corresponding dermatomes
2. Wasting and weakness of the muscles supplied by L4, L5, S1 and S2 roots (commonly glutei, hamstrings, tibialis anterior)
3. Sensory loss over the saddle area extending into the L4, L5 and S1 segments
4. Absent ankle reflexes (S1) and plantar responses (S2)
5. Urinary urgency, incontinence or acute retention and constipation
6. Loss of anal and bulbocavernosus reflexes
7. Impotence

It is often impossible clinically to distinguish between a tumour of the conus from one arising within the cauda equina.

General Examination

In addition to the detailed neurological examination described above a careful systems examination must be made including the breasts and pelvic structures when appropriate. Café-au-lait patches may signify neurofibromatosis and iris hamartomas (Lisch nodules) have the same significance. Deformities of the spine such as kyphosis, scoliosis and torticollis can be associated with spinal neoplasms due to the imbalance of muscular activity. The presence of a tuft of hair, pigmented naevus, skin dimple or sinus in the lumbosacral area indicates the presence of spina bifida which in turn can be associated with tumours such as lipomas, dermoid and epidermoid cysts. The extraspinal portion of a neurofibroma may be palpable in the neck and occasionally the paravertebral extension of a metastatic deposit in the spine is palpable as a mass. Anterior wedge collapse of the vertebral body due to a metastatic tumour, myeloma or lymphoma may be recognized posteriorly by tenderness over the corresponding spinous process which is often more prominent or sunken giving the impression of a "step" when the palpating finger is run gently along the spines.

Spinal Tumours

In 1753, Lecat made the first surgical attempt to remove an intraspinal tumour (Lecat 1765). Over a century later, in 1887, Sir Victor Horsley performed the first successful operation to remove a spinal intradural tumour which had caused cord compression (Horsley and Gowers 1888). The tumour was probably a meningioma or neurofibroma although reported as a "fibromyxoma" at the time. The patient who was severely paralysed prior to surgery made a remarkable recovery even by modern-day standards and walked again. Yet, in the ensuing 100 years significant advances have been seen in the diagnosis and treatment of spinal tumours. Positive contrast myelography came into use in 1921, CAT spinal scanning in the late 1970s and the advent of MRI techniques in the 1980s has revolutionized the radiological demonstration of spinal neoplasms. Safer, modern neuroanaesthesia combined with advanced micro-neurosurgical techniques has reduced the risks to the patient and considerably improved the prognosis.

This section will describe the basic pathology and special clinical features and treatment of individual spinal tumours. The methods of radiological diagnosis are mentioned briefly but are dealt with in more detail in Chapter 8. Similarly, vascular malformations and congenital tumours associated with spinal dysraph-ism have been excluded. Treatment is briefly dealt with under the individual tumour type and special aspects emphasized in the section on Management.

Incidence

Spinal tumours are less common than cerebral neoplasms, the reported ratios varying from 1:4 (Nittner 1976) to 1:9 (Gudmundsson 1970). It is difficult to establish their true incidence in the general population. A recent population-based survey carried out in Norway revealed the annual incidence of primary intraspinal neoplasms as 5 per million for females and 3 per million for males (Helseth and Mork 1989).

The relative frequency of different types of spinal tumour in a reported series is not necessarily an index of the natural order in the population, the figures being biased by the local patterns of case referral as well as the criteria of patient selection of the neurosurgical department concerned. The inclusion or exclusion of paediatric patients and/or those with spinal metastatic tumours appear to be the most important factors which determine the variations in incidence figures. The conclusions of an interesting and comprehensive review of 29 series by Nittner (1976) are compared to three large series within the analysis (Torma 1957; Sloof et al. 1964; Nittner 1968; Helseth and Mork 1989) in Table 23.1. Meningioma and neurofibroma are the most frequently en-countered primary intradural spinal neoplasms. Astrocytoma and ependymoma are the commonest of the intramedullary tumours. Metastatic tumour, myeloma and lymphoma are very frequent causes of extradural spinal cord compression encountered in ordinary neurosurgical practice.

Classification

The traditional method is to divide spinal tumours into extradural and intra-dural lesions, the latter being further subdivided as extramedullary or intra-medullary depending on whether the lesion is situated outside or within the spinal cord respectively. Mixed extradural/intradural and intramedullary/extramedullary tumours exist and will be described under the relevant sections.

Pathologists adopt a system of classification based on the tissue of origin of the tumour. The classification depicted in Table 23.2 is an attempt at regroup-ing spinal tumours in this traditional method. Relative incidences apply within each vertical category rather than in an overall context. Some tumour-like con-ditions which can cause spinal cord compression e.g., inflammatory granulomata, have been omitted as being outside the scope of this particular chapter. A histogenetic bias has been incorporated into the classification whenever poss-

Table 23.1. Incidence of adult spinal tumours (percentages corrected to the nearest whole number). The table has been devised from Nittner's composite analysis of 29 series (Nittner 1976). The figures in this analysis should be compared to the individual series. Note the absence of metastatic tumours in the series analysed by Sloof et al. and Helseth and Mork. The latter includes paediatric patients

	Torma (1957) 1119 cases	Sloof et al. (1964) 1322 cases	Nittner (1968) 513 cases	Nittner (1976) 4885 cases	Helseth and Mork (1989) 467 cases
Glioma and intramedullary tumour	17%	22%	9%	13%	32%
Ependymoma			6%	3%	
Neurinoma/neurofibroma	23%	29%	21%	23%	11%
Meningioma	30%	26%	22%	22%	47%
Vascular tumours and angiomas		6%	7%	7%	4%
Metastases	22%		9%	6%	
Sarcomas		12%	8%	8%	
Others	8%	5%	19%	18%	6%

Table 23.2. Classification of "tumours" causing cord compression in adults

	Extradural: Bone tumours	Others	Intradural: Extramedullary	Intramedullary
More common	Vertebral haemangioma Aneurysmal bone cyst Chordoma Metastases – Carcinoma Myeloma Lymphoma Germ cell tumour	Metastases – Carcinoma Myeloma Lymphoma Germ cell tumour Dumb-bell neurofibroma Meningioma	Neurofibroma Schwannoma Meningioma Ependymoma	Astrocytoma Ependymoma Dermoid cyst Epidermoid cyst Haemangioblastoma
Less common or rare	Chondroblastoma Chondrosarcoma Osteochondroma Osteoblastoma Osteoblastoma Osteosarcoma Osteoclastoma	Metastases – Sarcoma Melanoma Neuroblastoma* Congenital – Lipoma Arachnoid cysts Meningocele Enterogenous cyst Calcifying pseudoneoplasm True lipoma Epidural hibernoma	Metastases (all types) Congenital – Lipoma Arachnoid cysts Enterogenous cyst Paraganglioma True lipoma	Metastases (all types) Oligodendroglioma Ganglioneuroma Neurofibroma Teratoma Dermoid cysts* Epidermoid cyst* Enterogenous cyst True lipoma*

* These tumours are seen more commonly in children (see text).

ible, but grouping is by no means inflexible because the cellular origin of some tumours is disputed.

Radiological Diagnosis

A brief general account of the important radiological findings will be helpful prior to the description of individual tumour types. Plain X-rays of the spine may reveal pathological fractures of the vertebral body and/or erosion of the pedicles in extradural metastatic disease. Benign tumours and longstanding intramedullary tumours may cause enlargement of the canal diameter with scalloping of the posterior vertebral border and widening of the interpedicular distance. A dumb-bell neurofibroma expands the intervertebral foramen. Congenital vertebral abnormalities are associated with intradural dermoids, epidermoids, lipomas and enterogenous cysts. An X-ray of the chest is essential, especially in the investigation of metastatic disease.

Conventional myelography using contrast medium may outline a tumour as a filling defect. An intramedullary tumour causes expansion of the spinal cord with the contrast thinning out around the narrow subarachnoid gutters. The contrast is held up ("blocked") either completely or partially at the polar end of a tumour. The pattern displayed is very useful in identifying whether the lesion is extradural, intradural or intramedullary (see Figs. 23.6–23.8 and 23.10.) When a complete block is evident, a second study with contrast inserted above the obstruction is needed to identify the opposite pole of the tumour. This will also exclude other tumours in the spine in conditions where multiple lesions are possible.

CAT scans are not very useful in demonstrating the morphology of intradural tumours. The bone destruction and paravertebral extensions of extradural lesions, primary osseous tumours and calcified intradural tumours are well demonstrated. CAT combined with conventional myelography yields information which is very useful to the neurosurgeon. The direction and pattern of contrast displacement will indicate whether the tumour is situated lateral, posterior or anterior to the spinal cord. In a partial block and even in an apparently complete block, some contrast will trickle around the tumour to the opposite poles. This can be used to demonstrate the total longitudinal extent of the tumour by axial CAT scans performed within six hours of the myelogram, thus obviating the need for a second myelographic study with contrast inserted from above. Finally, contrast medium may be seen seeping into a tumour cyst or syrinx.

MRI is most useful in the diagnosis of intramedullary tumours. The site and extent of the solid and cystic components are best demonstrated by this method. Intravenous gadolinium is used to enhance the solid component. MRI is the most convenient and non-invasive method of studying the entire length of the spine and spinal cord. Isotope bone scans always demonstrate the presence of benign and malignant tumours involving the vertebral column even when they are not visualized on the plain X-rays of CAT scans.

It is conventional for the radiologist to mark the skin of the back denoting the level of the tumour demonstrated by myelography in order to assist the surgeon. It is far more accurate to identify the relevant vertebral level by inserting a needle into the relevant spinous process under X-ray control immediately prior to the operation.

Metastatic Tumours

Virtually all metastatic (secondary) deposits involving the spine are situated in the extradural, vertebral/paravertebral compartments. Intradural metastatic lesions are extremely rare. However, tumours such as medulloblastoma, ependymoma and cerebral lymphoma can produce spinal subarachnoid space seedlings spread by the CSF pathways. These most often lodge in the lumbosacral canal due to gravitational forces.

The increased life expectancy of cancer patients has enhanced the prevalence of spinal metastatic disease. About 5% of all cancer patients develop spinal extradural metastases and about 20% of these patients suffer the effects of neural compression. Extradural malignant tumour is the commonest neoplasm encountered in the spinal epidural space. The resulting clinical syndrome of spinal cord compression is one of the commonest emergency conditions referred to a neurosurgical department.

Some tumours exhibit a selective spread into bone (osteotropism) and the common sites of primary disease are lung (17%), breast (16%), prostate (11%) and kidney (9%) but thyroid and gastrointestinal tract malignancy as well as malignant melanoma are also well recognized sources. Lymphoma (5%) also accounts for a significant number (see below). Myeloma in the spine is grouped under metastatic lesions in most studied series and is an important cause of extradural spinal cord compression (Gilbert et al. 1978; Connolly 1982).

The commonest mode of spread into the epidural tissues is via the blood stream, either through the arterial system or the vertebral extradural venous plexuses, the latter being especially incriminated in the dissemination of prostatic cancer into the spine. Direct spread to the vertebrae can occur from mediastinal, retroperitoneal and pelvic growths. Occasionally the neoplastic cells spread from the paravertebral tissues via the intervertebral foramen into the epidural space traversing along the lymphatics and/or the perineurium.

The anatomically long thoracic region is most commonly affected (60%) followed by the lumbosacral segment (26%) and cervical region (14%). The tumour may lie entirely within the extradural space in many cases (15%–40%) but most often the vertebral segment/s is involved with or without extension into the spinal canal (50%–85%). The vertebral body and pedicle are the sites commonly affected but the laminae and spinous processes can be occasionally affected. One to three contiguous vertebrae are usually diseased but multiple separate sites are known to occur. The disc and vertebral end plates are unaffected and this is an important diagnostic feature on plain films to distinguish the bone destruction of metastatic disease from that of osteomyelitis. Collapse of the vertebral body (pathological fracture), erosion of pedicles and a paraspinal soft tissue mass are important radiological features.

The extradural tumour is occasionally entirely posterior to the cord or encircles the dural sheath circumferentially (Fig. 23.6). In the majority of

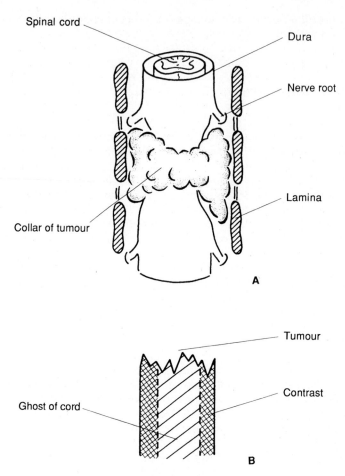

Spinal cord

Dura

Nerve root

Lamina

Collar of tumour

A

Tumour

Contrast

Ghost of cord

B

Fig. 23.6. A Extradural tumour. **B** Myelography appearance.

instances however, the tumour mass is sited anterior, anterolateral or lateral to the spinal canal. This feature determines the direction of the compression force on the spinal cord or cauda equina. Vertebral collapse can propel a fragment of bone into the spinal canal causing further neural embarrassment. These pathologic concepts dictate the modern surgical approaches designed to excise the tumour and decompress the neural structures.

Some vertebral metastases are asymptomatic in the early stages. However, spinal neural compression may be the initial manifestation of the malignant process. In other words, the primary site may be unknown at the time of first presentation with cord symptoms and may remain so even after systemic investigations. Whilst no age is exempt, the disease is more common in the high cancer risk ages of 40–65 years. The onset of symptoms can be acute or insidious. Back pain is the commonest initial symptom and is present in virtually all patients at the time of diagnosis. Radicular pain is less common but is always of localizing value. Neurological symptoms commence about 6–8 weeks after onset of pain but may be earlier or later. At the time of diagnosis nearly 80% of patients have weakness, 50% have sensory symptoms and 50% sphincter dysfunction. Anterior cord compression is associated with weakness and loss of spinothalamic function with preservation of posterior column sensation. The predominant loss of the latter modality signifies a posteriorly situated tumour mass. When the cord compression is in a lateral direction the neurological deficits are asymmetrical and a Brown-Séquard pattern is recognized. With an acute onset of paralysis (i.e. within 24 hours) flaccidity may be a feature even though the cord itself is affected. About 50% of patients have a severe neurological disability on presentation and are unable to walk, and 15% are paraplegic. The neurological findings depend on the spinal region affected and conform to the general description given earlier in the chapter. It is important to mention that in 20% of patients neurological deterioration occurs during the time which elapses between diagnosis and definitive treatment.

In addition to the radiological investigations mentioned previously, the ESR, serum protein electrophoresis, serum acid phosphatase and bone marrow biopsy will yield very useful diagnostic information. Treatment is by surgical decompression and/or biopsy combined with radiotherapy and/or chemotherapy (see Management).

Lymphoma

This tumour is now encountered more frequently than before because of increased awareness of the entity and the increased frequency of immune deficiency states. A current method of classification is:

1. Primary central nervous system lymphoma
2. Systemic non-Hodgkin's lymphoma
   a) Nodular type
   b) Diffuse type
3. Hodgkin's lymphoma

Primary Central Nervous System Lymphoma (PCNSL)

There is no true lymph tissue within the brain or spinal cord. Probably the commonest effect of lymphoma on the CNS is a paraneoplastic syndrome without the presence of a true neoplasm. PCNSL arises from the microglial cells which are the equivalent of lymphoreticular cells elsewhere. The tumour occurs in multiple sites within the CNS and is much more common in the brain than in the spinal cord. Occurrence is commoner in immune deficiency states (congenital or acquired) and an association with Epstein-Barr virus infection has also been recognized. The tumours represent proliferating B cells of the immune system in the absence of T-cell suppression which is normally present. Spinal tumours can occur either as intramedullary tumours which expand the cord or as diffuse meningeal seedlings from a cerebral lymphoma (Hochberg and Millar 1988). They cause weakness and sensory symptoms in the lower limbs. Myelography reveals an expanded cord or a filling defect or block in the subarachnoid space. It is unusual to find evidence of lymphoma elswhere in the viscera or lymph nodes. The CSF may show lymphoma cells on careful cytological examination. There is a dramatic clinical and radiological improvement with corticosteroids. The tumour is radiosensitive.

Systemic Non-Hodgkin's Lymphoma (SNHL)

This type primarily involves viscera, bone marrow and lymph nodes. It occurs mostly unrelated to PCNSL but the two can coexist. SNHL incorporates tumours previously called giant follicular lymphoma, lymphosarcoma, reticulum cell sarcoma and lymphoblastic lymphoma. Foci of intramedullary parenchymatous lymphoma may occur in the spinal cord but are very infrequent. A diffuse lymphomatous leptomeningitis can occur as a result of which the spinal nerve roots become thickened. Of SNHL cases, 5% are associated with extradural spinal tumours which invariably cause cord compression (Grant et al. 1986). The tumour may be confined to the extradural space with no evidence of vertebral involvement in two-thirds of patients. The "metastatic" origin of the lymphoma in the extradural space is disputed. There is no well-recognized lymph tissue in the extradural compartment. The tumour may arrive by haematogenous spread into the fat or from direct extension of adjacent vertebral disease. Paravertebral lymphoma may extend into the spinal canal via the intervertebral foramen (Haddad et al. 1976). In a few instances (termed primary spinal epidural lymphoma) there is no evidence of visceral or nodal disease and the extradural tumour is the only manifestation of lymphoma. Systemic involvement can develop later but cord compression is the first sign of the disorder. SNHL is histologically different to PCNSL usually. The tumour does not transgress the dura and the clinical features are those typical of extradural cord and nerve root compression. In extradural lymphoma the vertebral involvement may be confined to the laminae and spinous process rather than to the vertebral body. SNHL has a relatively good prognosis because the tumour is often of low grade malignancy and is radiosensitive. *This emphasizes the importance of establishing a histological diagnosis by biopsy in any unknown neoplastic cause of extradural cord compression.* Treatment is by surgical decompression or biopsy combined with steroids and radiotherapy.

Neural compression from an extradural metastatic tumour can occur in Hodgkin's lymphoma. It is always secondary to disease in the vertebrae, mediastinum or retroperitoneal lymph nodes.

Table 23.3. Tumours and "tumour-like" conditions of the spinal column

Benign	Malignant	"Tumour-like" conditions
Chondroma	Metastases (carcinoma)	Vertebral haemangioma
Osteochondroma	Lymphoma	Aneurysmal bone cyst
Osteoid osteoma	Myeloma: solitary multiple	Eosinophilic granuloma
Benign osteoblastoma	Osteosarcoma	Calcifying pseudoneoplasm
	Chondrosarcoma	
	Chondroblastoma	
Osteoclastoma	Chordoma (notochord)	

Vertebral Myeloma

Myeloma is characterized by malignant proliferation of plasma cells chiefly in the bone marrow. The disease involves marrow-containing parts of the skeleton such as the spine, skull, sternum and ribs (multiple myeloma). Solitary myeloma (plasmocytoma) in a vertebra is uncommon and invariably develops into multiple myeloma later. Neoplastic cells produce abnormal gamma globulins which can be detected in the serum and/or urine (Bence-Jones protein). It affects adults, there is no sex predilection and, despite treatment, the average survival after diagnosis is about two years. The affected bone undergoes osteolytic change and pathological fractures occur causing severe back pain due to wedge collapse of vertebrae. The tumour mass can extend into the spinal canal by direct extension and is a well-recognized cause of malignant extradural spinal cord compression. The lower dorsal and lumbar segments are more often affected and the condition is associated with anaemia, markedly elevated ESR, uraemia, proteinaemia and hypercalcaemia. Treatment consists of excision (total or partial), combined with radiotherapy and chemotherapy.

Tumours of Spinal Column

The notochord appears in the fourth week of embryonic life and the spinal column develops almost entirely from condensations of mesenchyme formed around the notochord. The only remnant of the notochord represented in adult spine is the centrum of the nucleus pulposus. Tumours arising primarily from the vertebrae can be benign or malignant (Table 23.3).

Primary osseous tumours whether benign or malignant are important causes of back pain in adults, adolescents and children. Certain conditions, e.g., aneurysmal bone cyst, benign osteoblastoma, Ewing's sarcoma and eosinophilic granuloma are commoner in the younger age groups. The likelihood of a neoplasm involving the vertebrae must always be considered in patients with persistent undiagnosed back pain. Most of the tumours have characteristic plain X-ray appearances but are better demonstrated with isotope bone scans or CAT scans, the former is a particularly good screening test for both benign and malignant vertebral neoplasms. Whilst the vertebral body is the commonest part affected, pedicles, laminae, spines and transverse processes can be involved. With continued growth these tumours can extend to the spinal canal or intervertebral foramen and cause extradural neural compression. Primary bone tumours are usually the province of the orthopaedic surgeon but when the spine is involved and neurological features are present, a combined orthopaedic and neurosurgical team effort is essential. A few common examples are described below.

Vertebral Haemangioma

This is one of the commonest tumours affecting the spinal column. It is usually sited in the dorsal or lumbar region and may be a chance finding on X-ray or at autopsy. The tumour is commoner in women over 40 years of age. Usually, only a single vertebra is involved and the disc is unaffected pathologically and radiologically. It is a cavernous haemangioma, effectively an arteriovenous shunt fed by the intercostal and lumbar arteries. The typical plain X-ray appearance consists of vertical trabeculae in the vertebral body which is reduced in height but has preserved end plates. All the components of the vertebra can be affected. The clinical presentation is back pain, paraparesis or radicular symptoms. Angiography, myelography and CAT scanning are all helpful diagnostic tests. Excision is extremely hazardous due to the intense vascularity of the tumour. Preoperative embolization of the tumour mass with small particles helps to reduce the blood flow facilitating surgical removal. Radiotherapy is not a very effective method of treatment.

Chordoma

This tumour arises from remnants of the primitive notochord. It is a slow growing, locally invasive mass which can extend into the extradural space causing cord compression (Sundaresan et al. 1979). It has recently been recognized to have the capacity to metastasize to distant sites. The majority of spinal chordomas occur in the sacrococcygeal region or cervical spine. Despite the embryonic origin, the tumour is symptomatic usually between 40–60 years of age. Sacral tumours present chronic low back pain, or urinary/bowel symptoms due to a pelvic mass. The tumour is palpable on rectal examination. Other vertebral chordomas manifest as chronic spinal pain later associated with paraparesis or radicular symptoms. Plain X-rays show an expanding, destructive lesion within the bone often with calcification and a paraspinal soft tissue mass. CAT scans can demonstrate the extent of bone involvement, extradural extension or the size of a pelvic tumour component. The extent of the tumour at the time of diagnosis invariably precludes total excision. Surgery is therefore confined to partial excision and achieving some degree of decompression of the neural structures. The tumour is known to be radioresistant.

Aneurysmal Bone Cysts

This is a rare but interesting lesion. Its aetiology is uncertain and it is probably not a true neoplasm. There is a soft, fleshy, trabeculated highly vascular mass within the vertebra any component of which can be affected. The "cyst" contains engorged vascular spaces lined by endothelium. The sufferer is usually under 20 years old and the sexes are equally affected. It can occur in any region of the spine and the commonest extraspinal sites are the ends of long bones. The usual symptoms are back pain, paraparesis and radicular complaints. Plain X-rays show a rounded, rarefied area with septa within an expanded vertebra. Surgery is fraught with hazard due to severe bleeding but decompression with partial excision is usually possible. Radiotherapy has been described as effective.

Benign Osteoblastoma

This is an unusual tumour (Myles and Macrae 1988). About 40% occur in the spine and the presentation is predominantly in the first and second decades. The tumour affects the posterior elements of the vertebra rather than the body. It is a cause of back pain, scoliosis and sciatica as well as limb weakness. The tumour may be missed on plain X-ray and an isotope scan is essential for diagnosis. Myelography will reveal the extent of neural compression. Complete excision will relieve symptoms and remove the risk of possible malignant change later. Partial removal and radiotherapy is an alternative but the tumour is not very radiosensitive.

Osteochondroma

This is probably the commonest benign tumour of bone. It occurs at multiple sites, has a familial tendency and is therefore called hereditary multiple exostoses. The lesions occur most commonly at the ends of long bones and are often bilateral and symmetrical. The vertebral lesions can encroach into the spinal canal causing neural compression and/or back pain (O'Connor and Roberts 1984). The disease is transmitted as an autosomal dominant and there is a strong male preponderance. If symptomatic, the only treatment is excision because the tumour is radioresistant.

Sacrococcygeal Masses

A variety of neoplastic and non-neoplastic lesions can present as a mass in this region. The capacious sacral canal and presacral space accommodates the "tumour" allowing it to reach a large size before symptoms occur. The commonest complaint is low back pain, sciatic pain, constipation, rectal symptoms or fullness in the perineum. The mass may be visible as a unilateral swelling of the buttock or palpable on rectal examination. Neural compression within the sacral canal or the sacral plexus outside the canal causes features of a low cauda equina lesion. Plain X-rays of the sacrum though usually abnormal are difficult to interpret. CAT is the most useful radiological examination. In adults, the common lesions encountered are: chordoma, schwannoma, ependymoma, osseous tumours of all types and anterior sacral meningocele. In neonates and children, teratomas, meningoceles, lipomas and neuroblastoma are common causes. Meningoceles communicate with the CSF space and therefore increase in tension on straining or crying.

Schwannoma (Syn: Neurinoma) and Neurofibroma

The neurofibromatoses are genetically determined disorders (Barker et al. 1987). Two types are recognized with distinct genetic, clinical and pathological features. Neurofibromatosis type I (NF type I) is the entity classically described by von Recklinghausen (1882) and also termed the peripheral variety. It is characterized by multiple café-au-lait spots, multiple cutaneous tumours (neurofibromas), plexiform neurofibromas, axillary/inguinal freckling and iris hamartomas (Lisch nodules). It is an autosomal dominant disease with a prevalence of 60 per 100 000 population. There is no family history of the disease in half the affected individuals indicating a high incidence of spontaneous mutation. The gene for NF type I has been identified on the long arm of chromosome 17.

Neurofibromatosis type II (NF type II) also known as the central variety is characterized by multiple cranial or spinal intradural tumours, the commonest being bilateral 8th nerve tumours (schwannomas). It is also an autosomal dominant disease with a prevalence of only 0.1 per 100 000 population and therefore much less common than NF type I. The locus for NF type II is on the long arm of chromosome 22. Benign spinal intradural nerve sheath tumours commonly occur sporadically or in individuals with either NF type I or II (Halliday et al. 1991). Curiously the sporadic variety is the commonest group seen in routine clinical practice. Therefore, solitary spinal intradural nerve sheath tumours occur in patients with no evidence of NF type I or II although the occasional patient may show one or two cutaneous stigmata typical of NF type I.

The clinician is not usually inclined to differentiate between schwannoma and neurofibroma. Both tumours originate from the Schwann cell but their microscopic features are distinct. The schwannoma has a mixture of packed and loose cellular elements but is devoid of nerve fibres whilst a neurofibroma has a loose myxoid stroma containing nerve fibres. Spinal nerve sheath tumours usually arise from dorsal (sensory) roots and less commonly from anterior (motor) roots. The peripheral, plexiform and the occasional cranial and spinal nerve sheath tumours seen in NF type I are invariably neurofibromas. In contrast, the spinal nerve sheath tumours seen as sporadic cases or in association with NF type II are invariably schwannomas.

In addition to nerve sheath tumours, both NF types I and II show a predilection for the development of tumours of glial and meningeal origin. This tendency is less apparent in NF type I where the classical association is optic nerve glioma. NF type II is however frequently associated with cranial and/or spinal meningiomas, astrocytomas and ependymomas or a diffuse gliomatosis of the pia-arachnoid of the brain or spinal cord. The neural sheath tumours associated with NF type I can undergo sarcomatous degeneration and even metastasize into distant sites.

In the following account the term neurofibroma is used to denote all spinal nerve sheath tumours as it is commonly used in clinical practice and the older literature. In adults, neurofibromas represent 23% of primary spinal tumours (Nittner 1976). The incidence is equal to or only slightly higher than that of spinal meningiomas. Both sexes are equally affected although a slight female preponderance has been suggested by certain authors. Over a third of patients are 25–40 years at diagnosis and the mean age of presentation is less in men and in those with cervical region tumours.

Over half the tumours occur in the dorsal region and the others are equally distributed between the cervical and lumbar regions, sacral regions being extremely rare. This distribution is compatible with a uniform incidence irrespective of region when considering the relative length of each area of the spine. Cervical and lumbar region tumours have the longest duration of symptoms prior to diagnosis. This may reflect the relatively smaller space available for tumour expansion in the dorsal region before causing cord compression. About half the patients are diagnosed within two years of the onset of symptoms.

Most tumours (72%) are intradural/extramedullary and intramedullary have been described in a few rare instances (less than 1%). Intradural/extradural tumours of the dumb-bell or hourglass type are as common (13%) as the purely extradural lesions (14%) and the latter may extend into the paravertebral tissues. The waist of an hourglass tumour lies within the enlarged intervertebral foramen and a surgeon who encounters an apparently extradural tumour should open the dura to exclude any intradural extension. The extradural/paravertebral component can be larger than the intradural part and may be palpable in the neck. Some dorsal neurofibromas are associated with lateral extraspinal meningoceles which can be seen as a mediastinal mass on a chest X-ray.

Neurofibromas commonly arise from a dorsal root and are thus invariably sited posterolateral in relation to the cord dorsal to the plane of the dentate ligament (Fig. 23.7). Occasionally, a neurofibroma can arise from a ventral root and is then sited anterior or anterolateral to the cord. The root involved is very closely adherent or attached to the tumour and has to be divided to achieve radical excision of the lesion. The sensory root involved can be sacrificed with impunity but section of a ventral root may cause a significant motor deficit in the cervical or lumbar region. In practice, the surgeon is pleasantly surprised at the absence of even a sensory deficit after dorsal root division and this is probably due to the overlap of cutaneous supply by adjacent roots. If more than one root is sacrificed, sensory loss is invariable and this can be troublesome if the hand, foot or genital area are involved.

An intradural tumour is usually 2–3 cm in size, sausage-shaped and often a lobulated pinkish-yellow mass but some, especially those in the lumbar region, can be much larger. They have a firm consistency and the cut surface has a yellow fatty tissue appearance. Contrary to common belief, most are quite vascular making surgical excision difficult. A few contain tumour cysts but calcification is rarely found. The mass lies entirely in the subarachnoid plane and the nerve root of origin is attached to the rostral and caudal poles of the tumour. The spinal cord is displaced and moulded around the tumour and the adjacent nerve roots draped around it. Small tumours especially those in the cauda equina can be mobile but larger lesions are wedged firmly between adjacent tissues.

Radicular pain is the commonest early presenting symptom. However, severe cord compression and neurological disability can occur without pain. Weakness and pyramidal signs follow the onset of root pain and sensory symptoms occur thereafter. Sphincter disturbance is the last major symptom to appear (Levy et al. 1986). The lumbar CSF protein may exceed 5 g/litre, well in excess of that expected with a spinal block. This feature may cause impairment of CSF absorption and contribute to the occasional syndrome of raised intracranial pressure described in association with many spinal tumours (Ridsdale and Moseley 1978).

Plain X-rays may show an enlarged intervertebral foramen and/or widening of the interpedicular distance. These changes are more common in neuro-

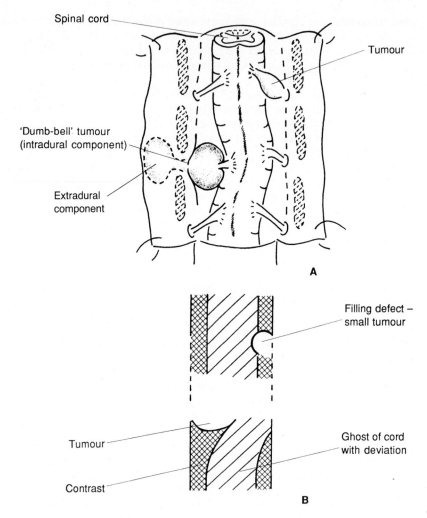

Fig. 23.7. A Intradural tumour: neurofibromata. **B** Myelography appearance.

fibromas than in spinal meningiomas. Myelography, CAT and MRI are the best means of diagnosis. The best treatment is excision. There is no place for radiotherapy unless the rare complication of sarcomatous change has occurred in a tumour.

Meningioma

Meningiomas also form nearly a quarter of all primary spinal neoplasms. They are of mesodermal descent and can arise from arachnoid cells situated in any meningeal layer. The tumour is therefore attached to the meningeal covering at

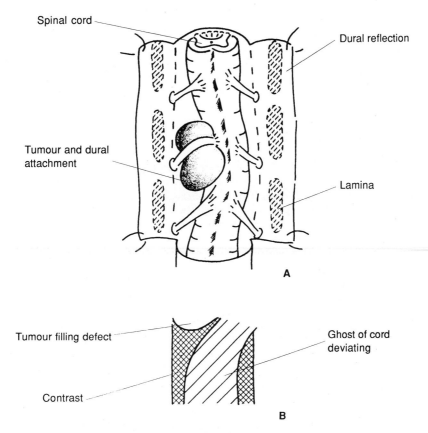

Spinal cord

Dural reflection

Tumour and dural
attachment

Lamina

A

Tumour filling defect

Ghost of cord
deviating

Contrast

B

Fig. 23.8. A Intradural tumour: meningioma. **B** Myelography appearance.

the point of origin (Fig. 23.8). The aetiology is unknown but the growth rate is related to sex hormones, perhaps explaining the marked female preponderance (80%) of the tumour. Oestrogen and progesterone receptors have been identified in these tumours and the rate of growth is known to increase with pregnancy (Davis 1990). Cranial meningiomas are four to five times commoner than their spinal counterpart probably due to the greater available dural surface for tumour origin.

Whilst they may occur in any part of the spine, 81% are found in the dorsal region. The tumour is uncommon in the lumbosacral area (2%). The age at presentation is 40–70 years with a peak incidence in the sixth decade. *Any middle-aged or elderly female presenting with features of gradual cord compression related to the dorsal area must be assumed to have a meningioma until proved otherwise.* The dorsal predilection is not observed in male patients. Most tumours are intradural/extramedullary in position. Intramedullary tumours have not been described. Intradural/extradural lesions occur (7%) and some of these can have a typical dumb-bell appearance. Meningiomas at the foramen magnum can have a similar shape with a waist-like union between the cranial and cervical portions. Purely extradural tumours are also well recognized (8%); they are more vascular, grow more rapidly and can erode the bone. The meningeal origin can be small or broad-based, the latter conferring a degree of immobility to the tumour. The main blood supply arises from enlarged extradural arteries and hypervascularity of the adjacent extradural space is usually near the insertion of the dentate ligament in proximity to the exit zone of the spinal root. Therefore, most meningiomas are sited lateral, posterolateral or anterolateral to the cord. Only a small proportion of tumours are truly anterior or posterior to the cord. A more interesting observation is that tumours sited above C7 are invariably anterior and those at or below C7 have a greater likelihood of being posterior to the dentate ligament (Levy et al. 1982). The classical en plaque tumour is a rare finding.

An intradural meningioma will enlarge displacing the arachnoid membrane towards the cord. This protective layer of arachnoid is very useful to the surgeon engaged in excision of the tumour. The pinkish-grey or purple mass is about 2–3 cm, either rounded or oval-shaped and lobulated only occasionally. The consistency is firm and numerous blood vessels are seen on the surface. The cut surface has a granular appearance and gritty areas of calcification occur. The occasional heavily calcified or even ossified tumour is an arduous challenge to the surgeon because the tissue cannot be fragmented by ordinary methods of tumour removal. Additional manipulation of the tumour and cord leads to a poor functional result after excision. Cyst formation and haemorrhage are uncommon but cord oedema, cystic change and myelomalacia may occur. Most meningiomas are totally benign tumours of the transitional or fibroblastic type but the occasional angioblastic variant is found in the pure extradural tumours.

Radicular pain occurs less commonly than in neurofibroma (21%). Midline back pain is the commonest early complaint. Vague sensory symptoms follow

Table 23.4. Comparison of clinical, pathological and radiological features of neurofibroma and meningioma

	Neurofibroma	Meningioma
Single/multiple	Usually single (multiple in NF 1 and 2)	Usually single (multiple in NF 1 and 2)
Age	25–40 years	40–70 years
Sex predilection	Equal	Female (×4) in dorsal tumours
Spinal level	Dorsal 50%. Cervical and lumbosacral equally affected	Dorsal 80%. Very uncommon in lumbosacral area
Relationship to cord	Invariably posterolateral	Commonly lateral
Dumb-bell tumour	Commoner	Possible
Calcification	Rare	Possible
Radicular pain	Very common 1st symptom	Less common
Motor features	Second symptom	Third symptom
Sensory features	Third symptom	First and second symptom
Bladder symptoms	Late symptom	Late symptom
Raised intracranial pressure	Rare	Very rare
CSF protein	Grossly elevated	Elevated
Abnormal plain X-rays	Up to 50%	Up to 20%

the pain and motor and bladder symptoms appear later. The average duration of symptoms is two years but about 50% come to surgery within a year of onset. About 65% of patients have motor or sensory features at the time of diagnosis. Misdiagnosis can occur in some who present with a fluctuating course when multiple sclerosis is naturally the first consideration. A rapidly growing angioblastic extradural meningioma with a short history of neurological evolution, pedicle erosion on plain X-ray and an extradural myelographic block can be mistaken for a metastatic deposit. The rare syndrome of raised intracranial pressure which has been described with spinal tumours occurs but is less likely.

Plain X-ray changes are found in 3%–20% of patients. Pedicle erosion is the commonest and calcification occurs in about 3%. Hyperostosis akin to the skull changes seen in cranial meningiomas does not occur in the spinal tumours. Conventional myelography combined with CAT scanning and/or MRI are the main methods of radiological diagnosis. A comparison of the main clinical and radiological features of neurofibroma and a meningioma is depicted in Table 23.4. The ideal treatment is surgical excision of the tumour and its dural attachment. Radiotherapy has a place following subtotal excision or in the aggressive angioblastic variety. In these situations tumour recurrence is possible.

Intramedullary Tumours

These tumours are not uncommon and comprise about 10%–20% of adult primary neoplasms (Sloof et al. 1964) but form less than 5% if metastatic tumours are also considered. There is a higher incidence of intramedullary tumours in children's series because neurofibroma and meningioma are less frequent in younger age groups. The commonest intramedullary tumours are astrocytomas and ependymomas both arising from cells of neuroepithelial origin and also included under the common term glioma. Their association with NF types 1 and 2 has already been mentioned. Other intramedullary tumours, though encountered less commonly, are haemangioblastoma, dermoid cysts, epidermoid cysts, lipomas and neurofibromas. The clinical features are similar and have been described already.

Astrocytoma

Intraspinal astrocytomas are rarer than their cerebral counterparts. In adults, they form about 8% of all primary spinal tumours (Sloof et al. 1964) and about 30% of intramedullary tumours. In children's series, astrocytomas are commoner comprising about 60% of intramedullary tumours (Reimer and Onofrio 1985; Rotisch et al. 1990). The tumour occurs mostly in the cervical and dorsal regions of the cord. Cervical tumours may extend or be an extension off a brain stem astrocytoma.

Astrocytomas are usually slow growing, histologically benign and akin to the Grade 1 and 2 fibrillary cerebellar astrocytomas. Therefore cyst formation is common (nearly 50%) and extends into several segments. The cyst may be situated at either end of a small solid tumour component and even extend to involve the entire length of the spinal cord (holocord tumours). Such lesions are commoner in children and young adults. The cysts contain xanthochromic proteinaceous fluid, have smooth walls and do not contain neoplastic cells. Macroscopically, the cord is enlarged but the tumour is not visible on the surface usually. The posterior nerve roots are wider apart and the cord may have a pale grey appearance. These benign astrocytomas are pale, relatively avascular tumours which may or may not have an identifiable plane of separation from the cord.

Symptoms run a slow, subtle course over months or years, often with remissions and relapses. This pattern may mimic the symptomatology of multiple sclerosis causing diagnostic error. There is a slight male preponderance with a peak incidence in the second and third decades. Scoliosis is a feature in children and adolescents. Midline spinal or central pain occurs in half the patients. Paraesthesiae eventually evolve into the typical dissociated sensory loss pattern. Limb paralysis is very subtle at first, perhaps affecting only one limb and progressing gradually to affect others sequentially.

Radiological appearances are as described before. It is very important to identify the presence and extent of a tumour cyst/s and the exact segmental location of the solid component. This can be achieved by MRI preoperatively or by ultrasonography peroperatively (see later). Treatment is by excision (total or subtotal) combined with cyst drainage and radiotherapy. The prognosis is good if significant tumour debulking can be achieved.

Malignant Astrocytoma

This neoplasm is seen only rarely and comprises about 7.5% of all spinal cord gliomas in adults and occurs even less frequently in children. The sexes are affected equally and the tumour is symptomatic within the first three decades of life. There is a rapidly progressive course of neurological deterioration with pain, paralysis and sensory impairment. The radiological evidence is similar to the benign variety. The solid tumour has a reddish colour, is more vascular and is not well demarcated from the cord. Tumour cysts containing xanthochromic fluid are present. Microscopic appearances are akin to Grade 3 or 4 cerebral astrocytomas. The tumour can spread to other areas along the CSF with leptomeningeal involvement of brain and spinal cord. Despite aggressive surgical treatment with resection, radiotherapy and chemotherapy, the prognosis is extremely poor (Cohen et al. 1989).

Ependymoma

Intraspinal ependymomas are also less common than the cerebral counterparts. They form about 5% of all primary CNS tumours, only a third occurring within the spinal canal. Nearly 60% of the spinal ependymomas occur in and around the cauda equina (Sloof et al. 1964). The remainder are intramedullary in the cervical and dorsal regions, the former being more frequently affected (McCormick et al. 1990). In adults, ependymomas comprise the majority of intramedullary tumours accounting for nearly 65%. It is the commonest primary tumour in the region of the conus/cauda equina (88%) (Norstrom et al. 1961). Some conus intramedullary ependymomas have an exophytic extra-medullary component extending into the lumbosacral spinal canal.

Males are more commonly afflicted. The mean age of presentation is about 35 years for both sexes but the tumour is uncommon below 20 years. It originates from the ependymal lining of the central canal or filum terminale and is histologically benign with a slow rate of growth and very little capacity to infiltrate the cord. A soft red or purple solid tumour mass expands the cord often separating the proprioceptive columns and presenting beneath the pial surface in the midline posteriorly. Rostral tumour cysts with xanthochromic fluid are described and the cyst wall is non-neoplastic. The tumour, though unencapsulated, has a layer of gliotic tissue around it which facilitates tumour excision. On microscopic examination the tumours around the conus and cauda equina are invariably of the benign myxopapillary variety. Malignant cerebrospinal ependymomas may produce subarachnoid seedlings via CSF dissemination.

The symptoms are of gradual onset and progress slowly. The average duration before diagnosis is about three years. There is good preservation of neurological function even with extensive tumours because of the protracted slow growth. Back pain, worse at night, and radicular pain, invariably of a sciatic distribution, are very common. Sudden haemorrhage into a tumour causes acute sciatic pain (Fincher's syndrome). The pattern of paralysis and sensory change will depend on the site of the tumour being either a central cord or cauda equina syndrome. Plain X-rays show an enlarged spinal canal in about one-third of patients. Myelography demonstrates either an enlarged cord or a filling defect in the cauda equina. CAT and MRI are extremely useful in identifying the morphology of the tumour including the presence of a cyst. Treatment is by total or subtotal excision combined in the latter instance with radiotherapy. The prognosis is very good in those in whom total excision is possible.

Haemangioblastoma

These tumours occur most commonly in the cerebellum either sporadically or as a manifestation of the von Hippel-Lindau syndrome (Neumann et al. 1989). They occur, although less frequently, in relation to the spinal cord mostly as intradural/intramedullary tumours or more rarely as pure extradural tumours (Murota and Symon 1989). Any part of the cord can be affected but thoracic lesions are commoner probably due to the anatomical extent of the region. The tumour is a reddish-orange mass with tortuous arterial channels on its surface and large draining veins situated in a polar position. This arrangement is very similar to that of an arteriovenous malformation and surgical removal is extremely difficult because of the intense vascularity. Associated tumour cysts are well described as in the cranial counterpart. They contain clear lemon-yellow fluid which is rich in erythropoietin. A family history of von Hippel-Lindau disease may be elicited and the patient may have been treated previously for a cerebellar tumour of the same type. Clinical features depend on the site of the lesion and usually consist of a progressive neurological disturbance with limb weakness and sensory deficit. Multiple tumours are common.

Plain X-rays are usually normal. Myelography will reveal the tumour mass as a filling defect with enlarged blood vessels around it. CAT and MRI will confirm these findings and the latter is very useful to screen the length of the spine as well as the cranial compartment for other lesions. Spinal angiography is extremely useful before contemplating surgical attack on these extremely vascular lesions. This may reveal tumour nodules in relation to a large cyst which may have been undetected with other radiology methods. Excision is the best treatment but the vascularity of the tumour renders the operation tedious. Yet, the results following excision are extremely favourable.

Spinal Cysts

A variety of neoplastic and non-neoplastic cystic extradural or intradural lesions of differing aetiology occur in relation to the spinal cord, nerve roots and meninges. Many of these are a result of maldevelopment and are therefore present at birth. They cause symptoms in childhood or in early adult life. Whilst some are harmless and invariably asymptomatic most cause neurological disease due to spinal neural compromise. The term cyst implies that the contents are fluid but certain notable exceptions contain solid material. Meningoceles, paracytic cysts and syringomyelic cysts are outside the scope of this chapter. Neoplastic cysts associated with spinal astrocytoma, ependymoma and haemangioblastoma have already been mentioned.

Dermoid and Epidermoid Cysts

These are invariably developmental lesions which are well recognized but relatively uncommon. They account for about 1%–2% of primary adult spinal tumours (Sloof et al. 1964). In paediatric series an incidence of 4.5% (Rand and Rand 1960) and 13% (Lunardi et al. 1989) has been reported. They arise from ectodermal tissue destined to become skin which is implanted within the neural tube during its closure. Such implantation can rarely occur following trauma or lumbar puncture. A small number of cases are therefore iatrogenic in origin and follow repeated spinal taps for the diagnosis and treatment of meningitis (Choremis et al. 1956).

Epidermoid cysts originate from epidermal elements only. The cyst has a glistening grey-white external surface thus acquiring the description of pearly tumour. The wall is lined with stratified squamous epithelium and the creamy-white, cheese-like material within arises from dead desquamated epidermal cells. Keratin breakdown produces an abundance of cholesterol and stearine-like compounds which produces shiny lipid droplets when the cyst contents float in water at operation. This tumour has also acquired the confusing misnomer cholesteatoma since the contents resemble the chronic inflammatory masses which occur in the middle ear.

Dermoid cysts originate from both epidermal and dermal elements. The wall has stratified squamous epithelium as well as hair follicles, sweat glands and sebaceous glands. The contents resemble an epidermoid but, in addition, hair is commonly seen and, very rarely, teeth are found. Both dermoids and epidermoids occur invariably as intradural lesions; extradural occurrence is rare. The intradural lesions are either intramedullary or juxtamedullary in situation. As a group they are more common in the region of the conus than elsewhere in the spine. Intramedullary epidermoids are more common in the thoracic region whereas intramedullary dermoids occur more often at the conus. The cervical region is relatively less affected by both tumours.

Being present at birth, initial presentation is usually in childhood but due to their slow rate of enlargement the diagnosis may be made only in adult life. A slight male preponderance is recognized for both lesions. There is an association with spina bifida occulta and the cutaneous stigmata of this condition (naevus, dimple, tuft of hair) may be present over the lumbosacral region. More importantly, dermoids can be associated with a dermal sinus which may communicate with the spinal subarachnoid space, lending a vulnerability to meningitis which may be the mode of initial presentation. The usual clinical picture is a gradually progressive neurological syndrome specific to the location of the cyst. The most common is a conus/cauda equina lesion with back pain, saddle anaesthesia, leg weakness and sphincter disturbance.

Plain X-rays may show localized enlargement of the spinal canal, congenital vertebral abnormalities and, rarely, teeth. Myelography reveals an extradural or intradural mass, the latter usually with cord enlargement. CAT and MRI show the tumour mass well due to the characteristic signal intensity of the fat content. MRI is useful to exclude associated congenital abnormalities of the spinal cord which may be present.

The best treatment is excision. However, total excision is often impossible and hazardous because the capsule is very adherent to the cord. The results of surgery are usually gratifying even with only partial excision creating sufficient tumour debulking to relieve neural compression. The edges of the cyst wall can be "marsupialized" to the dural surface so that tumour material which recurs does not cause cord compression. Recurrence only occurs after several years and with a prudent surgical approach the patient can be given years of independent mobility, continence and satisfactory sexual function. Radiotherapy is ineffective.

Teratomas

These developmental tumours of germ cell origin are less common than dermoid and epidermoid cysts. Their incidence is higher in children than in adults. The lumbar region is affected most frequently and the tumour is either intradural/extramedullary or intramedullary in position. The contents may be cystic or solid and histologically, cartilage, bone, smooth and skeletal muscle are recognized. The lining of the wall consists of columnar or cuboidal epithelium. The bony elements cause radiographic opacities which are diagnostic. Some tumours are malignant and produce remote seedlings via the CSF. Teratomas and seminomas (germ cell tumours) of the mediastinum can cause epidural metastatic deposits even due to direct or blood stream spread. Teratomas can occur anterior to the sacrum or coccyx often associated with a dermal sinus which opens near the anal verge. These so-called sacrococcygeal tumours are much commoner in children. The treatment is total or subtotal excision.

Neurenteric (Enterogenous) Cysts

The neurenteric canal joins the primitive yolk sac to the amniotic cavity. The canal splits the developing vertebrae and spinal cord in the early stages of fetal life. Persistence of any part of this canal in the fully-formed fetus is a developmental defect. In the worst type, the entire neurenteric canal is patent and the stomach and intestines herniate onto the dorsal surface of the fetus. The condition is very rare and survival is unknown. A persistent intradural (less commonly extradural) neurenteric canal can produce an expanding cystic lesion with resultant cord compression. The thoracic spine is most often affected. The cysts contain either clear colourless fluid or a viscous, mucoid material. Associated vertebral anomalies such as spina bifida occulta or anterior defects of the vertebral body occur in the region of the cyst. The tumour is commoner in young adult males and the usual presentation is back pain, root pain and a progressive neurological disturbance. The best treatment is excision but the tumour capsule is adherent to the cord and radical removal may be difficult and hazardous. Percutaneous or operative cyst drainage provides good symptomatic benefit in recurrent tumours. Radiotherapy is not effective.

Arachnoid Cysts

These are not true neoplasms but can cause cord or nerve root compression. Most are congenital and a result of meningeal maldevelopment but some may be traumatic in origin.

Extradural Arachnoid Cyst

These occur typically in the thoracic spine of adolescent males (Cloward and Bucy 1937). The cyst is situated either in the posterior midline or posterolaterally in relation to the dura covering the dorsal root. The cyst is essentially an evagination or herniation of the arachnoid layer and contains clear fluid (Gortvai 1963). It enlarges gradually probably due to a valve-like effect at the neck or pedicle which passes through the dural hiatus. Smaller cysts are often multiple and asymptomatic. Large lesions eventually cause neural compression, the characteristic feature of which is a spastic paraparesis and a sensory ataxia. A fluctuating course is possible because the cyst may empty intermittently. The contrast used in myelography usually fills the sac. Treatment is by excision with ligation of the pedicle.

Perineural Cysts

These are subarachnoid cysts wrapped around a nerve root. They occur in the lumbar and sacral regions in relation to the posterior roots and are usually multiple and bilateral (Tarlov 1938). The cyst contains clear fluid but there is usually no communication with the subarachnoid space. Therefore the cyst does not fill with contrast medium during myelography and some cysts occur in the lower sacral canal where no subarachnoid space is present. Most are asymptomatic but the associated root can become compressed causing sciatic pain and cauda equina symptoms. Treatment is excision but diagnosis can be difficult.

Other meningeal diverticula of congenital origin occur in the lumbosacral region. They communicate with the subarachnoid space and contrast used in myelography enters the cyst easily. Rarely, root pain or dysfunction occurs.

Intradural Arachnoid Cyst

These rare lesions occur in the posterior midline of the dorsal spine. They are intra-arachnoid cysts which contain clear fluid and cause cord compression if sufficiently large. The common symptom is back pain which increases on standing and is relieved on lying supine. Treatment is drainage with excision of the outer arachnoid covering.

Spinal Lipomas

Lipomatous tissue can occur within the spinal canal in two distinct conditions. The lipomyelomeningoceles are myelovertebral malformations which occur in association with spina bifida occulta. This condition is described elsewhere. Lipomas can also occur as true primary tumours in the spinal canal. They are usually intradural in situation and are uncommon tumours accounting for 0.5% of all primary spinal tumours and 2% of intramedullary tumours (Sloof et al. 1964). Their incidence is higher in children's series but the inclusion or exclusion of myelovertebral malformations skew the statistics. The sex incidence is equal. Symptoms begin in the first three decades of life but may be present even at birth. Usually there is about three years duration of symptoms before significant neurological disability occurs. Lipomas are common in the cervical and thoracic levels. They are either intramedullary or juxtamedullary in relation to the cord. The tumour capsule is very adherent to neural tissue and at operation, the intradural mass expands the thecal sac into a taut, non-pulsatile lump. The tumour itself is yellow, rubbery and lobulated. Multiple tumours may be present with other cranial or spinal lipomata. Associated malformations of the vertebrae are found in one-third of cases.

The typical clinical picture is a progressive spastic paraparesis and sensory ataxia. The latter is because the tumour is commonly situated in the posterior midline region. Root pain is rare. Plain X-rays of the spine reveal a widened canal and congenital vertebral anomalies may be seen. Myelography demonstrates an intradural tumour with or without cord expansion. Treatment is excision but total removal is rarely possible due to the adherence of the capsule to the spinal cord. Partial excision with tumour debulking is sufficient to obtain good symptomatic benefit. Radiotherapy is not helpful.

Extradural Lipomas

These tumours are very uncommon (Ehni and Love 1945). They form large extradural fatty lumps on the posterior aspect of the dura in the dorsal region.

The fat is reddish-yellow or brown in colour, loosely attached to the dura and can be removed easily at operation. The clinical history of cord compression is of short duration. Plain X-rays of the spine are usually normal. Excision produces good symptomatic benefit.

Some Unusual Tumours

Epidural Hibernoma

The lipomas described above commonly contain white or yellow adipose tissue. Brown fat is an important source of non-shivering heat production under cold stress in animals who hibernate. This tissue is relatively underdeveloped in man for obvious reasons. Fat cells contain steroid receptors and dexamethasone binds to these strongly. It depletes white fat by lipolysis but increases the mass of brown fat by the metabolism of glycogen and lipid. Patients on long-term steroid therapy are known to develop centripetal fat deposition. This increase may occur in the epidural space and the condition epidural lipomatosis is a recognized complication of steroid therapy (Perling et al. 1988). The excess fat can produce spinal neural compromise manifesting as a neurological syndrome of a myelopathy, radiculopathy, cauda equina syndrome or neurogenic claudication. Unless the aetiology is recognized the steroid dose may be increased when the cord syndrome occurs thus worsening the situation.

Paraganglioma

This neoplasm arises from cells of neuroendocrine origin associated with the autonomic nervous system. The nomenclature and classification is complex but currently the term paraganglioma is applicable to all tumours arising from chromaffin tissues of adrenal or extra-adrenal sites. They are related to phaeochromocytomas and chemodectomas. The extra-adrenal paragangliomas are usually benign and non-secretory. Common examples are carotid body tumour and glomus jugulare tumour. Paraganglioma is a well described tumour within the lumbosacral canal occurring as an intradural lesion which can produce a cauda equina syndrome (O'Sullivan et al. 1990). It probably arises from neuroblast cells which are capable of differentiating into chemoreceptor cells or ganglion cells. The sex incidence is equal and the tumour occurs in late adult life. It is attached to the filum terminale or a nerve root of the cauda equina, is well encapsulated and can be excised easily. It is not pharmacologically active but may contain dopamine, adrenaline and noradrenaline. Myelography reveals an intradural/extramedullary mass. The treatment is excision and results are excellent.

Calcifying Pseudoneoplasms

Recent literature has revealed unusual granulomatous fibrochondro-calcifying masses which can occur within the spinal canal causing neural compression

(Bertoni et al. 1990). Their aetiology is unknown and they are probably non-neoplastic lesions. There is neither a sex predilection nor an age pattern but the described cases have been in adults. Patients present with back pain and progressive neurological disturbance. Plain X-rays reveal a calcified mass within the spinal canal. Myelography and CAT confirm an intraspinal tumour which is difficult to distinguish from a prolapsed calcified disc protrusion. Treatment is by excision.

Extradural Haematopoiesis

In thalassaemia and myelosclerosis, compensatory haematopoiesis can occur in sites remote from the marrow, liver and spleen. Extradural masses of such haematopoietic tissue can produce spinal cord compression (Jackson et al. 1988). The diagnosis is by bone scan or MRI and treatment is excision and/or radiotherapy.

Paediatric Spinal Tumours

Incidence

Many of the spinal tumours seen in adult neurosurgical practice also occur in children. Moreover, the majority of intraspinal neoplasms seen in paediatric practice are benign in nature. Specific comment has already been made regarding the incidence of the different tumour types in children. Similar to adults, childhood spinal tumours are about five times less common than cerebral neoplasms. However, the relative incidence of the various tumours is different as shown in Table 23.5 (Till 1975; Matson 1969; Rand and Rand 1960). Metastases, neurofibromas and meningiomas occur less frequently. There is a relatively higher incidence of congenital tumours and intramedullary gliomas. Approximately 25% of childhood tumours are intramedullary in site and 30% either extradural or intradural/extramedullary. A small number are found in the subarachnoid space as seedlings from distant malignant neoplasms. The commonest lesions in the last category are medulloblastoma, ependymoma, pinealoma and choroid plexus papilloma. All areas of the spine are affected but congenital neoplasms are commoner in the lumbosacral or cervical regions.

Clinical Features

The basic neurological disturbances caused by a spinal neoplasm are similar to those described in adults. However, diagnostic difficulties arise for a variety of reasons. Most tumours being benign and slow growing produce a subtle and gradual neurological evolution. Very young children are unable to complain and even the older child is not usually prone to do so unless pain is a feature. Pain is not an early symptom of intramedullary tumours which are the commonest neoplasms seen in children. The low incidence of spinal tumours in

Table 23.5. Incidence of spinal cord tumours in children

	Rand and Rand (1960) (65 cases)*	Matson (1969) (135 cases)*	Till (1975) (68 cases)*
Intramedullary Astrocytoma Ependymoma Other gliomas	31%	22%	24%
Intradural Meningioma	3%	2%	3%
Neurofibroma	8%	4%	9%
Extradural Sarcoma Neuroblastoma Ganglioneuroma	25%	21%	33%
Arachnoid cyst			2%
Dermoid cyst	3%	10%	4%
Lipoma	6%	5%	
Teratoma	2%	10%	2%
Neurenteric cyst		1%	6%
Osteoblastoma	5%		
Vertebral haemangioma	3%	2%	
Aneurysm bone cyst	2%		2%
Ewing's sarcoma	3%		2%
Medulloblastoma	6%	3%	2%
Metastases		13%	
Others	3%	7%	2%

* See references.

children renders an element of impaired vigilance in the inexperienced clinician thus diagnostic errors are made, confusing the clinical picture with other neurological or orthopaedic disorders.

In an infant, the only manifestation of pain may be irritability, being off feeds or incessant crying. In older children, root pain may be mistaken for joint disease or visceral pain. A rigid spine with paraspinal spasm is always sinister. Weakness of a limb may only be noted by a parent as a limp, reluctance to run or play, or a sudden change of dexterity when an upper limb becomes weak. Sensory examination is difficult and requires tact and patience. Examination with a pin should be kept to the last in the routine. Incontinence in a child who had previously acquired sphincter training is significantly abnormal. Scoliosis, kyphosis, torticollis and foot deformities such as talipes should alert the clinician to the possibility of neuromuscular imbalance due to neurological dysfunction. Recurrent meningitis may be caused by infection of a dermal sinus communicating with the subarachnoid space. Symptoms of raised intracranial pressure or hydrocephalus may be the first sign of a spinal neoplasm (Ridsdale and Moseley 1978). When a family history of neurofibromatosis or von Hippel-Lindau disease is present there is a greater vulnerability to develop spinal tumours. The presence of cutaneous stigmata of spina bifida should alert the clinician to the potential possibility of an intraspinal tumour.

Diagnosis

The fundamental concepts are similar to those noted in adults. Plain X-rays will show canal widening, congenital anomalies or scoliosis. Myelography is difficult to perform and may require general anaesthesia. MRI is an extremely useful non-invasive examination which can be used to screen the entire central nervous system.

Malignant Epidural Tumours

A number of solid malignant neoplasms which are rare in adults can produce spinal metastatic disease in children. The commonest are Ewing's sarcoma and neuroblastoma (Klein 1991). The sarcoma group also includes osteogenic sarcoma, rhabdomyosarcoma and soft tissue sarcomata. Neuroblastoma is a malignant tumour of the adrenal medulla or sympathetic ganglia in the retroperitoneal tissues (Wilson and Draper 1974). It spreads by direct extension via the intervertebral foramen into the spinal canal to produce an extradural mass. Severe and rapidly progressive spinal neural compromise occurs. The majority of neuroblastomas arise in children less than four years old. It is probably the commonest malignant tumour in childhood. Treatment is by partial excision, radiotherapy and chemotherapy.

Medulloblastoma

This is a malignant neoplasm which occurs primarily in and around the fourth ventricle. Tumour cells can spread via CSF pathways into the spinal subarachnoid space. These seedlings are initially asymptomatic and often multiple. Back pain, root pain, weakness and a sensory loss are common symptoms. It is customary to perform a myelogram in all patients with a posterior fossa medulloblastoma following excision of the primary tumour. Most radiotherapists administer full craniospinal radiotherapy even if there is no clinical or X-ray evidence of metastatic disease in the spinal subarachnoid space. Recurrence, despite radiotherapy, can be treated with chemotherapy. Surgery has a place for discrete lesions which are causing severe cord compression.

Management

Spinal cord and/or cauda equina compression is one of the commonest conditions requiring emergency treatment in a neurosurgical department. Compression can evolve slowly or rapidly. Slow evolution is the usual pattern of a benign tumour but a rapidly progressive cord disturbance can be due to a benign or malignant lesion. When the time course is gradual there is greater opportunity for diagnostic assessment and the institution of definitive treatment to avoid the catastrophe of permanent neurological disability. A rapidly progressive compression syndrome is a surgical emergency and delay in the commencement of appropriate treatment will alter the prognosis significantly. The latter clinical scenario often exposes the inherent drawbacks of even the most comprehensive health care systems. Diagnostic error is the main cause of delay at the family doctor level. Failure of the patient to seek early medical help is not a significant factor. The main avoidable delays at the referring hospital consist of failure of diagnosis as a result of poor neurological assessment, misinterpretation of the clinical picture, the failure to realize the urgency of the condition or the delay in obtaining the appropriate medical opinion. Neurological deterioration, including worsening paralysis and loss of sphincter control, occurs during the process of diagnostic delay and lethargy of referral (Maurice-Williams and Richardson 1988).

The avoidance of these pitfalls is primarily achieved by the capability of family practitioners and hospital doctors to recognize, or at least suspect, the condition and then refer the patient to an appropriate department for further evaluation. In most instances this will be the local neurosurgical unit and all cases of spinal neural compromise should at least be initially referred for an opinion to a neurosurgeon. Constant clinical vigilance is essential. Back pain in a patient known to have a history of carcinoma must be investigated. Similarly, chronic back pain associated with lumbar paraspinal muscle spasm is always of sinister significance in a child. Vascular accidents of the cord are uncommon and demyelinating disease rarely produces a steady progressive cord disturbance in the initial stages. Neither condition is associated with back pain or radicular pain at the onset. If symptoms and signs cannot be explained on a rational clinical basis further investigation and opinion should be sought expediently. Careful documentation of neurological findings is important and a source of useful information to the attending neurosurgeon who must determine the rate of evolution of the neurological deterioration.

General Treatment

During the period of investigation, the control of pain is an important aspect of treatment. Pain can be severe especially in extradural tumours and regular opiate analgesia may be required. Strict bed rest is essential in these patients and electrically-operated beds minimize discomfort when nursing procedures are carried out. Patients with acute retention or dribbling incontinence require an indwelling urinary catheter. Active and passive physiotherapy to paralysed limbs will help maintain joint mobility and muscle tone. The general care of anaesthetic skin areas is essential to prevent pressure sores. A bed cradle will facilitate free lower limb movement which should be encouraged in the pre- and postoperative periods.

Dexamethasone is commonly used to gain neurological stability until definitive treatment is carried out and for a short while thereafter. Often a dramatic improvement to neurological function is seen within a few hours of commencing the medication. Dexamethasone reduces cerebral oedema (Yamada et al. 1979) and the mechanism of action on the compromised spinal cord may be similar. Very high doses of steroids have been shown to enhance spinal cord blood flow after injury (Braughler and Hall 1983). A specific antimitotic effect of steroids has also been postulated and the dramatic effect of dexamethasone in reducing the size of a lymphoma is well recognized. The standard dose used in routine practice is 16 mg per day given in divided doses but high bolus dose administration over a short period is feasible in severe cases of cord compression.

Rarely, neurological deterioration may be precipitated after myelography. In tumours of the cervical or cauda equina region, clinical worsening may be due to iatrogenic haemorrhage from the tumour. The removal of CSF may cause displacement of the tumour and alter the existing delicate balance between it and the cord. Some patients merely develop subjective sensory symptoms and others report an unexplained improvement of pain or paraesthesiae.

Surgical Treatment

The patient with a symptomatic spinal tumour has at least one of three main aspects of concern and disability. They are (1) pain, (2) difficulty in walking and (3) lack of sphincter control. The aims of treatment are therefore to relieve pain, restore mobility and normal sphincter function. Fortunately, many patients are ambulant and continent when the diagnosis is made and remain so after tumour excision.

The best and most effective treatment of a spinal tumour is total excision. This ideal cannot always be attained and the extent of possible excision is mainly determined by the relationship of the tumour to the neural contents of the canal or to the extent of involvement of the spinal column and paraspinal structures. It is relatively easy to excise an intradural/extramedullary neurofibroma or even to remove a well-encapsulated intramedullary astrocytoma but virtually impossible to achieve radical excision of an extensive extradural metastasis involving the vertebral column. The ambition to achieve a total excision must always be tempered by an awareness of the hazards of surgery with inevitable worsening of existing neurological function. Some of these limiting factors have already been indicated in the description of individual tumour types.

Surgical access to a spinal tumour is determined by the location of the lesion in relation to the spinal cord, meninges and vertebral column (Fig. 23.9). Posterior, posterolateral and some anterolateral tumours are approached by removal of the overlying spinous processes and laminae (laminectomy or hemilaminectomy). This is by far the commonest route of surgical access to a spinal tumour. Anterior and most anterolateral tumours are difficult to approach in this manner because the spinal cord intervenes between the surgeon and the tumour and tumour visualization involves excessive cord manipulation. These can be reached by a costotransversectomy involving excision of the relevant rib, transverse process and pedicle to gain access into the spinal canal. There are two hazards of this surgical approach. If the dura exposed at operation is damaged, a pneumothorax will develop in the postoperative period. In the thoracolumbar region, especially on the left side, the artery of Adamkiewicz is endangered. The resultant cord ischaemic disturbance can be catastrophic. Nevertheless this route is very useful especially to deal with extradural benign and malignant tumours. Those involving the vertebral body are best visualized and dealt with from an anterior approach. The commonly used routes are transoral (C1, C2 levels), transcervical (C3–C7 levels), transthoracic (T3–T10 levels) and extraperitoneal/transabdominal methods

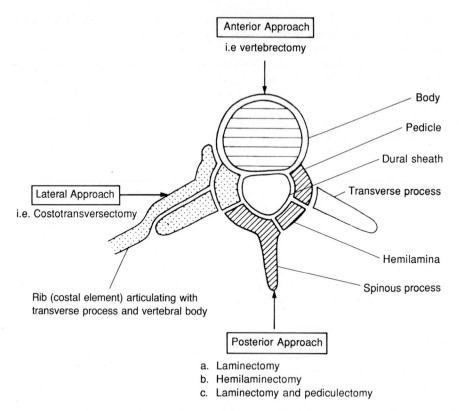

Fig. 23.9. Surgical approaches to tumours of the spine. Shaded areas represent bone removal necessary for access depending on the approach used. ▤ anterior approach; ▨ lateral approach; ▧ posterior approach.

to reach the anterior aspect of the lumbar vertebrae or sacrum. All these methods are most suitable for extradural tumours. If the dura is breached or deliberately opened, suture repair of the defect is very difficult and closure is best achieved by a patch graft using artificial dura or fascia sealed with tissue glue. If a water-tight closure is not obtained, CSF can leak into the wound with the potential risk of meningitis or extradural abscess. Whichever approach is used it is important to identify the level of the tumour in relation to the vertebrae so that the surgical incision is placed accurately.

The midline incision for laminectomy (or hemilaminectomy) is centred just above the tip of the spinous process corresponding to the vertebral level of the tumour, recognizing the slope of the spinous element to the laminae especially in the thoracic region. The laminectomy is extended to expose the cranial and caudal poles of the tumour and widened up to the vertebral facet joints. Usually, about three laminae are removed but more may be necessary depending on the size of the tumour. A posterior or posterolateral extradural tumour will be immediately visible. Absence of extradural fat in the region of any tumour is useful in recognizing the site and extent of the lesion. An intradural tumour will be seen as a tense, non-pulsatile localized expansion of the dura which is firm to gentle palpation. The dura is opened in the midline usually beginning below the lower pole of the tumour. When the arachnoid is opened a gush of CSF will occur from the subarachnoid space. The cord which is distorted and displaced will begin to pulsate gently after tumour debulking.

Removal of the tumour is best achieved by piece-meal excision. The central part of the lesion is debulked so that the peripheral portion and capsule can be systematically peeled away from the neural structures. It is important to avoid or minimize manipulation of the cord and nerve roots. An operating microscope is invariably used providing good lighting and adequate magnification for safe surgery. An ultrasonic aspirator will disintegrate and remove the tumour without causing significant disturbance to adjacent neural structures. Laser excision is extremely useful in dealing with spinal intramedullary tumours. The dural edges are sutured following tumour removal. The laminae and spinous processes are not usually replaced.

Neurofibroma. The excision of an intradural neurofibroma inevitably involves sacrifice of the nerve root which is attached to the tumour. When dealing with a dumb-bell neurofibroma the dural sleeve is opened well into the intervertebral foramen. A large extradural/extraspinal extension may be best tackled at a separate second stage procedure via a more lateral approach. When multiple tumours are present the aim should be to remove the tumour identified as being responsible for the current symptoms on the grounds of careful clinical assessment. If precise identification is impossible the largest tumour which is the most likely culprit should be removed. Prophylactic excision of other lumps in the vicinity at the same operation is sensible but the choice must be limited by the nature of the associated obligatory neurological deficit.

Meningioma. The aim is to remove the tumour as well as the portion of dura which lends attachment and origin. The latter minimizes the possibility of tumour recurrence. If the dural origin is in the posterior or posterolateral circumference of the dura, excision is not technically difficult. Anterior attachments are awkward to excise and are usually dealt with by heavy bipolar coagulation instead. The excised dura can be replaced by a patch of cadaver dural graft which can be sutured or glued into place. Water-tight repair will prevent the recurrence of a CSF leak from the wound or the formation of a pseudomeningocele. A calcified tumour can prove to be a tedious technical challenge especially when placed in the anterior quadrants of the canal. Often even the ultrasonic aspirator will fail to disintegrate a hard tumour. In these circumstances, cord manipulation is unavoidable and increases the hazard to existing neurological function.

Astrocytoma and Ependymoma. For many years, intramedullary astrocytomas and ependymomas were treated with a wide decompressive laminectomy, tumour biopsy, cyst aspiration and radiotherapy. In current neurosurgical practice, the primary treatment for these tumours is surgical excision of the solid tumour, cyst drainage and radiotherapy. This trend has evolved in the realization that excision is technically feasible, that radiotherapy has only little benefit to offer and that radical surgery improves neurological function and increases survival time (Epstein and Epstein 1982). The tumour is exposed by a

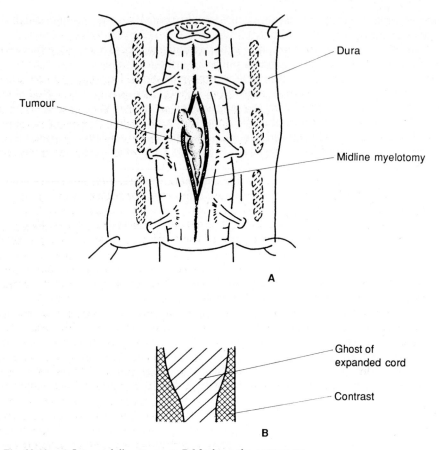

Fig. 23.10. **A** Intramedullary tumour. **B** Myelography appearance.

laminectomy which is limited to the extent of the solid tumour only. Polar cystic components can be drained whilst dealing with the solid part without extending the laminectomy. The tumour is reached by an incision on the dorsal midline of the cord (myelotomy) (Fig. 23.10). Eventually, the myelotomy can be extended over the entire length of the tumour which is excised by debulking the central core and then gradually separating it from the surrounding expanded cord leaving a shallow trench-like tumour bed. The capsule of a dermoid, epidermoid cyst, enterogenous cyst or lipoma can be very adherent to the spinal cord making radical excision difficult and dangerous.

Extradural Malignant and Metastatic Tumours

The management of these patients presents a multitude of controversies including the role of surgery in the treatment. The clinician is invariably confronted with a patient who has developed pain, paralysis and incontinence or retention. The expected survival time is short, being determined by the nature, extent and response to treatment of the primary tumour rather than the secondary deposit in the spine.

Primary lung carcinoma has a notoriously bad prognosis whereas lymphoma, prostatic and breast cancer patients have better outcomes and longer survival. The goals of treatment are to return the patient to a pain-free, ambulant and continent status. The attainment of these ideals is especially relevant to a patient with malignant disease because quality of life is paramount when longevity is reduced. The method of treatment used must be judged primarily in terms of possible benefit in improving symptoms but modulated by the risk of producing neurological deterioration as well as the discomfort and the distress caused to the patient.

Many patients with malignant cord compression are elderly with either cardiorespiratory compromise, other systemic diseases or malignant cachexia. They are poor surgical risks, prone to postoperative infections as well as impaired wound healing. Therefore the physical age (rather than the actual age), and general medical condition of the adult patient may dictate the choice of treatment method. In children, an aggressive policy of treatment is more readily accepted. After an overall assessment of the patient and the primary disease, a certain group will be much better served with conservative treatment. These are usually patients with complete cord transection, multiple levels of spinal metastatic disease and those with advanced and widespread disseminated tumour. Pain control is the mainstay of treatment combined with good basic nursing care usually in a hospice or home environment.

All methods of treatment aimed at the malignant metastatic tumour are palliative rather than curative. The main options of aggressive treatment are surgery, radiotherapy and chemotherapy used singly or in combination. Rapidly progressive neurological deterioration due to extradural metastatic compression has a very poor prognosis whatever method of treatment is adopted.

It seems reasonable to accept the concept that neural structures which are being mechanically compressed will benefit from the surgical procedure which achieves a decompression. This is best achieved by excision of the tumour, as in the case of benign intradural tumours. However, most malignant extradural lesions are extensive at clinical presentation and total excision is not possible. Traditionally, decompression was achieved by a laminectomy at the tumour site. This procedure is relatively simple technically and therefore quickly performed, thus conferring an advantage when dealing with poor-risk, elderly patients. In most instances however, the tumour is sited anteriorly or anterolaterally and only a limited excision or diagnostic biopsy is possible at the operation. Being considered a neurosurgical emergency, these decompressive laminectomy (DL) operations were often carried out late at night by junior surgeons on poor-risk patients. Not surprisingly, the operation gradually became unpopular for a variety of reasons. Although neurological improvement occurred, less than 5% of those who were unable to walk before surgery became ambulant. More importantly, only 50% of those who were able to walk before operation retained this ability after surgery (Findlay 1984). An important cause of neurological deterioration following DL was anterior vertebral collapse due to removal of posterior supporting elements when the anterior spinal column was already diseased by tumour (Brice and McKissock 1965). Nevertheless, DL is still the ideal surgical approach when the tumour is situated in the posterior or even posterolateral quadrants of the canal. Results were better when DL was combined with radiotherapy although about 30% of patients deteriorated despite the treatment (Findlay 1984). Several studies have shown that radiotherapy combined with steroids has a similar beneficial response as DL plus radiotherapy, with ambulation rates of 46% and 40% respectively (Black 1979; Barcena et al. 1984; Findlay 1984). This overall benefit with radiotherapy is applicable to relief of pain as well as to preservation or restoration of neurological function.

When the site of the primary cancer is unknown it is important to obtain a diagnostic biopsy before deciding on the method of definitive treatment. A percutaneous needle biopsy will provide excellent diagnostic material. A hemilaminectomy will achieve the dual purpose of tumour decompression and diagnostic biopsy without jeopardizing spinal stability significantly.

Since most extradural metastases are sited anterior or anterolateral to the cord the more logical method of tumour debulking is via a costotransversectomy or anterior approach to the spinal column (Fig. 23.9). The tumour can be removed under direct vision and a greater extent of debulking can be achieved. In solitary vertebral body disease almost a total excision is possible. Ambulation rates of 70%–80% have been reported (Siegal et al. 1985) by this method and the recovery to ambulation of paraplegic patients is far higher than with DL (Findlay 1984). As in DL, anterior decompression produces a potentially unstable spinal column. Therefore most of these patients require a spinal stabilization procedure (see below). The operation is thus a major surgical exercise and not easily tolerated by poor-risk patients. The correct choice of patient is therefore all important in achieving the therapeutic goals whichever method is used. The indications for surgery can be summarized as follows:

1. Diagnosis – when primary tumour is unknown (options hemilaminectomy or needle biopsy)
2. Decompression of cord when
   a) Tumour is radioresistant
   b) When deterioration occurs during radiotherapy
   c) When vertebral collapse has caused bone fragments to collapse into spinal canal causing cord compression
   d) Recurrent cord compression by tumour after maximal radiotherapy doses
   e) Single body disease with significant anterior cord compression (anterior decompression ideal)
3. Spinal stabilization

The definite indications for radiotherapy are:

1. Radiosensitive tumours (especially without significant anterior collapse or cord compression) e.g., lymphoma, neuroblastoma, Ewing's sarcoma, myeloma
2. Stable, ambulant patients with known primary tumour who present with pain and/or minor neurological deficit
3. Postoperatively in de novo cases
4. Advanced, generalized disease
5. Refusal of, or medically unfit for, major surgery

Spinal Stabilization

Whatever method of cord decompression and tumour removal is used, it is sound surgical practice to aim for stability of the spinal column. If anterior disease is absent and posterior bone removal did not involve bilateral facet joint excision, the stability will be acceptable without added instrumentation. In most other instances, a stabilization procedure must complement the decompressive operation. A variety of complex spinal instrumentation methods are now available. Essentially, they are metal rods or rectangular metal prostheses which are fixed to the weakened area of the spinal column with wires or screws in order to achieve both vertebral distraction (to correct kyphosis) and stabilization. Also, acrylic vertebral body prostheses are available to support the column anteriorly after excision of a single vertebral body involved with tumour (Moore and Uttley 1989).

In children, severe spinal deformities (kyphosis/scoliosis) can occur as a result of laminectomy for spinal tumours. This is common in children under two years of age or when the laminectomy involves more than three consecutive vertebral levels. The cervical spine is especially vulnerable. The cause is muscle weakness due to neurological deficit, loss of posterior support to the vertebral column and radiation growth arrest of the vertebral body. External supports do not usually help and eventually anterior or posterior internal fixation becomes necessary (Holmes and Hall 1978). These deformities can be prevented by limiting the laminectomy to the level essential for tumour excision, preservation of facet joints at surgery or performing en bloc excision and replacement of the laminae. It is better to perform the stabilization procedure as part of the initial surgical exercise when it is anticipated that spinal deformity may occur as a result of the bone and tumour excision.

Radiotherapy and Chemotherapy

Radiotherapy plays an important role in the treatment of primary and metastatic tumours of the spinal column and cord. The vast majority of benign intradural/extramedullary tumours can be excised totally and do not require additional treatment. In the case of intramedullary tumours radiotherapy is used when tumour excision is incomplete and/or when the neoplasm is malignant. In the former, postoperative irradiation therapy increases the recurrence-free survival time but in malignant tumours the outcome is altered only slightly. The role of radiotherapy in extradural malignant and metastatic lesions has already been described. Meningiomas of the aggressive type or those treated with partial excision or when the dural origin is not removed, can be administered local irradiation treatment in order to reduce the likelihood of recurrence. In medulloblastomas, spinal irradiation is used as a prophylactic measure or when seedlings are known to be present. A number of spinal tumours are relatively radioresistant. Radionecrosis of the cord is an uncommon but recognized complication.

Chemotherapy is becoming increasingly relevant in the control of certain malignant spinal tumours. Optimistic results are being reported especially in intramedullary malignant ependymomas. There is no evidence of a superior survival when chemotherapy is used in malignant astrocytomas of the cord.

Immunotherapy with intrathecal monoclonal antibodies may become useful in the treatment of subarachnoid seedlings of medulloblastoma and other primitive ectodermal tumours. Antimitotic chemotherapy is used as standard treatment in the management of myeloma and lymphoma. There has been optimistic speculation about administering progesterone agonists or antagonists in the treatment of inoperable cerebral meningiomas and the same concept made applicable to the small number of surgically unresectable spinal counterparts.

Recovery

Following successful tumour excision neurological recovery is dependent on several factors, the most important of which is the degree of initial disability. Patients with mild deficits recover better and complete reversal of paraplegia is very uncommon. Children and young adults show a greater potential for regaining normal function. The general health of the patient is important and poor nutrition and intercurrent infections impair recovery. Those who show signs of regaining function in the early stages are more likely to continue to do so. It is reasonable to allow about 18–24 months for the recovery process to continue before accepting that the residual neurological disability is unlikely to improve further.

During this period there is immense benefit in intensive, supervised physiotherapy. Formal programmes of rehabilitation are ideal and should include bladder retraining if necessary. Control of pain, spasticity and dysaesthesiae may require regular medication and provide a significant improvement in the quality of life. The vast majority of patients who undergo excision of a benign intradural tumour return to a normal independent life. The key to successful therapy is early diagnosis and prompt surgical treatment.

Acknowledgements. I am indebted to Mr. A.J. Keogh FRCS, Marion Dela-Rosa and Debbie Clowes for the tables and illustrations and to Barbara Tomlinson for secretarial assistance. I am also grateful to Dr. R.H. Gurusinghe for much helpful advice.

References

Barcena A, Lobato RD, Rivas JJ, et al. (1984) Spinal metastatic disease: analysis of factors determining functional prognosis and the choice ofreatment. Neurosurgery 15:820–827

Barker D, Wright K, Nguyen L (1987) Gene for von Recklinghausen's neurofibromatosis is in the pericentric region of chromosome 17. Science 236:1100–1102

Bertoni F, Unni MK, Dahlin D (1990) Calcifying pseudoneoplasms of the neural axis. J Neurosurg 72:42–48

Black P (1979) Spinal metastases: current status and recommended guidelines for management. Neurosurgery 5:726–746

Braughler JM, Hall ED (1983) Lactate and pyruvate metabolism in injured cat's spinal cord before and after a single large intravenous dose of methylprednisolone. J Neurosurg 59:256–261

Brice J, McKissock W (1965) Surgical treatment of malignant extradural spinal tumours. Br Med J i:1341–1344

Choremis C, Oelonomos D, Papadatos P, Gargoulas A (1956) Intraspinal epidermoid tumours (cholesteatomas) in patients treated for tuberculous meningitis. Lancet 2:437–439

Cloward RB, Bucy PC (1937) Spinal extradural cyst and kyphosis dorsalis juvenalis. Am J Roetgenol 38:681–706

Cohen AR, Wisoff JH, Allen JC, Epstein F (1989) Malignant astrocytoma of the spinal cord. J Neurosurg 70:50–54

Connolly ES (1980) Spinal cord tumours in adults. In: Youman JR (ed) Neurological surgery vol 5. Saunders, Philadelphia, pp 3196–3214

Davis C (1990) Meningiomas and sex hormones. Eur J Cancer 26(8):859–860

Ehni G, Love JG (1945) Intraspinal lipomas. Report of cases: review of the literature and clinical and pathologic study. Arch Neurol Psychiatry 53:1–28

Epstein F, Epstein N (1982) Surgical treatment of spinal cord astrocytomas of childhood. A series of 19 patients. J Neurosurg 75:685–689

Findlay G (1984) Adverse effects of the management of malignant spinal cord compression. J Neurol Neurosurg Psychiatry 47:767–788

Gilbert RW, Kim JH, Posner JB (1978) Epidural spinal cord compression from metastatic tumours. Diagnosis and treatment. Ann Neurol 3:40–51

Gortvai P (1963) Extradural cysts of the spinal cord. J Neurol Neurosurg Psychiatry 26:223–230

Grant JW, Kaech D, Jones DG (1986) Spinal cord as the first presentation of lymphoma: a review of 15 cases. Histopathology 11:1191–1202

Gudmundsson KR (1970) A survey of tumours of the central nervous system in Iceland during the 10 year period 1954–1963. Acta Neurol Scand 46:538–552

Haddad P, Thaell JF, Kielly JM, et al. (1976) Lymphoma of the spinal extradural space. Cancer 38:1862–1864

Halliday AL, Sobel RA, Martuza RL (1991) Benign spinal nerve sheath tumors: their occurrence sporadically and in neurofibromatosis types 1 and 2. J Neurosurg 74:248–253

Helseth A, Mork SJ (1989) Primary intraspinal neoplasms in Norway 1955 to 1986 – a population-based survey of 467 patients. J Neurosurg 71:842–845

Hochberg FH, Millar DC (1988) Primary CNS lymphoma. J Neurosurg 68(6):835–853

Holmes JC, Hall JE (1978) Fusion for instability and potential instability of the cervical spine in children and adolescents. Orthop Clin North Am 9:923

Horsley V, Gowers WR (1888) A case of tumour of the spinal cord. Trans R Med Chirurg Soc Glasgow 70:377

Jackson DV, Randall ME, Richards F (1988) Spinal cord compression due to extramedullary haematopoiesis in thalassaemia: long term follow up after radiotherapy. Surg Neurol 29:389–392

Klein SL (1991) Pediatric spinal epidural metastases. J Neurosurg 74:70–75

Lecat CNL (1765) Traite de l'existence, de la nature et des propriétés du fluide des nerfs et principalement de son action dans le mouvement musculaire. Ouvrage coutonne en 1753, par l'Academie de Berlin; suivi des dissertations sur la sensibilité des meninges, des tendons, etc., l'insensibilité du cervaux, la structure des nerfs, l'irritabilité hallerienne. Berlin

Levy WJ, Bay J, Dolm D (1982) Spinal cord meningiomas. J Neurosurg 57:804–812

Levy WJ, Latchew J, Halm JF, et al. (1986) Spinal neurofibromas. A report of 66 cases and a comparison with meningiomas. Neurosurgery 18:331–334

Lunardi P, Missori P, Gagliardi FM, Fortuna A (1989) Long term results of the surgical treatment of spinal dermoids and epidermoid tumours. Neurosurgery 25:860–864

Matson D (1969) Neurosurgery of infancy and childhood, 2nd edn. Thomas, Springfield, Illinois

Maurice-Williams RS, Richardson PW (1988) Spinal cord compression: delay in the diagnosis and referral of a common neurosurgical emergency. Br J Neurosurg 2:55–60

McCormick PC, Torres R, Post KD, Stein B (1990) Intramedullary ependymomas of the spinal cord. J Neurosurg 72:523–532

Moore A, Uttley D (1989) Anterior decompression and stabilisation of the spine in malignant disease. Neurosurgery 24:713–717

Murota K, Symon L (1989) Surgical management of haemangioblastoma of the spinal cord. A report of 18 cases. Neurosurgery 25:699–708

Myles ST, Macrae ME (1988) Benign osteoblastoma of spine in childhood. J Neurosurg 68:884–888

Neumann HPH, Eggert HR, Weigel K, et al. (1989) Hemangioblastomas of the central nervous system. J Neurosurg 70:24–30

Nittner K (1968) Discussion zu den Vortragen von Jellinger U. von Piscol. Bericht über die Jahresfagung der Dtsch. Ges für Neurochirugie (13–16 Sept 1967 Bad Harzburg) Loew F (ed) Acta Neurochir (Wien) 19:91

Nittner K (1976) Spinal meningiomas, neurinomas and neurofibromas and hour-glass tumours. In: Vinken PJ , Bruyen BW (eds) Handbook of clinical neurology, vol 20. Elsevier, Amsterdam, pp 177–322

Norstrom CW, Kernohan JW, Love JG (1961) One hundred primary caudal tumours. JAMA 178:1071–1077

O'Connor GA, Roberts TS (1984) Spinal cord compression by osteochondroma. J Neurosurg 60:420–423

O'Sullivan MG, Keohane C, Buckley TF (1990) Paraganglioma of the cauda equina: a case report and review of the literature. Br J Neurosurg 4:63–68

Oppenheim H (1923) Lehrbuch der Nervenkrankheiten für Arzte und Studierende, vol 1. Karger, Berlin

Perling LH, Laurent JP, Cheek WR (1988) Epidural hibernoma as a complication of corticosteroid treatment. J Neurosurg 69:613–616

Rand RW, Rand CW (1960) Intraspinal tumours of childhood. Thomas, Springfield, Illinois

Reimer R, Onofrio M (1985) Astrocytomas of the spinal cord in children and adolescents. J Neurosurg 63:669–675

Ridsdale L, Moseley I (1978) Thoracolumbar intraspinal tumours presenting features of raised intracranial pressure. J Neurol Neurosurg Psychiatry 41:737–745

Rotisch E, Zeidman SM, Burger PC, et al. (1990) Clinical and pathological analysis of spinal cord astrocytomas. Neurosurgery 27:193–196

Siegal T, Topya P, Siegal T (1985) Vertebral body resection for epidural compression by malignant tumours. Results of 47 consecutive operative procedures. J Bone Joint Surg 67A:375–382

Sloof JL, Kernohan JW, McCarty CS (1964) Primary intramedullary tumours of the spinal cord and filum terminale. Saunders, Philadelphia, pp 124–129

Sundaresan N, Galicich JH, Chu FCH, Huvos AG (1979) Spinal chordomas. J Neurosurg 50:312–319

Tarlov IM (1938) Perineural cysts of the spinal nerve roots. Arch Neurol Psychiatry (Chicago) 40:1067–1074

Till K (1975) Paediatric neurosurgery for paediatricians and neurosurgeons. Blackwell Scientific, Oxford

Torma T (1957) Malignant tumours of the spine and the spinal extradural space: a study based on 250 histologically verified cases. Acta Chir Scand (suppl) 225:1–176

von Recklinghausen F (1882) Uber die multiplen Fibrome der Hant und ihre Bezichung zu den multiplen Neuromen. Festschrift zur Feier des funfundzwanzigjahrigen Bestehens des pathologischen Instituts ze Berlin, (Herrn Rudolf Virchow dargebracht). Hirschwald, Berlin

Wilson LMK, Draper GJ (1974) Neuroblastoma – its natural history and prognosis: a study of 487 cases. Br Med J 3:301–307

Yamada K, Bremer AM, West CR (1979) Effects of dexamethasone on tumor induced brain edema and its distribution in the brain of monkeys. J Neurosurg 50:361–367

Chapter 24

Trauma and Paraplegia

K.A. Tucci, H.J. Landy, B.A. Green and F.J. Eismont

Epidemiology

Spinal cord injury (SCI) is a multibillion dollar annual health care problem in the United States and throughout the world (Green et al. 1987). Paralysing SCI represents a catastrophic disease associated with high morbidity and mortality. There are an estimated 250 000–300 000 spinal cord injured patients living in the United States. Approximately 10 000–12 000 new injuries occur annually, a rate of 5 per 100 000 population (Thomas 1979; Kalsbeek et al. 1980). The majority of injuries occur in the second to third decade of life, with 80% of patients being less than 40 years of age and male (Young and Northrup 1979). Automobile accidents represent the most common mechanism of injury, with a growing number each year from motorcycle accidents. Injuries from falls, industrial, gunshot, agricultural and sporting accidents account for the remainder of these injuries. In recent years, however, there has been an increase in the number of hand-gun wounds, particularly in metropolitan areas (Green et al. 1981). The most frequently injured level is the mid to low cervical, with the thoracolumbar area ranking second. These represent the areas of greatest mobility of the spinal column. The National Spinal Cord Injury Data Research Center in Phoenix, Arizona reported that 53% of spinal cord injuries result in quadriplegia and 47% in paraplegia (Green et al. 1981). The mortality rate is estimated at 6% within the first six months of injury for patients treated at major SCI centres (Bracken et al. 1990). The morbidity is greater than 100%, since each SCI victim experiences one or more systemic complications associated with their paralysis.

Pathophysiology

Victims of non-penetrating SCIs suffer lesions of the spinal cord and nerve roots by fractures, subluxation, or stretching distraction injuries of the vertebral column. Compression and contusion of the cord, causing haemorrhage, oedema, and biochemical sequelae lead to neurological compromise. Haematomyelia and areas of necrosis and cystic changes may be present within the

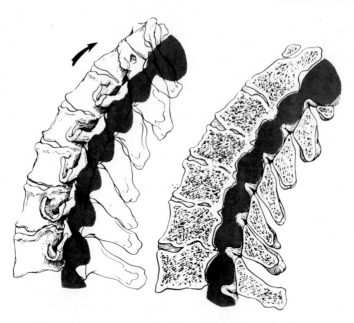

Fig. 24.1. Spondylosis with a hyperextension injury. Cord compression from spurs and infolding of the ligamentum flavum. (Reproduced with permission from *Post's radiographic evaluation of the spine*, © 1980 Masson Publishing USA, Inc.)

cord. Non-penetrating trauma rarely produces complete anatomical transection, but it is common to have a physiological transection of the cord. Instances of SCI without bony fracture or subluxation may be found in older patients who have a pre-existing cervical spondylosis and stenosis (Fig. 24.1). With sudden flexion or extension of the neck, the spinal cord is stretched over spondylitic bars and buckling of the ligamentum flavum further narrows the canal. In younger patients with a normal calibre canal, SCIs from blunt concussive forces can occur without actual fracture or subluxation. In children, the entity of SCI without radiological abnormality (SCIWORA) has been well classified and is believed to be due to a distraction stretching type of mechanism due to the relatively lax spinal ligamentous support (Pang and Wilberger 1982). Spinal cord and/or nerve root injury may also occur due to intervertebral disc herniation with or without fracture and/or subluxation.

Neurological Assessment and Spinal Cord Syndromes

A spinal cord injury is termed complete if there is no sparing of motor or sensory function below the level of injury. The level of injury, by convention (Landy and Tucci 1991), is defined as the last intact functioning spinal cord level. If a patient has preserved normal function at the C5 level with no preservation of function below this level, the patient will be classified as a C5 complete quadriplegic. Most patients have a "zone of injury" so the same C5 complete patient may have some partially preserved function of C6, and would be described as a C5 incomplete/C6 complete. Some of the zones of injury may span two or more levels with no motor or sensory preservation distally. If the patient shows no signs of recovery of function below the level of injury during the first 24 hours post injury, there is only a 3%–4% chance that the patient will demonstrate distal motor recovery (Suwanwela et al. 1962). During the acute phase of the complete injury, the patient, in addition to absence of motor and sensory function, will also demonstrate loss of all reflex activity including sphincter function. This state is termed spinal shock and usually spans 6–16 weeks or more. It is not to be confused with neurogenic shock which refers to the loss of sympathetic input below the level of injury (brain stem to T4) and presents as a triad of hypotension, bradycardia, and hypothermia. The end of spinal shock is heralded by increased muscle tone with hyperreflexia and spasticity.

An incomplete SCI has distal sparing of some motor or sensory function. In recent years, an increasing proportion of spinal cord injured patients who arrive in the emergency room present as incomplete lesions (Green et al. 1987). The majority of these patients will demonstrate some degree of improvement in their neurological function (Suwanwela et al. 1962). Incomplete lesions usually demonstrate sparing of sensation in the sacral dermatomes along with some volitional control of the anal sphincter. This is referred to as sacral sparing and implies an incomplete lesion. An SCI that demonstrates complete recovery of neurological function within 24 hours is rare and is classified as a spinal cord concussion (Zwimpfer and Bernstein 1990). These patients will frequently have unremarkable radiographic and MRI studies.

The phenomenon of neuropraxia of the cervical cord with transient quadriplegia has been described in young male athletes who have forced hyperextension or hyperflexion of the neck. Sensory changes include burning pain, numbness, tingling, and loss of sensation. The motor changes have been reported to range from mild weakness to complete paralysis. These deficits are transient, lasting from a few minutes to hours, followed by complete recovery of motor and sensory function. Neck pain is rare at the time of injury and upon resolution of deficits the patient may have full and pain-free range of motion of the neck. Radiographic evaluation of these patients can disclose pre-existing spinal stenosis, congenital cervical fusion, cervical instability, or intervertebral disc herniation. In a review of these cases, Torg et al. (1986) found no evidence that an episode of neuropraxia of the cervical spine predisposes the athlete to permanent neurological injury, unless instability or chronic degeneration is present. Other authors disagree with their conclusions and advise patients with neuropraxic episodes to discontinue participation in contact sports as there is strong evidence that pre-existing canal dimensions have a significant effect on the occurrence and severity of paralysis associated with spinal injuries (Eismont et al. 1984b; Ladd and Scranton 1986).

Incomplete lesions are categorized into syndromes depending on the anatomical structures involved. However, a significant number of incomplete patients exhibit a mixed motor and sensory deficit rather than one of the clinically described syndromes. Patients who present with loss of motor and pain and temperature function below the level of injury with sparing of crude touch, vibration and proprioception are classified as anterior spinal cord

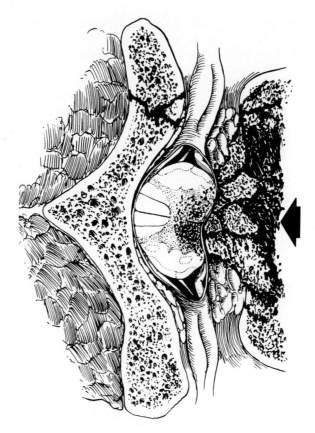

Fig. 24.2.   Anterior spinal cord syndrome involving the central grey area and the tracts of the anterior and lateral funiculus. The posterior columns are spared.

syndrome (Schneider 1955). The corticospinal and spinothalamic tracts are involved, with sparing of dorsal column fibres (Fig. 24.2). This is frequently caused by a flexion mechanism with vertebral body fracture or subluxation or by a herniated disc with compression of the anterior portion of the cord. The distribution of clinical findings is similar to an infarction of the anterior spinal artery (Schneider 1959). The prognosis for improvement in motor function is poor and is similar to that of a complete SCI.

The posterior cord syndrome is a rare entity and involves injury only to the dorsal columns. The patient presents with loss of vibratory, crude touch, and position sensation, with preservation of motor function and of pain and temperature sensation (Fig. 24.3). This syndrome may occur in patients who demonstrate fractures of the lamina. Dorsal column sensory input is necessary for adequate motor control, and an injury to this area can be as disabling as a motor deficit.

The Brown-Séquard syndrome presents as an ipsilateral loss of motor and dorsal column function with contralateral loss of pain and temperature sensation. This is usually described in rotational injuries or penetrating injuries

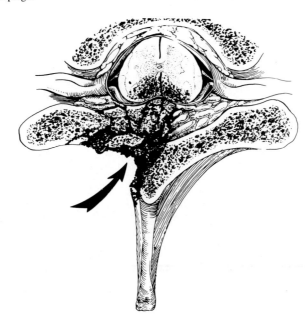

Fig. 24.3.   Posterior cord syndrome; injury involving the dorsal column fibres.

to the spinal cord with a resultant functional hemisection of the cord. Stab wounds are the most common cause. These patients, in general, have an excellent prognosis, with a 90% chance of good functional recovery (Mesard 1978).

The central cord syndrome is frequently seen in older men who have suffered a hyperextension injury of the neck (Schneider et al. 1954), most often without evidence of fracture or subluxation but with cervical spondylosis and stenosis. The picture frequently seen is that of an elderly man with a bruise on his forehead and quadriparesis with weakness of the distal upper extremities being the more severe. Although bowel and bladder control may be retained (Schneider et al. 1958), it is not uncommon for these patients to present with sphincter control dysfunction or loss. The sensory deficit in these patients is variable, with the usual picture of most severe loss in the hands and fingers and an associated painful hyperaesthetic state (Fig. 24.4). Proprioceptive loss in the lower extremities is involved with spasticity, often making walking difficult in spite of relatively well spared motor function. The prognosis for recovery adequate for independent ambulation is approximately 50%, with variable recovery of distal upper extremity function (Mesard 1978). A recent study in our centre of central cord syndrome points to a diffuse white matter injury instead of the central grey haemorrhage. Thoracolumbar junction injuries can present with a mixed conus medullaris and cauda equina lesion. These patients often present as cord complete with "saddle" distribution loss of sensation and flaccid sphincters but with cauda equina (nerve root) incompleteness. In our centre, we treat these patients aggressively with regard to surgical decompression and stabilization in order to maximize the chance

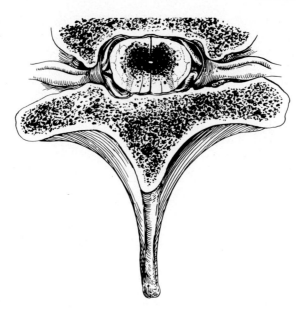

Fig. 24.4. The central cord syndrome; injury to the central grey area and the medial fibres to the corticospinal tract.

of functional nerve root (lower motor neurone) recovery, but treatment remains quite controversial.

Injuries of the lumbar spine below the conus medullaris produce cauda equina injuries with lower motor neurone findings. The paralysis is flaccid, with loss of reflexes. There are also varying degrees of bowel and bladder dysfunction and impotence. The sensory loss involves the lumbar and sacral dermatomes to varying degrees. The cauda equina is composed of nerve roots and, if adequate decompression is achieved, the prognosis for recovery in cauda equina injuries is better than in SCIs.

Hysterical paralysis may present a difficult dilemma from a management and liability standpoint. These patients must be differentiated from the malingering patient who is feigning paralysis for economic gain following an accident or potentially compensable injury. Both types of patients may present following an accident stating that they are unable to move or feel below the umbilicus. Very often they will not move their limbs even to painful stimuli. The hysterical patient may also present with complaints involving part or all of one limb, particularly with lack of movement at a single joint. The diagnosis of hysterical paralysis rests on several findings (Brain and Walton 1969). Since most patients are not knowledgeable of the nervous system, their paralysis does not correspond to that which may be produced by organic or traumatic lesions of the nervous system. It is common that these patients, in an attempt to move the paretic limb, will contract both the agonist and antagonist muscles about a joint. For example, on attempted flexion of the knee there will be associated contraction of the quadriceps. Radiographic evaluation is always negative. Deep tendon reflexes are normal, which contradicts the claim of complete flaccid paralysis. However, in able-bodied people, for many reasons, deep tendon reflexes may be absent. Although the patient may deny rectal sensation, their rectal tone will be normal, as will the anal wink reflex. The hoover sign (DeJong 1962) is elicited when a patient, placed in the recumbent position, is asked to flex the thigh and elevate one leg as the examiner supports the heels in the palms of his hands. In a normal subject there is a downward movement of the opposite leg as the patient elevates the contralateral leg. In a hemiplegic patient, when asked to elevate the paretic leg, the downward pressure of the opposite leg is accentuated. With hysterical hemiplegia, this phenomenon is absent in the normal leg as the patient attempts to raise the supposed paretic leg, although when elevating the normal leg the patient will depress the "paretic" leg. Once the diagnosis of hysterical paralysis is made, the physician is advised not to take a confrontational approach to the patient. The patient is given assurance that his condition is temporary and is admitted to the hospital where the nursing staff is instructed to carefully document movement of the limbs as the patient sleeps.

Systemic Sequelae to SCI

Injuries to the spinal cord produce profound general systemic effects, as all organ systems suffer from loss of neural control. Cardiovascular instability as a result of loss of sympathetic tone produces hypotension, bradycardia and hypothermia. Patients with high thoracic/low cervical lesions have compromised respiratory states with loss of intercostal and abdominal accessory respiratory musculature. Injuries at the levels of C3–C4 or above may involve loss of phrenic nerve innervation of the diaphragm, rendering the patient dependent upon mechanical respiratory support. Atelectasis and pneumonia are common occurrences in the spinal cord injured patient. Lower extremity paralysis aggravated by immobility predisposes these patients to deep vein thrombosis and the risk of pulmonary embolus. The gastrointestinal tract responds to acute cord injury with paralytic ileus, gastric hyperacidity and dysfunction of the pancreatic sphincter. The patients are then at risk of bowel impaction, vomiting, aspiration, stress ulcers and pancreatitis. Loss of normal bladder function leads to urinary stasis which, in turn, predisposes the patient to cystitis, pyelonephritis, hydronephrosis, urinary tract stones and renal failure. Most often, when the period of spinal shock subsides, patients may develop a spastic bladder which may lead to reflex emptying. Bladder distension, rectal distension, infection, decubitus ulcers, and almost any type of noxious stimulus in sympathectomized patients can trigger an autonomic dysreflexia producing hypertension, severe headaches, flushing, palpitations and abnormal sweating, and in extreme cases may even be fatal.

The spinal cord injured patient can develop contractures across joint spaces and heterotopic bone formation may develop near or within major joints. Mobilization of skeletal calcium results in osteoporosis placing these patients at risk of pathological fractures. The deafferented and immobilized patient can also develop decubitus ulcers at pressure points most often overlying bony prominences. These bedsores occur most commonly at the sacrum, buttocks, hips, and heels. It only requires a pressure of 50–60 mmHg to compromise cutaneous blood supply, and in a period of 6–12 hours, an ulcer can form (Campbell and Delgado 1977). If neglected, the ulcer may become secondarily infected and large lesions may even require skin flap or grafting. Osteomyelitis may also complicate pressure sores, especially in severe ulcers.

Progressive post-traumatic cystic myelopathy is a delayed sequela of SCI (Barnett et al. 1966) seen in 1%–2% of spinal cord injured patients (Eismont et al. 1984a). These lesions present from 3 months to 23 years post injury with a mean of 4.7 years (Eismont et al. 1984a). These cavities are most often found at the level of injury with extension in the caudal or cephalad direction. They usually form in the ventral aspect of the dorsal columns and in the medial regions of the dorsal horn where ischaemic myelomalacia undergoes cavitation by lysosomal and cellular enzyme action (Kao et al. 1977; Williams et al. 1981). Tethering of the posterior aspect of the cord at the site of the lesion in conjunction with movement of the cervical spine causes progressive shearing forces accounting for extension of the cavity (Barnett and Jousse 1976). The cyst can be unilateral or bilateral and may be multiple, separated by glial or collagenous septations (Quencer et al. 1990). Patients with post-traumatic syringomyelia present with unilateral or bilateral loss of motor and sensory function, intractable pain which may be local or radicular, hyperhydrosis, increased spasticity, autonomic dysreflexia, Horner's syndrome, and respiratory compromise. The diagnostic procedure of choice is MRI. It can be, at times, difficult to differentiate a cyst on MRI from an area of myelomalacia; however, the addition of gadolinium DTPA enhancement can increase diagnostic accuracy. Cardiae-gated cine-MRI can demonstrate the pulsatile nature and dynamics of the cavity, indicating that gradual cyst expansion is occurring with dissection into the cord (Quencer et al. 1990). Cine-MRI will also show the septated character of a cyst reflecting the fibroglial septations causing variations in the flow pattern within the cord lesion (Quencer et al. 1990).

Surgical treatment of these lesions includes a posterior laminectomy over the site of injury with untethering of the spinal cord. Intraoperative ultrasound will demonstrate the cystic lesion and its pulsatile nature (Post et al. 1988). Shunting of these cysts with a special silastic tube into the subarachnoid space (Tator et al. 1982) or to the peritoneal space is performed. If treated in a timely fashion the motor and sensory losses, as noted by the senior authors, are reversible as well as the hyperhydrosis and dysreflexia related to the cysts. Dorsal column sensory loss may be noted postoperatively from the posterior myelotomy performed; however, in most cases the loss is transient and resolves within several weeks to months.

Virtually all SCI patients experience stages of psychological adjustment similar to terminally ill patients. They pass through periods of denial, anger and depression before they become able to "cope" with their disability. This "coping phase" heralds the beginning of effective rehabilitation and may occur in certain cases shortly after injury, and in others it never may become apparent.

The Systems Approach

Prevention

A national prevention programme is gaining momentum across the USA after demonstration of success of the "feet first first time" diving injury prevention programme. However, we as physicians have failed to institute a serum containing "commonsense" with which we can inoculate the American public. Hand-gun control and alcohol and drug use and abuse remain the major issues, especially in metropolitan areas of our country.

Pre-hospital Treatment

With the increasing sophistication of emergency medical systems and paramedics, the percentage of patients with incomplete injuries has increased. If an SCI is suspected at the scene, the priorities of respiratory and cardiovascular stabilization are followed by immobilization of the spinal column in an anatomically neutral supine position. One should never attempt to free-lift a potential spinal cord injured patient. The log-rolling technique will minimize the chance of a secondary neurological injury. The patient should be immobilized and prepared for transfer by being placed on a spine board in the supine position with sandbags and adhesive tape securing the cervical area. Cervical collars are not recommended at this stage as they most often do not provide adequate immobilization (Johnson et al. 1977), and can give the rescue team a false sense of security. They also can act as a tourniquet if there is neck swelling from an associated vascular or other soft tissue injury, and may hide tracheal deviation or subcutaneous emphysema (Green and Hall 1976) from view. A new generation of trauma collars (Ducker 1990) offers a greater degree of stability and can be opened anteriorly to monitor the status of the soft tissues. A loose strap is also placed over the chest and one over the pelvis and knees and the patient is transported in a Trendelenberg position to minimize the risks of the aspiration and haemodynamic shock which are the major causes of pre-hospital mortality.

Emergency Room Management

The multidisciplinary trauma team approach is the key to emergency room care since many of these victims have associated multiple injuries. A thorough general physical assessment accompanies a complete neurological examination. One must always suspect a concomitant head injury in these patients. Baseline laboratory and X-ray studies must be complete and promptly available. Serial vital signs and neurological signs should be monitored and well documented. Venous access with central and peripheral lines, a Foley catheter and a sump nasogastric tube should be inserted.

Any patient suspected of having an SCI should have X-rays of the entire spine. The cervical spine series should include anteroposterior (AP), lateral and odontoid views since 15%–20% of spinal injuries occur at multiple levels.

The cervicothoracic junction and upper thoracic spine are sometimes difficult to visualize with routine views, and a swimmer's view may be necessary. If review of the spinal X-rays demonstrates a cervical fracture or subluxation, cervical traction is applied via tongs or an external halo device for immobilization and anatomical realignment. Traction is contraindicated if the initial injury resulted in a severe spinal column disruption or distraction which is most commonly seen at the occipitocervical junction. Approximately five pounds of traction per interspace is generally sufficient as a starting level (Crutchfield 1954). For example, if a patient presents with a subluxation at the C5–6 area, it will require about 25–30 pounds of traction for reduction and the weight may be adjusted up or down as indicated by serial X-rays or real-time fluoroscopy monitoring. If increasing the weight does not provide adequate reduction, muscle relaxation with intravenous diazepam may be helpful. If still not reduced, the patient may require endotracheal intubation and pharmacological paralysis to allow realignment. If all of these manoeuvres prove unsuccessful, one must consider open reduction and fusion in the operating room. With each manoeuvre and adjustment, a neurological and radiological reassessment must be performed and documented. Overdistraction of the cervical spine should be avoided. The objective of cervical traction is to provide decompression of the neural elements by restoring normal spinal alignment. Thoracic and lumbar injuries should not be treated with traction. If indicated, surgical reduction is required.

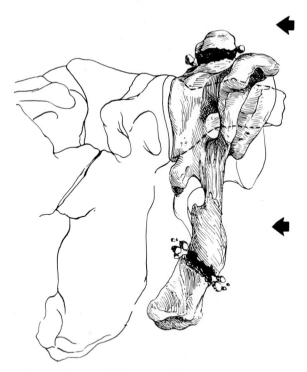

Fig. 24.5.   Jefferson fracture; fracture of the anterior and posterior arch of the atlas. (Reproduced with permission from *Post's radiographic evaluation of the spine*, © 1980, Masson Publishing USA, Inc.)

A recent multicentre randomized double-blind placebo-controlled study has shown a degree of benefit in the administration of high dose corticosteroid treatment in the acute spinal cord injured patient (Bracken et al. 1990). Ideally, the steroid treatment is initiated within the first 8 hours of injury, with a loading intravenous bolus of 30 mm/kg of methylprednisolone, followed by 5.4 mg/kg per hour of methylprednisolone over the next 23 hours. This study showed a statistically significant benefit for potential long-term neurological improvement in the acute spinal cord injured patients but is not purported to "cure" SCI or reverse paralysis. Although not the panacea for acute SCI victims, even the limited improvement experienced in the study population has the potential to affect meaningfully the quality of life of these paralysis victims.

Radiologic Evaluation and Surgical Treatment

After the emergency room X-rays, computerized tomography (CT) is the test of choice for the bony detail of the spine. A sagittal reconstruction can provide further visualization of spinal column alignment. MRI provides optimal visualization of the soft tissues, intervertebral discs, and the cord itself but lacks the bony detail that CT offers. MRI was not feasible in acute SCI victims if the patient was unstable or required mechanical ventilation until the development and availability of new low-field MRI machines. If not available, myelography with water-soluble contrast followed by a post-myelogram CT scan may be performed, with good visualization of the spinal canal, and the status of its contents. Complex motion tomography in certain selected cases can provide additional detail of the bony injury and is especially useful in assessing facet relationships and alignment at the lower cervical or upper thoracic spine.

Bilateral lines of fracture of both the anterior and posterior arches of C1 constitute a *Jefferson fracture* (Fig. 24.5). This is a result of axial loading which causes bursting of the atlas (Jefferson 1920; Hinchley and Bicker 1945). On an AP view, the lateral masses of C1 will be displaced laterally. It is rare for this type of fracture to cause neurological compromise. Treatment with halo-vest immobilization for six weeks is sufficient in most cases (Zimmerman et al. 1976).

There are three types of odontoid fractures. The first type is an oblique fracture through the tip of the odontoid due to avulsion at the alar ligament. Type II, the most common, is a tranverse fracture at the base of the odontoid. An oblique fracture from the base of the odontoid extending into the body of C2 is designated a Type III fracture (Osgood and Lund 1928; Aymes and Anderson 1956). These patients can also frequently be managed with halo-vest immobilization. Many Type II fractures, especially in older patients, will not heal with halo-vest immobilization alone and require surgical fusion (Dunn and Seljeskog 1986). Fractures across the pedicles of C2 from hyperextension type injuries are called hangman's fractures (Fig. 24.6). The bilateral fractures of the pedicles widen the spinal canal and frequently no SCI occurs. Cervical traction followed by halo-vest immobilization is usually adequate treatment (Schneider et al. 1958).

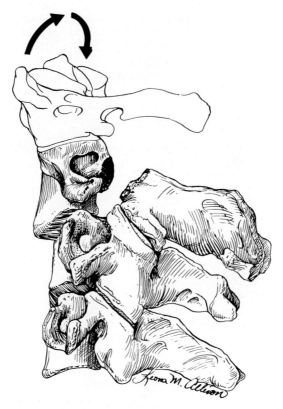

Fig. 24.6. Hangman's fracture; transpedicle fracture from a hyperextension injury. (Reproduced with permission from *Post's radiographic evaluation of the spine*, © 1980 Masson Publishing USA, Inc.)

Cervical injuries with a horizontal subluxation of greater than 2.5 mm or angulation between adjacent bodies of greater than 11 degrees or with severe disruption of the anterior and/or posterior elements are considered unstable. A sagittal subluxation of about 25% is usually associated with perched facets, facet fractures or a unilateral locked facet. When bilateral facets are locked in subluxation, there is generally at least a 50% vertebral subluxation (Landy and Tucci 1991). These patients require cervical traction to realign the spinal canal, and will ultimately require operative fusion of the unstable segment.

Adult patients can present with a cervical cord injury deficit with no initial evidence of fracture or subluxation. These patients are initially placed in 5–10 pounds of cervical traction. MRI or myelogram/CT is performed to rule out disc herniation. If no disc herniation is present, under controlled circumstances, flexion and extension films are later obtained to check for occult instability. It is not uncommon for the patient to have muscle spasms acutely which, after a period of time, relax to disclose a cervical instability. If unrecognized, this instability can lead to aggravation of neurological deficits.

There is greater mobility and therefore greater chance of injury at the thoracolumbar junction that at thoracic spine levels. A certain degree of

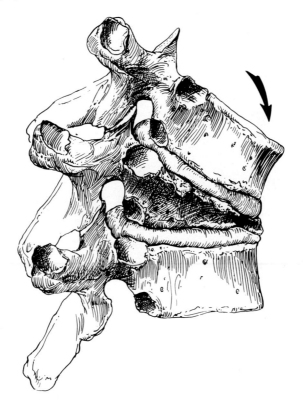

Fig. 24.7. Wedge compression fracture. (Reproduced with permission from *Post's radiographic evaluation of the spine*, © 1980 Masson Publishing USA, Inc.)

stabilization is afforded the T1–T11 area by the rib cage, intercostal muscles and sternum. Thoracolumbar injuries can present as wedge fractures, burst fractures or fracture/dislocations (Hinchley and Bicker 1945; Holdsworth 1970). A wedge fracture is produced when axial compression is combined with flexion (Fig. 24.7). Injuries with greater than 50% anterior wedging can lead to a kyphotic angulation instability (Hinchley and Bicker 1945; Holdsworth 1970). More severe injuries can involve fractures of the pedicles, laminae and facets. A burst fracture is the result of axial compression and is seen as a decrease in height of the vertebral body (Figs. 24.8 and 24.9). With either wedge or burst fractures the spinal cord and cauda equina can be compressed by posterior protrusion of the fractured vertebral body. Passengers in a motor vehicle accident who wear lap seat belts can suffer extreme flexion injuries to the thoracolumbar area (Smith and Kaufer 1969) with disruption of the posterior ligaments and dislocation of the vertebral bodies. Fractures of the vertebrae may be horizontal and split the spinous process, neural arch and vertebral body; this is called a Chance fracture. These patients most often present with cauda equina injuries with the majority having intra-abdominal injuries (Chance 1948; Smith and Kaufer 1969) as well.

If the patient has an incomplete thoracic injury, operative decompression and stabilization may be necessary. Complete injuries of the thoracic spine

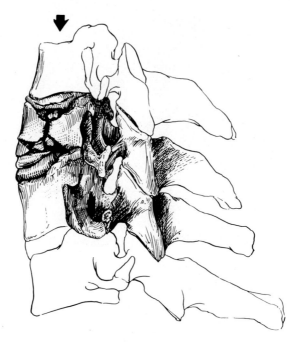

Fig. 24.8. Comminuted vertebral body fracture. (Reproduced with permission from *Post's radiographic evaluation of the spine*, © 1980 Masson Publishing USA, Inc.)

are considered for surgical stabilization only if the spine is mechanically unstable, as the prognosis for significant neurological recovery following decompression is poor.

Thoracolumbar junction and lumbar injuries represent more of a lower motor neurone injury and these patients have a somewhat better prognosis. Surgical decompression and stabilization are performed as an emergency with hopes of a greater degree of root recovery. Spinal instrumentation with Harrington (Dickson et al. 1973; Jacobs et al. 1980) rods produces realignment of the spine which contributes to decompression of the neural elements (Eismont and Green 1986), although additional decompressive manoeuvres may be necessary. Intraoperative sonography is useful to visualize cord and cauda equina compression from vertebral body fractures, soft tissue or other compressive elements and can be performed through a laminectomy or laminotomy defect (Montalvo et al. 1985). Recording of somatosensory motor evoked potentials can also be helpful intraoperatively as a monitor of neurological status and function. More recently our group has found real-time electromyography integrated with the evoked responses to be most useful.

Spinal cord injuries from gunshot wounds are best managed by a team approach. These patients frequently have serious injury to other organ systems. The majority of civilian injuries in the United States are low velocity injuries from hand-guns. High velocity injuries from automatic and semi-automatic weapons are seen in some areas of the United States, but more commonly are military injuries. The spinal cord may be injured directly by

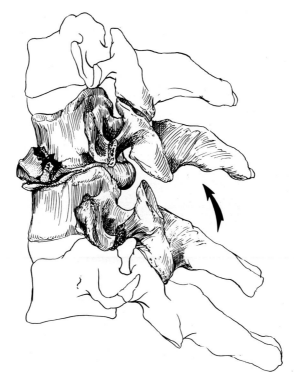

Fig. 24.9. Comminuted fracture of the vertebral body with a small anteroinferior detached bone fragment and an abnormal widening between the spinous process. (Reproduced with permission from *Post's radiographic evaluation of the spine*, © 1980 Masson Publishing USA, Inc.)

a bullet, soft tissue, or by bone fragments driven in by the missile (Fig. 24.10). Intramedullary haemorrhage is common, particularly in the grey matter, whereas epidural and subdural haematomas sufficient to cause cord compression are rare. A high velocity missile passing through adjacent tissue produces shock waves which can cause physiological disruption of the cord without direct contact. These patients may demonstrate the clinical picture of spinal cord concussion with resolution of neurological deficits within several hours to days after injury. If emergency surgery is not required for other life-threatening injuries, the patient is taken for CT scan of the involved area of the spine. CT will demonstrate the extent of bony injury, location of intraspinal bone and bullet fragments, and the rarely-occurring extra-axial haemorrhage causing cord compression. The treatment of patients with complete injury from a gunshot wound remains controversial. A retrospective review of more than 100 cases of complete injury treated surgically at the University of Miami showed no improvement in neurological outcome when compared to non-surgically treated patients (Landy and Green 1988). The surgically treated group showed higher morbidity and mortality than the non-surgical group. If there is no evidence of CSF leakage or bony instability, patients with complete cervical and thoracic injuries should be treated with

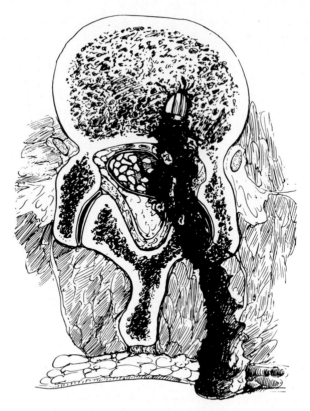

Fig. 24.10. Gunshot injury to the neural canal. (Reproduced with permission from *Post's radiographic evaluation of the spine*, © 1980 Masson Publishing USA, Inc.)

local wound debridement only. Incomplete injuries of the cervical and thoracic regions with significant bone or bullet fragments in the canal are treated with operative decompression. Cauda equina injuries are usually incomplete and operative decompression, with removal of significant-sized bone and metal fragments, is performed. Every patient with a gunshot wound to the spine should be treated with 10–14 days of intravenous antibiotics (Landy and Green 1988). The steroid protocol outlined above did not include penetrating wounds, and therefore has not been shown to be of benefit to the gunshot injured patient (Bracken et al. 1990).

Intensive Care Unit Management

After stabilization in the emergency room or postoperatively, the patients are taken to the intensive care unit (ICU). Each patient is placed on a kinetic nursing bed with continuous rotation. Rotation can be interrupted for testing, physiotherapy, bathing, bowel and bladder care, respiratory therapy, diagnostic tests and X-rays. The kinetic treatment table adequately immobilizes the spine while the continuous rotation decreases the complications associated with immobility (Green et al. 1985), for example improving drainage of pulmonary secretions and decreasing lower extremity venous stasis. Patients are placed on the steroid protocol for the first 24 hours. A nasogastric sump tube is maintained at low constant suction until ileus resolves with gastric pH monitored and kept above 4.5 by the use of antacids. Foley catheters are used until haemodynamic stability is achieved, then are discontinued and replaced by an intermittent catheterization programme. A central venous line is placed for venous access, monitoring of central venous pressure, and hyperalimentation. Central venous hyperalimentation is started within two days of admission in all cases. Older individuals and complicated multiple injury cases may require a Swan-Ganz catheter. Daily spinal and chest X-rays are performed along with blood and urine analysis as indicated.

SCI Rehabilitation

The rehabilitation phase actually begins in the ICU, with physical and occupational therapy and psychology rehabilitation interventions. Formal rehabilitation begins when the patient is transferred to the SCI rehabilitation centre. The rehabilitation phase is provided by a multidisciplinary team of physicians from disciplines such as physical medicine and rehabilitation, neurosurgery, orthopaedic surgery, internal medicine, psychiatry, urology, and plastic surgery. The allied health staff includes rehabilitation nurses, physical therapists, occupational therapists, recreational therapists, psychologists, social service specialists, vocational rehabilitation counsellors, sex counsellors, dieticians, and administrative personnel. The goals of treatment during this phase are to preserve neurological function, maximize neurological recovery, assure spinal stabilization, and expedite mobilization to the rehabilitation centre. Placement in a comprehensive dedicated SCI rehabilitation centre is most important. The duration of rehabilitation is related to the level of injury, age of the patient, severity of injury, type and number of complications. The average rehabilitation time is 3–4 months for a paraplegic and 4–6 months for a quadriplegic patient (Stauffer 1989). Patients with adequate rehabilitation support groups and good family support can be successfully and productively integrated back into society. Often transitional living facilities and communal living facilities can be most beneficial. Essential to a relatively normal life expectancy, however, is biannual preventive check-ups in a comprehensive SCI outpatient clinic. SCI victims dynamically change throughout their lives, physiologically, neurologically and emotionally, and require this close monitoring to prevent and minimize complications as well as to identify and take advantage of potential areas for functional improvement.

References

Aymes EW, Anderson FM (1956) Fractures of the odontoid process. Arch Surg 72:377–386
Barnett HJM, Jousse AT (1976) Post-traumatic syringomyelia. In: Vinken PJ, Bruyn GW (eds) Injuries of the spine and spinal cord, part II. Handbook of clinical neurology, vol 26. North-Holland, Amsterdam, pp 113–157

Barnett HJM, Bottersell EH, Jousse AT, Wynn-Jones M (1966) Progressive myelopathy as a sequel to traumatic paraplegia. Brain 89:159–174

Bracken MB, Shepard MJ, Collins WF, et al. (1990) A randomized control trial of methylprednisolone or Naloxone in the treatment of acute spinal cord injury. N Engl J Med 322:1405–1411

Brain L, Walton JN (1969) Hysteria. In: Brain L, Walton JN (eds) Brain's diseases of the nervous system. Oxford University Press, Oxford, pp 998–1001

Campbell RM, Delgado JP (1977) The pressure sore. In: Converse M (ed) Reconstructive plastic surgery. Saunders, Philadelphia, pp 3763–3799

Chance GQ (1948) Note on a type of flexion fracture of the spine. Br J Radiol 21:452–453

Crutchfield WG (1954) Skeletal traction in the treatment of injuries of the cervical spine. JAMA 155:32–41

DeJong R (1962) Case taking and the neurologic examination. In: Baker AB (ed) Clinical neurology, vol I. Hoeber-Harper, Philadelphia, pp 1–98

Dickson JH, Harrington PR, Erwin WD (1973) Harrington instrumentation in the fractured, unstable thoracic and lumbar spine. Tex Med 69:91–98

Ducker TB (1990) Restriction of cervical spine motion by cervical collars. Presented at the Scientific Exhibit of the 58th Annual Meeting of the AANS, 4/28–5/3/90, Nashville, TN

Dunn ME, Seljeskog EL (1986) Experience in the management of odontoid process injuries: an analysis of 128 cases. Neurosurgery 18:306–310

Eismont FJ, Green BA (1986) Technical considerations in the management of the unstable lumbar spine. In: Dunsker SB, Schnidels HH, Frymoyer J, et al. (eds) The unstable spine. Grune and Stratton, Orlando, pp 153–190

Eismont FJ, Green BA, Quencer RM (1984a) Post traumatic spinal cord cyst: a case report. J Bone Joint Surg 66A:614–618

Eismont FJ, Clifford S, Goldberg M, Green B (1984b) Cervical sagittal spinal canal size in spine injury. Spine 9(7):663–666

Green BA, Hall WJ (1976) Recognition and accident care for spinal cord injured patients. Paraplegia Life 5:5–11

Green BA, Callahan RA, Klose KJ, De la Torre J (1981) Acute spinal cord injury: current concepts. Clin Orthop 154:125–145

Green BA, Green KL, Klose KJ (1985) Kinetic therapy for spinal cord injury. Spine 8:722–728

Green BA, Eismont FJ, O'Heir JT (1987) Pre-hospital management of spinal cord injuries. Paraplegia 25:229–238

Hinchley JJ, Bicker WH (1945) Fractures of the atlas. Ann Surg 121:826–832

Holdsworth F (1970) Fractures, dislocations and fracture/dislocations of the spine. J Bone Joint Surg (Am) 52A:1534–1551

Jacobs RR, Asber MM, Snider RK (1980) Thoracolumbar spinal injuries: a comparative study of recumbent and operative treatment in 100 patients. Spine 5:463–471

Jefferson G (1920) Fractures of the atlas vertebra. Br J Surg 7:407–418

Johnson RM, Hart DL, Simmons, RF, et al. (1977) Cervical orthosis: a study comparing their effectiveness in restricting cervical motion in normal subjects. J Bone Joint Surg 59A:332–339

Kalsbeek WD, McLaurin RL, Harris BSH, Miller JD (1980) The national head and spinal cord injury survey: major findings. J Neurosurg 53:519–531

Kao C, Chang LW, Bloodworth JMB (1977) The mechanism of spinal cord cavitation following spinal cord transection. J Neuropath Exp Neurol 36:140–156

Ladd AL, Scranton PE (1986) Congenital cervical stenosis presenting as transient quadriplegia in athletes. J Bone Joint Surg 68A:1371–1374

Landy, HJ, Green BA (1988) Gunshot wounds of the spine. In: Ordog G (ed) Management of gunshot woulds. Elsevier, New York, pp 267–282

Landy HJ, Tucci KT (1991) Non-penetrating spinal cord injury. In: Weiner W (ed) Neurologic emergencies. (in press)

Mesard L (1978) Survival after spinal cord trauma. Arch Neurol 35:78–86

Montalvo BM, Quencer RM, Green BA, et al. (1985) Intraoperative sonography in spinal trauma. Radiology 153:125–129

Osgood RB, Lund CC (1928) Fractures of the odontoid process. N Engl J Med 198:61–72

Pang D, Wilberger JE (1982) Spinal cord injury without radiographic abnormalities in children. J Neurosurg 57:114–118

Post MJD, Quencer RM, Green BA, et al. (1988) The role of cine-MR in the evaluation of the pulsatile characteristics of post-traumatic spinal cord cysts. Presented at the 26th Annual Meeting of the ASNR, paper #6, 15/5/88, Chicago, IL

Quencer RM, Post MJD, Hinks RS (1990) Cine-MR in the evaluation of normal and abnormal CSF flow: intracranial and intraspinal studies. Neuroradiology 32:371–391

Schneider RC (1955) The syndrome of acute anterior spinal cord injury. J Neurosurg 12:95–122

Schneider RC (1959) Chronic neurological sequelae of acute trauma to the spine and spinal cord. Part II. The syndrome of chronic anterior spinal cord injury or compressed herniated intervertebral discs. J Bone Joint Surg 41A:449–456

Schneider RC, Cherry G, Pentek H (1954) The syndrome of acute central cervical spinal cord injury. J Neurosurg 11:546–577

Schneider RC, Thompson JM, Bebin J (1958) The syndrome of the acute cervical spinal cord injury. J Neurol Neurosurg Psychiatry 21:216–227

Schneider RC, Livingston KE, Cave AJE, Hamilton, G (1965) Hangman's fracture of the cervical spine. J Neurosurg 22:121–154

Smith WS, Kaufer H (1969) Patterns and mechanisms of lumbar injuries associated with lap seat belts. J Bone Joint Surg (Am) 51A:239–254

Stauffer ES (1989) Rehabilitation of post-traumatic cervical spinal cord quadriplegia and pentaplegia. In: Sherk HH (ed) The cervical spine, 2nd edn. Lippincott, Philadelphia, pp 317–322

Suwanwela C, Alexander E, Davis CH (1962) Prognosis in spinal cord injury, with special reference to patients with motor paralysis and sensory preservation. J Neurosurg 19:220–227

Tator CH, Kooto M, Rowed DW (1982) Favorable results with syringosubarachnoid shunts for treatment of syringomyelia. JNRS 56:517–523

Thomas JP (1979) Rehabilitation of the spinal cord injured: the model systems approach. SCI Digest 1:3–10

Torg JS, Pavlov H, Genuario SE, et al. (1986) Neuropraxia of the cervical spinal cord with transient quadriplegia. J Bone Joint Surg 68A:1354–1370

Williams B, Terry AF, Jones F, McSweeny T (1981) Syringomyelia as a sequel to traumatic paraplegia. Paraplegia 19:67–80

Young J-S, Northrup NE (1979) Statistical information pertaining to some of the most commonly asked questions about SCI – Part I. SCI Digest 1:11–23

Zimmerman E, Grant J, Vise WM, et al. (1976) Treatment of Jefferson fracture with a halo apparatus. Report of two cases. J Neurosurg 44:372–375

Zwimpfer TJ, Bernstein ME (1990) Spinal cord concussion. J Neurosurg 72:894–900

Rehabilitation, Walking Aids, Functional Electrical Stimulation and Overcoming Spasticity

R.J. Weber and B. Pentland

Injuries to the vertebral column resulting in damage to the spinal cord are uncommon with an annual incidence at about 2/100 000 in the United Kingdom (Swain et al. 1985). While small in number, the cost in personal terms to the injured, his family and to society in health, social and other resources is immense. Due to the pioneering work of Riddoch and Guttman in Britain and Munro and Bors in the United States (Collins and Chehrazi 1982), management of spinal cord injury (SCI) has become established as a medical specialty in its own right. It also provides one of the clearest examples of modern rehabilitation practice.

Rehabilitation implies the restoration of individuals to their fullest capability in physical, psychological and social terms after trauma or an episode of disease. This encompassing of both physical and psychological elements in an integrated, transdisciplinary team manner is termed comprehensive re-habilitation to distinguish it from a physical restoration approach. All health care is a continuum of services involving prevention, acute care and reha-bilitation, none of which exists in isolation. Thus in addition to its primary emphasis, rehabilitation includes considerable acute care and education to prevent secondary disabilities associated with SCI. The medical problems and psychosocial concerns of individuals with disease of the spinal cord from whatever cause are similar and most centres will accept patients with spinal paralysis from whatever cause.

To be effective, rehabilitation must include not only the patient but also the family unit and must be provided in a milieu which supports the patient's special needs and promotes success. Effective management also requires a unified rather than a fragmented treatment programme. Each involved health professional must simultaneously address both the physical and the psycho-social aspects of the patient's needs in an approach integrated with that of colleagues – supporting and extending colleagues' efforts while adding his/her particular contribution. This transdisciplinary approach to rehabilitation is effected through the Comprehensive Rehabilitation Team. The composition of this team is likely to vary in detail but usually includes medical and nursing staff, physical, occupational, speech, and recreational therapists, clinical psychologists and medical social workers with bioengineers, orthotists and other specialists recruited as necessary. The team works by coalescing the specific assessments and impressions of all members into a joint management approach. The identification of problems expands beyond the simple documentation of clinical signs and physical disabilities to include the psychological impact on individuals and their families, and the implications of the functional disturbance for housing, vocation and leisure activities.

The frequent failure of services adequately to identify these broader issues resulted in the development of the International Classification of Impairments, Disabilities and Handicaps (ICIDH) (WHO 1980). The principal categories are defined as follows: an impairment is any loss or abnormality of psychological, physiological or anatomical structure or function; a disability is any restriction or lack (resulting from an impairment) of ability to perform an activity in the manner or within the range considered normal for a human being; and a handicap is a disadvantage for a given individual (resulting from an impairment or a disability) that limits or prevents the fulfilment of a role that is normal for that individual (depending on age, sex, social and cultural factors). These definitions are imprecise; however, they do provide a framework to understand that there is a hierarchical structure to the effect that a change of ability has on an individual and that the intensity of this effect will vary with the individual's goals or tasks.

The Spectrum of Problems

The rehabilitation management issues raised by a SCI derive principally from the spinal level of the compromise, but are also affected by the patient's age, sex, health, associated injuries, psychosocial and fiscal resources. They can be conceptually grouped as arising from the paralysis, the alteration of physiological function or from psychosocial disruption. The mobility and self-care (i.e. activities of daily living) disruptions of paralysis are the most visibly addressed during comprehensive rehabilitation: positioning in bed, transferring to chair, toilet, bath or standing, development of strength and balance, special techniques for dressing, bathing and grooming must all be mastered.

Perhaps the most pervasive physiological disruption comes from compromise of the autonomic nervous system which influences most organ systems. Loss of sympathetic drive increases with more cephalad placement of the lesion: absent peripheral vasoconstriction produces general and orthostatic hypotension; cardiovascular response to exercise is lost; temperature regulation, sweating, sexual function are disrupted. In lesions above T6 the sympathetic system may be reflex triggered to over-respond (infection, bowel or bladder distension, pressure, etc.) resulting in profuse sweating, hypertension and reactive bradycardia. Patients must be trained to recognize and manage all these difficulties. Learning self-management of neurogenic bowel and bladder is a major rehabilitative element. The patient must become adept at regulating stool bulk and hardness and controlling evacuation with stimulation of the rectal ampulla and the judicious use of bowel stimulants. Bladder management through intermittent self-catheterization is preferred but requires adequate hand function. Reflex voiding, indwelling catheters and urinary diversions all have roles. Muscle spasms from altered spinal cord reflex activity can impair function and disrupt rehabilitation progress.

More than most difficulties, sexual dysfunction presents both physiological and psychological challenges. The young, trauma SCI patient is most vulnerable to the psychological aspects of self-image, worth and role loss and the threat to established interpersonal relationships. Erectile and ejaculatory problems of the male are more obvious than analogous difficulties of the female. Both must deal with the problem of positioning, physical performance and psychogenic arousal. Additional rehabilitation psychological issues are those posed by challenges to the general self-concept, family role change, vocational loss and the impact of variations of dependency. The rehabilitation process must address all these, enabling the patient and family to gain a new accommodation with their lives.

Mobility Aids

Depending upon the extent and severity of paralysis, patients with spinal lesions often require aids to achieve mobility. These fall into three principal categories: wheelchairs, walking aids and orthoses. Irrespective of which one or combination of them is supplied, it is essential that it is selected through adequate assessment of the individual's needs and that he receives careful instruction to ensure safe and proficient use. A device which seems ideal in hospital may be impractical in the patient's home or of limited value in the wider environment of work place or local shopping centre. There is often a psychological barrier to the acceptance of mobility aids which may be seen as obvious symbols of disability. Sensitive presentation of the aid with counselling as to its potential value is usually necessary.

Society places tremendous value on personal appearance and freedom. It is not surprising, then, that often the first concern of newly spinal injured individuals (and their families) is how to regain ambulation since standing and mobility seem to exemplify normality and independence. When this goal is appropriate and properly directed, it can be a positive motivating tool in the overall rehabilitation programme. When circumstances preclude independent ambulation, a critical responsibility of the rehabilitation team is to help refocus motivation and energy on alternative means of mobility. When this process of redirection with its attendant adjustment to disability fails, it can disrupt not only the acute rehabilitation programme but also affect the longer-term prospects of the patient for success.

All individuals with SCI can regain self-directed mobility. The rehabilitation team must be able to predict accurately the orthotic needs of each individual in order to help set patient goals and expectations and to allocate treatment resources. For individuals who experience immediate and complete paralysis at the time of injury, neurological recovery is unlikely. Therefore, mobility needs for these patients can be more confidently predicted at the outset of rehabilitation since the level of the lesions is the principal factor which determines their ultimate residual functional capability. There are two transition levels of injury at which the assistance needed varies considerably among individuals. Preservation of C7 provides elbow extension and some wrist control leading to independence in a manually propelled chair. At the L3/4 injury level the preservation of an effective quadriceps permits energy-efficient, independent and fully functional ambulation using ankle-foot orthosis (short leg braces) and canes.

Wheelchairs

Wheelchairs can be broadly categorized into four types: manually propelled, attendant propelled, indoor powered and outdoor powered. Many factors will determine the choice of chair and some patients will need more than one model to serve different functions. Basic considerations include the height, weight and buttock circumference of the patient. The stage of recovery or, alternatively, progression in deteriorating conditions, influences the model chosen and the prescription may need to be changed over time. Depending upon the individual's basic mobility, front or sideways entry and exit from the wheelchair may be more suitable. Environmental factors such as storage and transport of the chair are often a major concern. The demands to be made upon the chair in use will differ considerably between patients. Young paraplegics often need a model which is capable of robust and varied use while an elderly patient may require a less sophisticated one. The majority of spinal cord damaged individuals use standard chairs with rear propelling wheels, but young or active paraplegics with good upper limb function may prefer special chairs with the axle moved forward for easier propulsion and greater ease in climbing curbs, etc. Sports chairs which are light and highly manoeuvrable are popular with this group. Virtually all users benefit from use of lightweight chairs the cost of which is now similar to that of standard chairs.

In addition to the wheelchair itself, attention must be given to accessories such as the seat cushion, back, arm and footrests. Again, a range of these and more specialized accessories are available, and in some instances a bio-engineer may make special adaptations to a chair to meet an individual's particular needs.

Power wheelchairs are the norm for injury above C7 and appropriate for many at C7 or even lower. The SCI level for respirator dependence varies due to the multiple root supply to the diaphragm. Most C4 (C4 root functioning) injuries can eventually be weaned from respirators while most C2 injuries cannot. Needle electromyography of the diaphragm and phrenic nerve conduction studies can help predict the potential for diaphragmatic pacing. Although respirator-dependent individuals do require an assistant to be available full time who could, in theory, push a manual chair, such dependency is severely limiting to both the assistant and the SCI individual. Power chairs with appropriate modifications for a portable respirator including increased battery capacity, power recline, and computer-based communication and environmental control devices permit an important degree of self-direction. They open some vocational and avocational options and permit much more flexibility for the care giver. This is of critical importance in permitting home care by family members. Power chairs require a van with suitable ramp or power lift for transport.

In very high SCI, head control is diminished. Although the intact spinal accessory and facial nerves provide for some cervical motor activity, it may be insufficient to permit wheelchair or other device activation in very high cervical SCI. The presence of a tracheostomy and respirator tubes further complicates the situation. These individuals require special head supports, power recline features and special control switches.

Walking Aids

Walking aids are partially weight-relieving devices in contrast to wheelchairs which are completely weight-relieving. Aids can be grouped into walking sticks or canes, crutches and walking frames (walkers). Walking sticks may be made of wood or metal alloy and may be three-legged (tripod) or four-legged (quadruped) to provide greater stability. The height of a walking stick is of paramount importance: the handle should be level with the greater trochanter when the patient is standing erect in shoes. As most patients with spinal lesions have bilateral lower limb weakness it is often necessary for them to use two sticks.

Crutches also come in various types suitable for different purposes. Axillary crutches are only suitable for short-term use. They put considerable strain on upper limb joints and muscles, particularly the shoulder joints, which can lead to osteoarthrosis or brachial neuropathy. Elbow (Lofstrand) crutches put less strain on the joints than axillary crutches but are less stable and usually need stronger arms. They are essentially walking sticks with a vertical extension to the vertical component with an arm clip. This needs to be correctly aligned and well padded to prevent pressure over the ulna. A third form of crutch is the forearm support or gutter crutch. The length of the crutch is adjusted so that the forearm rests in the gutter. This demands less of the upper arm joints. It is particularly suitable for those with weakness of the hands and wrists. They tend, however, to be heavier and less stable and manoeuvrable than axillary or elbow crutches.

Walking frames (walkers) provide more support and stability than sticks or crutches but are of more limited application for spinal patients. The types available in addition to the standard model include gutter frames which, like gutter crutches, take weight through both forearms which can be useful in early mobilization stages, and models with wheels or rollators. Rollators may have brakes and folding models are available.

As a patient recovers from a lesion of the spinal cord, the physiotherapist may use any combination of these devices after the patient graduates from parallel bars or walking devices which provide considerable support to the trunk. They should also determine when it is appropriate and safe for the individual to use the walking aid in the ward or at home once they are confident that the patient is proficient in its use.

Orthoses

With orthotic support, healthy young individuals with complete paraplegia can stand and ambulate. That is not to say that this is an effective answer to their mobility needs. Two orthotic approaches are available for individuals with complete, high level lesions. Long leg braces (LLB), sometimes attached to a pelvic band to control abduction/adduction and rotation of the limb, provide knee and ankle locking necessary for weight bearing. Once standing with the brace joints locked, the individual must elevate the body using the arms and a walker or crutches and advance by swinging or dragging the legs forward to a new weight-bearing location.

The other approach exemplified by the Louisiana State University reciprocating gait orthosis (RGO) (Beckmann 1987) is to place the individual into a device similar in appearance to a parapodium or to locked LLB with pelvic bands but with the hip joints also controlled and connected to each other by a cable. The standing user can tilt weight from one leg and, by shifting body weight, cause it to advance due to the cross-leg control cable attachment to the weight-bearing leg. This multiarticulated system is more rigid and stable than LLB and permits easier pacing of ambulation and better freedom of the hands during standing. Individuals with cervical or midthoracic lesions usually require a spinal orthotic extension for back stabilization. Truly adequate trunk control requires abdominal muscle function which is fully present at T12. This and similar systems such as the ParaWalker (Butler and Major 1987) require motivated patients and considerable training to use. In a follow-up study, 17 of 20 patients were still regularly using their ParaWalker on average 20 months from the date of issue (Butler and Major 1987).

LLB ambulation requires reasonable trunk control and strong shoulder depressors to lift the body forward over the braces. This is very difficult to accomplish with upper dorsal level lesions. LLB require good balance despite absent lower body proprioception, high upper extremity strength and very high work capacity. High level paraplegics have impaired respiration and cardiovascular responses which contribute to fatigue in high work situations. Doffing and donning the orthoses are difficult and time-consuming; repair and adjustment are frequent. Spasticity can make donning and use more difficult. LLB can be a source of skin pressure injury, mobility in them is very much slower than in a chair and availability of the hands for functional tasks limited. Nevertheless, they provide a means of standing, weight bearing and ambulation which have important benefits for a selected group of individuals and, for some, can provide a functionally critical capability necessary to resume life tasks.

Although adding functional spinal levels through the thoracic and upper lumbar levels improves performance, basic orthotic factors are unchanged (other than elimination of spinal extensions). Adding L2/3 improves hip stabilization and leg swing with LLB ambulation and provides a motor (rectus femoris, iliopsoas) to actively drive the RGO, improving efficiency.

The addition of L4 permits a fundamental change. Strong knee extension sufficient to support the body (plus active hip flexion) permits energy-efficient walking. Shifting weight of the body behind the hip axis permits passive hip locking (support by anterior ligaments) and thus weight bearing on the leg by actively locking the knee with the quadriceps. The opposite side is then actively flexed at the hip and passively at the knee to generate a forward step (swing phase). Energy requirements are very greatly reduced since it is no longer necessary to elevate the whole body to advance the flexed limb. Ankles are stabilized by plastic ankle foot orthoses. Setting the ankle in slight dorsiflexion permits the body to roll forward over the foot during late stance phase (weight bearing) of gait. The gait is waddling due to poor hip stabilization and canes are used to compensate by providing medial-lateral stability. The addition of L5 greatly improves gait through additional hip, knee, and partial ankle control and may permit elimination of all bracing. The S1 root level is necessary, however, to gain full hip and knee stability along with good push-off for a fully normal gait.

The situation is very different in incomplete SCI. Here some neurological improvement is almost certain but its ultimate extent is utterly unpredictable. The course of recovery is sometimes delayed for months and often extends more than a year beyond injury. With the pressure to shorten hospital stays, patients may still be showing considerable neurological improvement at discharge. In such circumstances, although the spinal level of the SCI remains important in determining ambulation capability and appropriate orthotic needs, the extent of sensation, proprioception, motor control and spasticity below the lesion is also critically important.

These individuals often are managed best by a strategy of cardiovascular reconditioning and strengthening of functional muscles linked to an initial goal of wheelchair independence – if possible, using a stand pivot transfer technique. From this point, hospital discharge can occur when adjustment and home support status permit, and efforts toward ambulation or other advanced mobility goals pursued at the appropriate pace.

Features which influence whether individuals with incomplete SCI will become community ambulators include: trunk control, lower extremity proprioception, sensation, motor control of one knee, spasticity, upper extremity strength. When a number of these factors are favourable early post injury, an initial goal of independent ambulation at discharge may be elected rather than that of phased management.

An individual with incomplete SCI can require considerable orthotic aid and still be an effective community ambulator. Balance assistance from walkers, forearm crutches or canes is frequently required. Bracing with single or bilateral ankle foot orthoses (to provide ankle dorsiflexion and/or to control plantar spasms) often permits effective walking. A single knee ankle foot orthosis (KAFO) can also prove effective. Orthotic needs beyond this level such as bilateral KAFOs or KAFOs with pelvic bands to control the hips and spinal extensions may permit ambulation but they impose a severe energy consumption and speed penalty. Again, functional needs must be considered in selecting the method of routine mobility. Ageing may require revision of a previously successful strategy if developing osteoarthritis or cardiovascular problems begin to interfere with performance.

Automobile Driving

Next to walking, the ability to drive may be the most valuable tool for resuming independent living after SCI. Happily all new public transportation in the United States must be wheelchair accessible; however, most of the US is not served by public transport. Even in cities where it is available, the layout and density of the city limits its use. Driving is usually necessary for vocational access, health care, shopping and normal social contact.

Power-equipped vans including power wheelchair lifts and automatic wheelchair tie downs are now readily available for about $25 000. They permit driving from the individual's own wheelchair and can be handled by some individuals with C5 and most with lower level injuries.

There is considerable variation in the SCI level which permits personal automobiles equipped with hand controls to be utilized. Manipulating the automobile controls is the easiest of the tasks. Trunk control behind the wheel can be aided by seating but remains compromised even in thoracic level lesions. Independent transfer into the car and, as importantly, the ability to load the wheelchair are also necessary for independent automobile use. These improve at lower levels of injury but usually can be accomplished with injury below T1.

Functional Electrical Stimulation

Electrical shocks have been used to cause muscle contraction since antiquity, and many newly invented electrical sources found a momentary application as a medical treatment for paralysis (Licht 1971). Modern clinical research has focused on electrical stimulation as a means of preserving muscle "viability" pending reinnervation and on developing orthotics such as an electrical "drop foot brace" for hemiplegics. These efforts have had only limited success in producing clinically applicable devices. Research into electrical stimulation as a means of restoring motion in paralysis has been resurgent for the past decade. Public interest has centred on the possibility of restoration of ambulation. Interest among knowledgeable physicians is perhaps keenest concerning its effect on the physiology of spinal cord-injured individuals. How its use alters cardiovascular deconditioning, osteoporosis, muscular atrophy, spasticity, pressure sore frequency and other sequelae of paralysis may ultimately define its usefulness as importantly as its effectiveness as a mobility aid.

Clinicians have long appreciated the principles of muscle response to electrical stimulation in paralysis. When the lower motor neurone (LMN) is intact, i.e., upper motor neurone (UMN) paralysis, a short or long duration electrical stimulation applied over the muscle triggers a muscle twitch through depolarization of the associated intramuscular nerves, i.e., a nerve mediated response. When the LMN is lost, i.e., LMN injury as in a cauda equina injury, a long duration stimulus will produce a twitch by direct muscle cell depolarization but there is no response to a short duration pulse.

Although a muscle twitch can be produced by applying an appropriate duration and intensity of shock in either upper or lower motor neurone paralysis, a single twitch does not result in a functional muscle contraction. Effective contraction occurs only during a continuous train of twitches which can sustain tension in the muscle adequately between stimulations in order to produce muscle shortening. This is easily accomplished in UMN paralysis since the intact motor nerves respond with distinct depolarizations to the high frequency (20–100 Hz) stimuli. Stimulation of a single motor point results in spread of the depolarization signal through the branching nerve network to the whole muscle. By contrast, the isolated muscle fibres of LMN paralysis must be individually stimulated throughout their full length, requiring a much larger stimulating field. Denervated muscles may respond to an electrical stimulation pulse with a tetanic contraction (low twitch to tetany ratio) rather than a single twitch. Denervated muscle has been considered unsuitable for use as a motor for electrobracing because of the difficulties in effectively stimulating it and in controlling and sustaining its response.

Conversely, steady interest in functional electrical stimulation (FES) in UMN paralysis has resulted in numerous electrical orthotic applications utilizing brief, rapid stimulation of the peripheral nerve. Most commonly this has involved peroneal nerve stimulation to control foot drop in hemiplegia. Past research on electrical stimulation in SCI as a means of causing muscle conditioning and on its effect on the physiology of spinal man showed limited changes. The high frequency stimulation used in many of these studies to produce a strong, tetanic contraction rapidly exhausted the muscle, blocking the contraction. The high frequency electrical stimulations applied did not emulate the normal neuromuscular functional pattern in which each motor unit fires at its own sustainable rate and in which force of contraction is increased by both the recruitment of additional units and firing rate increases for individual units. Instead it cycled all motor units at the same high, un-sustainable frequency similar to normal maximal recruitment conditions. Exhaustion usually was reached before significant muscle work i.e., exercise, was accomplished. Since muscle must be metabolically stressed, i.e., worked in order to increase its strength or endurance, the studies often showed little physiological effect from the stimulation programme.

Crudeness of stimulation control also limited progress in orthotic applications: the force of sustained contraction the stimulated muscle could produce was limited; the force of tetanic contraction could not be graduated; it was difficult to coordinate stimulated contractions of several muscles to produce functional limb motions. These difficulties were significantly reduced with the introduction of the microprocessor (Petrofsky 1979; Petrofsky et al. 1983a) to control stimulation and the rotary stimulation approach by Petrofsky in the late 1970s (Petrofsky 1978; Petrofsky and Phillips 1979). In rotary stimulation each muscle is stimulated at multiple sites non-simultaneously. By stimulating each muscle at, for instance, three sites each site can be stimulated at a sustainable rate of 15–20 Hz; while by stimulating each site out of phase from the others the effect on the muscle as a whole is that of a fused contraction equivalent to that of a 45–60 Hz stimulation. The microcomputer permits complex manipulation of the stimulation parameters. Stimulation rates can be easily ramped up or down as can stimulation intensity, more closely mimicking natural muscle recruitment. Similarly, stimulation parameters can be based on real-time environmental factors such as limb position and movement, and the stimulation of many muscles can be coordinated.

While developing applications for the rotary stimulation technique, the Wright State University group followed two important FES concepts. One was to re-emphasize the critical role that work, i.e. resistance, plays in reconditioning paralytic as well as normal muscle. By utilizing progressive resistive exercise techniques coupled with sustainable electrical stimulation, they produced significant muscle bulk and strength improvement (Petrofsky and Phillips 1984). This "improved" muscle in turn increases the functional capabilities of FES orthotic systems.

The second concept was that of real-time, feedback control of stimulation in FES (Petrofsky et al. 1984b; Phillips et al. 1984). The closed loop approach immediately improves the efficiency and safety of FES powered exercise equipment (Petrofsky et al. 1984c). Here motion/position sensors can be built into the equipment. The microcomputer monitors performance (work) vs. stimulation intensity and is programmed to detect the gradual decline of work caused by muscle fatigue. It then compensates by increasing stimulation rates and intensity – ensuring a maximal muscle work programme prior to halting the exercise programme at a predetermined fatigue (stimulation intensity) level. The monitoring system can also detect a sudden change in performance indicative of system trouble such as electrode failure or limb disconnection from the system and prevent injury by instituting an emergency shutdown. The same approach can be applied to FES gait systems, although the placement and maintenance of sensors along with the control logic needed to safely and effectively operate such a system is far more complicated (Petrofsky and Phillips 1983; Petrofsky et al. 1984b).

Once strong and easily controlled muscle was available through electrical stimulation, its application to power functional tasks was an obvious goal. Paralytic muscle-powered weight lifting machines (Petrofsky et al. 1984c), exercise bicycles (Petrofsky et al. 1983b, 1984a) muscle-powered wheelchairs Glaser (1983), standing, ambulation (Kralj and Grobelnik 1973; Marsolais and Kobetic 1983; Petrofsky and Phillips 1983) and ambulation via muscle-powered orthoses have followed.

The following general approaches to clinical utilization of FES as an ambulation aid have received the most study to date. Kralj and Grobelnik (1973) described a simple system which combined tetanic muscle stimulation of the quadriceps to power standing and stance with the triggering of a mass flexor response through peroneal nerve stimulation to initiate gait swing phase. Gluteal stimulation during stance can be used to help the opposite side leg swing by preventing forward pelvic rotation. The system is manually cycled by the subjects using buttons on the walker and neither rotary stimulation nor a feedback loop to adjust stimulation intensity is employed. Implantable or surface electrodes can be used; however, individuals with sensory sparing may not be able to tolerate the discomfort of surface stimulation. A recently reported modification uses surface electrodes positioned in an elasticized garment which simplifies the set up process (Patterson et al. 1990). Similar systems offer promise as an alternative to LLB for supervised, therapeutic standing or ambulation.

Complex FES systems utilize multiple muscle groups with stimulation co-ordinated by a microprocessor. These systems control all or virtually all aspects of gait via FES including joint motion and stabilization. Closed loop systems, i.e. self-monitoring with feedback supplied by joint position and movement sensors, can adjust the stimulation intensity to smooth gait and to compensate for muscle fatigue or obstacles (Petrofsky and Phillips 1983; Petrofsky et al. 1984b; Phillips et al. 1984). The feedback-driven, closed-loop FES system has considerable theoretical advantage over the open-loop system's fixed stimulation pattern in generating an efficient and safe gait. However, its requirement for a reliable, complex sensor system and control logic has hindered its development. On the other hand, Marsolais and Kobetic (1983, 1987) have made steady progress using an open-loop approach and have developed implantable electrodes which are fairly reliable (Marsolais and Kobetic 1986). They have been able to demonstrate stair climbing as well as level surface ambulation. Either of these "full" FES approaches requires improved reliability and user friendliness before moving from research to clinical use.

The coupling of the reciprocating gait orthosis (RGO) and FES is clinically promising. The orthosis provides a reliable, safe platform to support standing and ambulation. RGO ambulation can usually be sustained for sufficient distance to be functional in certain situations and a hand can be free while standing to perform desired tasks. FES can be utilized to power standing up, i.e., quadriceps stimulation as well as hip flexion for forward stepping. Energy consumption using FES to power ambulation in the RGO is favourable compared to the RGO alone at most speeds and energy consumption with the RGO-FES combination is much less than that of LLB or pure FES at all gait speeds (Hirokawa et al. 1990; Nene and Patrick 1990).

The clinical use of FES is not yet established. It can unequivocally reverse muscle atrophy and maintain cosmetically acceptable muscle bulk in UMN paralysis. This muscle-strengthening application of FES is the greatest beneficiary of the rotary stimulation technique since that stimulation technique permits extended, heavy resistance exercise without exhaustion from excessive stimulation rates.

Improved muscle bulk may protect against pressure sores through better weight distribution but this can only be demonstrated through extensive trials. FES of the gluteal muscles during sitting appears to improve blood flow in the muscle and adjusts the gluteal contour to a more normal one (Levine et al. 1990a,b). The combination of maintaining muscle bulk with a long-term FES resistance exercise programme and phasic gluteal FES during sitting is promising as a means of pressure sore prevention.

Although FES can slow the demineralization process in SCI (Flores 1985) it does not reverse established osteoporosis of SCI when administered at levels used for routine muscle conditioning by a commercially available FES bicycle ergometry system (Leeds et al. 1990).

Spasticity may be briefly reduced following an FES exercise session but use of FES appears to intensify the overall difficulty of spasticity management in some SCI patients rather than reduce it as initially hoped (Petrofsky et al. 1984c). Unfortunately, strong spasms remain a contraindication to FES since the spontaneous spasm during the use of FES could cause injury by suddenly resisting the FES contraction. This study suggests that using FES may cause some individuals, who were initially appropriate, to become inappropriate for use of FES exercise because of strengthening of their spasms.

FES-powered exercise including bicycle ergometry does provide a modest cardiac conditioning challenge (Glaser 1986; Hooker et al. 1990). It is more effective in direct proportion to the degree of sympathetic innervation preserved, i.e. paraplegics show a greater cardiac response than quadriplegics. FES coupled with voluntary upper extremity exercise is more effective than FES exercise alone for cardiovascular conditioning.

FES remains investigational as an ambulation aid. Operational complexity, electrode and system reliability and cost remain impediments. For individuals using a RGO, the addition of FES seems a logical advancement. In a clinic setting, simple FES systems to permit therapeutic standing and ambulation similar to those described by Kralj and Grobelnik (1973) may become practical if inexpensive elasticized garments to simplify electrode management become commercially available. In the clinic the electronics can be shared to reduce costs and close supervision is available to prevent injury in case of system failure.

At present a single FES-based exercise system is commercially available for bicycle ergometry. It is hoped that we will gain a full understanding in the coming years of its long-term benefits and costs. It will be of considerable benefit to individuals with SCI if the introduction of future commercial application is preceded by a clear exposition of their benefits, limits and long-term costs.

Overcoming Spasticity

Spasticity is a motor disorder characterized by a velocity-dependent increase in tonic stretch reflexes with exaggerated tendon jerks, resulting from hyper-excitability of the stretch reflex, as one component of the upper motor neurone syndrome (Kalz and Rymer 1989). The spinal reflex area below the level of the spinal lesion must be intact. In acute spinal cord injuries, flexor spasticity gradually emerges over the first few weeks to six months after the initial spinal shock when the characteristic flaccidity ends. This is followed more slowly by extensor spasticity which predominates in most cases (Marsden 1988).

Spasticity can produce contractures and can interfere with preserved voluntary movement, positioning in bed or chair producing pressure ulcers, transfers, driving or activities of daily living. It can be triggered by movement, i.e. stretch, and increased by noxious stimuli such as bladder distension. Conversely, treatment with severe loss of tone may reduce existing weight-bearing capability in an incomplete lesion (Marsden 1988).

Prevention of Spasticity

The first measures to be considered are those directed at avoiding or treating triggering factors which provoke spasms. This includes provision of good skin, bladder and bowel care and prevention of pressure sores, urinary tract infections, bladder or renal stones, constipation and perianal conditions such as fissures. Other intercurrent problems such as infections, deep venous thrombosis and localized lesions such as ingrowing toenails may exacerbate spasms and require prompt and thorough treatment.

Physiotherapy with passive stretching of the spastic muscles prevents joint and muscle contractures, which themselves provoke spasms, and has a positive, direct effect on spasticity. Evidence is also accumulating that proprioceptive facilitation in the early stages of spinal shock may reduce the eventual degree of spasticity (Marsden 1988).

Drug Treatment

Baclofen, dantrolene sodium and benzodiazepines are the principal drugs used orally to relieve spasticity. All have a tendency to cause drowsiness although patients may develop tolerance to this side-effect. They can all also lead to hypotonia to an extent that is counterproductive in that, while the patient may be relieved of spasms, he loses the extensor tone which aids his stance.

Baclofen is a gamma-amino-butyric acid (GABA) analogue which selectively acts on the GABA-B receptor. It primarily restricts calcium influx into the presynaptic terminal thus reducing presynaptic transmitter release, but is also thought to have a postsynaptic action as well, depressing neuronal activity (Ochs et al. 1989). In general it is well tolerated although in addition to drowsiness, it can cause nausea. It occasionally results in a toxic confusional state with hallucinations and seizures, but this is usually associated with large doses. Baclofen is usually given on a thrice daily basis with a total daily dose range of 15 to 100 mg. Baclofen is usually the more effective of these medications and often is used in combination with a diazepam.

Dantrolene sodium acts on muscle, depressing calcium ion release from the sarcoplasmic reticulum. As it acts on muscle rather than centrally it can be used in conjunction with baclofen or benzodiazepines. It can cause minor gastrointestinal symptoms such as anorexia, nausea or alteration of bowel habit as well as drowsiness. Of more significance is the risk of hepatic damage, rarely resulting in liver failure. For this reason careful monitoring of liver function is essential. It too is given in divided dose with a range of about 25 to 400 mg daily, starting with only 25 mg a day and building up the dose over several weeks.

Benzodiazepines such as diazepam, clorazepate and medazepam have a place in the treatment of spinal spasticity due to partial cord lesions as they appear to increase presynaptic inhibition of stretch reflex mechanisms. The sedative action and habit-forming tendency of these agents tend to limit their usefulness (Grundy and Russell 1986). The hypotensive effect of benzodiazepines may also cause difficulty in individuals who have significant autonomic dysfunction in association with their spinal lesion.

The alpha-2 adrenergic agonist, clonidine, has been shown to have an antispasticity effect in SCI patients that is recognized subjectively and demonstrable neurophysiologically by restoration of vibratory inhibition of the H reflex (Nance et al. 1989). Because of its tendency to cause postural hypotension it has been used with desipramine. Further work is needed before clonidine is recognized as an agent for routine use.

When oral drug therapy is not tolerated or found to be ineffective, there may be a place for the use of intrathecal baclofen. Recent reports have described sustained beneficial effect on spinal spasticity with few adverse effects when baclofen is given by infusion via a permanent intrathecal catheter (Ochs et al. 1989; Parke et al. 1989).

Invasive Measures for Treatment of Spasticity

It is sometimes necessary to try to relieve localized spasticity by interrupting the nerve supply to the muscles affected by chemical or surgical means. The motor point of a muscle can be identified neurophysiologically and it can be injected with the local anaesthetic bupivacaine to give a short-lived relaxation. If this procedure is successful, a more lasting effect can be achieved with the motor point injection of 6% aqueous phenol or 45% ethyl alcohol (Grundy and Russell 1986). Alternatively, the nerve supply to the muscle may be interrupted by a neurectomy, the commonest example being obturator neurectomy for severe hip adductor spasm. These limited procedures seldom are effective in altering generalized spasms.

Dorsal rootlet rhizotomy is a promising means of controlling intractable, disabling spasms. It consists of section of selected dorsal rootlets in the lumbosacral area which interrupts the reflex arc. After laminectomy, rootlets are stimulated and those noted to produce extensive spread of reflex muscle response (monitored via multichannel electromyography) are sectioned. The technique has been most utilized in cerebral palsy where it has been well tolerated and is thought to be effective (Brown 1990). Other neurosurgical procedures such as anterior rhizotomy, cordectomy and myelotomy have largely been abandoned for, although they had variable efficacy, they led to problems with subsequent skin care (Marsden 1988).

Rarely, in the presence of severe spasticity, intrathecal phenol or alcohol may be used to destroy nerve roots of the cauda equina. This technique is, however, unselective, converting an upper motor neurone lesion to a lower motor neurone disturbance with resulting interference with bladder and bowel function together with sensory loss which increases the risk of pressure sores.

When spasticity results in contractures, procedures such as tenotomy, tendon lengthening or muscle division may prove necessary.

References

Beckmann J (1987) The Louisiana State University reciprocating gait orthosis. Physiotherapy 73:386–392

Brown E (1990) Dorsal rhizotomy for spastic cerebral palsy: report of diagnostic therapeutic technology assessment panel of the American Medical Association. JAMA 264:2569–2574

Butler PB, Major RE (1987) The ParaWalker: a rational approach to the provision of reciprocal ambulation for paraplegic patients. Physiotherapy 73:393–397

Collins WP, Chehrazi B (1982) Concepts of the acute management of spinal cord injury. In: Matthews WB, Glasor CH (eds) Recent advances in clinical neurology. Churchill Livingstone, Edinburgh, pp 67–82

Flores JL Jr (1985) Electrically induced isometric exercise as a means of preventing muscle atrophy and bone demineralization. MSc thesis, Wright State University, Dayton, OH

Glaser RM (1983) Locomotion via paralyzed leg muscles: feasibility study for leg propelled vehicle. J Rehabil R D 20:87–92

Glaser RM (1986) Physiologic aspects of spinal cord injury and functional neuromuscular stimulation. Cent Nerv Syst Trauma 3:49–62

Grundy D, Russell J (1986) ABC of spinal cord injury: medical management in the spinal injuries unit. Br Med J 292:183–187

Hirokawa S, Grimm M, Le T, et al. (1990) Energy consumption in paraplegic ambulation using reciprocating gait orthosis and electric stimulation of the thigh muscles. Arch Phys Med Rehabil 71:687–694

Hooker SP, Figoni SF, Glaser RM, Rodgers MM, Ezenwa BN, Faghri PD (1990) Physiologic responses to prolonged electrically stimulated leg-cycle exercise in the spinal cord injured. Arch Phys Med Rehabil 71:863–869

Kalz RT, Rymer WZ (1989) Spastic hypertonia, mechanisms and measurement. Arch Phys Med Rehabil 70:144–155

Kralj A, Grobelnik S (1973) Functional electrical stimulation – a new hope for paraplegic patients? Bull Prosthet Res 10–20:75–102

Leeds EM, Klose KJ, Ganz W, Serafini A, Green BA (1990) Bone mineral density after bicycle ergometry training. Arch Phys Med Rehabil 71:207–209

Levine SP, Kett RL, Cederna PS, Brooks SV (1990a) Electrical muscle stimulation for pressure sore prevention: tissue shape variation. Arch Phys Med Rehabil 71:210–215

Levine SP, Kett RL, Gross MD, Wilson BA, Cederna PS, Juni JE (1990b) Blood flow in the gluteus maximus of seated individuals during electrical muscle stimulation. Arch Phys Med Rehabil 71:682–686

Licht S (1971) Electrodiagnosis and electromyography, 3rd edn. Elizabeth Licht, New Haven, CT

Marsden CD (1988) Spasticity. In: Goodwill CJ, Chamberlain MA (eds) Rehabilitation of the physically disabled adult. Croom Helm, London, pp 455–464

Marsolais EB, Kobetic R (1983) Functional walking in paralyzed patients by means of electrical stimulation. Clin Orthop 175:30–36

Marsolais EB, Kobetic R (1986) Implantation techniques and experience with percutaneous intramuscular electrodes in the lower extremities. J Rehabil R D 23:1–8

Marsolais EB, Kobetic R (1987) Functional electrical stimulation for walking in paraplegia. J Bone Joint Surg 69A:728–733

Nance PW, Shears A, Nance DM (1989) Reflex changes induced by clonidine in spinal cord injured patients. Paraplegia 27:296–301

Nene AV, Patrick JH (1990) Energy cost of paraplegic locomotion using the ParaWalker-electrical stimulation "hybrid" orthosis. Arch Phys Med Rehabil 71:116–120

Ochs G, Stuppler A, Meyerson BA, et al. (1989) Intrathecal baclofen for long-term treatment of spasticity: a multicentre study. J Neurol Neurosurg Psychiatry 52:933–939

Parke B, Penn RD, Savoy SM, Coreas D (1989) Functional outcome after delivery of intrathecal baclofen. Arch Phys Med Rehabil 70:30–32

Patterson RP, Lockwood JS, Dykstra DD (1990) Functional electric stimulation system using electrode garment. Arch Phys Med Rehabil 71:340–342

Petrofsky JS (1978) Control of the recruitment and firing frequencies of motor units in electrically stimulated muscles in the cat. Med Biol Eng Comput 16:302–308

Petrofsky JS (1979) Digital analogue hybrid 3-channel sequential stimulator. Med Biol Eng Comput 17:421–424

Petrofsky JS, Phillips CA (1979) Constant-velocity contractions in skeletal muscle by sequential stimulation of muscle efferents. Med Biol Eng Comput 17:583–592

Petrofsky JS, Phillips CA (1983) Computer controlled walking in the paralyzed individual. J Neurol Orthop Surg 4:153–164

Petrofsky JS, Phillips CA (1984) The use of functional electrical stimulation for rehabilitation of spinal cord injured patients. Cent Nerv Syst Trauma 1:57–73

Petrofsky JS, Heaton HH, Glaser RM, Phillips CA (1983a) Applications of the Apple as a microprocessor controlled stimulator. Collegiate Microcomputer 1:97–104

Petrofsky JS, Heaton HH, Phillips CA (1983b) Outdoor bicycle for exercise in paraplegics and quadriplegics. J Biomed Eng 5:292–296

Petrofsky JS, Phillips CA, Heaton HH, Glaser RM (1984a) Bicycle ergometer for paralyzed muscle. J Clin Eng 9:13–19

Petrofsky JS, Phillips CA, Heaton HH (1984b) Feedback control system for walking in man. Comp Biol Med 14:135–149

Petrofsky JS, Heaton HH, Phillips CA, Glaser RM (1984c) Leg exerciser for training of paralyzed muscle by closed loop control. Med Biol Eng Comput 22:298–303

Phillips CA, Petrofsky JS, Hendershot DM, Stafford D (1984) Closed loop control for restoration of movement in paralyzed muscle. Orthopedics 7:1289–1302

Robinson CJ, Kett NA, Bolam JM (1988) Spasticity in spinal cord injured patients: 2. Initial measures and long-term effects of surface electrical stimulation. Arch Phys Med Rehabil 69:862–868

Swain BN, Grundy D, Russell J (1985) ABC of spinal cord injury: at the accident. Br Med J 291:1558–1560

WHO (1980) International classification of impairments, disabilities, and handicap. World Health Organisation, Geneva

Subject Index